The Science of Mindfulness: A Research-Based Path to Well-Being

Ronald D. Siegel, Psy.D.

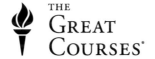

THE
GREAT
COURSES

PUBLISHED BY:

THE GREAT COURSES
Corporate Headquarters
4840 Westfields Boulevard, Suite 500
Chantilly, Virginia 20151-2299
Phone: 1-800-832-2412
Fax: 703-378-3819
www.thegreatcourses.com

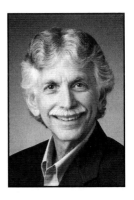

Ronald D. Siegel, Psy.D.

Assistant Clinical Professor of Psychology
Harvard Medical School/
Cambridge Health Alliance

D r. Ronald D. Siegel is an Assistant Clinical Professor of Psychology at Harvard Medical School/Cambridge Health Alliance, where he has taught for more than 30 years, and an Adjunct Clinical Assistant Professor of Psychiatry at the University of Massachusetts Medical School. He received his Doctor of Psychology degree from Rutgers University and completed his clinical internship and postdoctoral fellowship at Harvard Medical School.

Dr. Siegel is a longtime student of mindfulness meditation and serves on the board of directors and faculty of the Institute for Meditation and Psychotherapy. He teaches internationally about mindfulness and its application to psychotherapy and other fields, has worked for many years in community mental health with inner-city children and families, and maintains a private clinical practice in Lincoln, Massachusetts.

Dr. Siegel is an author or editor of a number of important publications relating to physical and mental health, including the following.

- *The Mindfulness Solution: Everyday Practices for Everyday Problems* (author), a guide for clinicians and general audiences

- *Positive Psychology: Harnessing the Power of Happiness, Mindfulness, and Inner Strength* (medical editor), a Harvard Medical School Special Health Report

- *Back Sense: A Revolutionary Approach to Halting the Cycle of Chronic Back Pain* (coauthor), a self-treatment guide that integrates Western and Eastern approaches for treating chronic back pain

- *Sitting Together: Essential Skills for Mindfulness-Based Psychotherapy* (coauthor), a new professional skills manual

- *Mindfulness and Psychotherapy, Second Edition* (coeditor), a critically acclaimed textbook

- *Wisdom and Compassion in Psychotherapy: Deepening Mindfulness in Clinical Practice* (coeditor), a collection of the work of leading scholars with a foreword by the Dalai Lama

Dr. Siegel is also a contributor to other professional books and publications, including *Psychotherapy Networker* and *Contemporary Psychology*, and is a codirector of the annual Harvard Medical School conference Meditation and Psychotherapy. His recent work focuses on identifying which mindfulness practices are most effective for treating particular conditions and populations.

Dr. Siegel has taught workshops for diverse organizations, including Kripalu Center for Yoga & Health, NASA, the National Institute for the Clinical Application of Behavioral Medicine, Kaiser Permanente, Psychotherapy Networker, the Massachusetts Collaborative Law Council, and numerous state psychological and social work associations. Topics have included integrating mindfulness practices into psychotherapy, advances in positive psychology, mindfulness for dispute resolution, mindfulness in education, and treating chronic back pain and other psychophysiological disorders. His work has been featured on National Public Radio and on local radio and television programs. ■

Disclaimer

This series of lectures is intended to increase your understanding of how doctors diagnose and treat diseases and how you can improve your own health by being an active and informed patient. However, these lectures are not designed for use as medical references to diagnose, treat, or prevent medical illnesses or trauma, and neither The Teaching Company nor the lecturer is responsible for your use of this educational material or its consequences. Furthermore, participating in this course does not create a doctor-patient relationship. The information contained in these lectures is not intended to dictate what constitutes reasonable, appropriate, or best care for any given health issue, nor does it take into account the unique circumstances that define the health issues of the viewer. If you have questions about the diagnosis, treatment, or prevention of a medical condition or illness, you should consult your personal physician. The opinions and positions provided in these lectures reflect the opinions and positions of the relevant lecturer and do not necessarily reflect the opinions or positions of The Teaching Company or its affiliates.

The Teaching Company expressly DISCLAIMS LIABILITY for any DIRECT, INDIRECT, INCIDENTAL, SPECIAL, OR CONSEQUENTIAL DAMAGES OR LOST PROFITS that result directly or indirectly from the use of these lectures. In states that do not allow some or all of the above limitations of liability, liability shall be limited to the greatest extent allowed by law.

Table of Contents

INTRODUCTION

Professor Biography i
Course Scope 1

LECTURE GUIDES

LECTURE 1
Why Mindfulness Matters 4

LECTURE 2
Our Troublesome Brains 23

LECTURE 3
Informal, Formal, and Intensive Practices 43

LECTURE 4
Who Am I? The Perils of Self 62

LECTURE 5
Mindfulness or Psychotherapy? 82

LECTURE 6
Attention and Empathy in Relationships 103

LECTURE 7
The Science of Compassion and Self-Compassion 123

LECTURE 8
Tailoring Practices to Fit Changing Needs 143

LECTURE 9
Modifying Our Brain Function and Structure 165

LECTURE 10
Solitude—An Antidote to Loneliness 187

Table of Contents

LECTURE 11
Connecting with Children and Adolescents 208

LECTURE 12
Seeing Sadness and Depression in a New Light 228

LECTURE 13
Befriending Fear, Worry, and Anxiety 249

LECTURE 14
Transforming Chronic Pain...268

LECTURE 15
Placebos, Illness, and the Power of Belief 289

LECTURE 16
Interrupting Addiction and Troublesome Habits..............................310

LECTURE 17
Overcoming Traumas Large and Small..331

LECTURE 18
Groundbreaking Mindfulness Programs...353

LECTURE 19
The Neurobiology of Self-Preoccupation...374

LECTURE 20
Growing Up Isn't Easy—Facing Impermanence.............................396

LECTURE 21
Toward a Science of Wisdom 416

LECTURE 22
The Promise of Enlightenment 438

LECTURE 23
Mindful Ethics as a Path to Freedom..459

Table of Contents

LECTURE 24
The New Science of Happiness 481

SUPPLEMENTAL MATERIAL

Mindfulness Practices..502
Obstacles to Mediation Practice...506
Breath Awareness Practice 507
Loving-Kindness Practice..511
Mountain Meditation 515
Breathing Together 518
Stepping into Fear 524
Bibliography..527

The Science of Mindfulness:
A Research-Based Path to Well-Being

Scope:

Mindfulness—awareness of present experience with acceptance—is a deceptively simple way of relating to the contents of our minds that has been successfully practiced to alleviate psychological suffering and enhance emotional well-being for over 2,500 years. Cutting-edge scientific research and rapidly accumulating clinical experience are now validating what ancient wisdom traditions have long taught: that mindfulness practice is an effective antidote to our hardwired propensity for psychological distress and is a reliable pathway to increased wisdom, compassion, and fulfillment.

Neurobiologists are learning that mindfulness practice changes brain structure and function in meaningful, desirable ways, while mental health professionals are enthusiastically discovering that mindfulness practice holds great promise not only for their own personal development, but also as a powerful tool to augment virtually every form of psychotherapy. Studies indicate that it can be effective in alleviating a remarkably wide range of psychological difficulties, including anxiety, depression, stress-related medical problems, addictions, eating disorders, interpersonal problems, and even the challenges of aging.

Mindfulness is not, however, a one-size-fits-all remedy. Practices need to be tailored to fit our individual needs. Furthermore, to incorporate mindfulness into our work and personal lives, we need an intuitive, visceral understanding of the practice as well as an intellectual one. So, we need to learn how to actually practice mindfulness ourselves in order to reap its benefits.

Through lectures, experiential exercises, case examples, and presentations of scientific research, this course will provide practical skills that anyone can use to deal more effectively with everyday psychological challenges and live a richer, happier, more fulfilling life. Once you understand the core components of mindfulness practices and how they work to alleviate psychological distress, you will be able to creatively adapt them to meet the needs of changing conditions. You will develop a solid theoretical understanding of mindfulness from both ancient wisdom and modern scientific perspectives. You will also receive instruction and guidance in how to develop a regular mindfulness practice and how to work with obstacles and challenges that may arise as you pursue it.

This course will begin by examining the common elements in mindfulness practices, how they address everyday psychological distress, and how we can begin integrating mindfulness practice into a busy life. It will then investigate the evolutionary and neurobiological processes that scientists believe predispose us to psychological suffering and how mindfulness practices can help us interrupt them.

You will then learn and practice a variety of informal mindfulness techniques that can be incorporated throughout a busy day, as well as formal meditation techniques that, while requiring some dedicated practice time, have been demonstrated to change brain structure and function.

Having begun practicing mindfulness, you will use ecological and cognitive models to understand the fluid nature of the self that is revealed in mindfulness practice and its implications for well-being. These will be compared and contrasted with traditional Western psychological models of health and distress as you explore the similarities and differences between mindfulness practice and Western psychotherapy as paths to happiness.

The use of mindfulness practices to enhance our interpersonal relationships generally at home and at work, as well as specifically with children and adolescents, will be explored. Exercises will also be presented to help young people practice mindfulness themselves.

The course will devote considerable attention to what has been discovered about using mindfulness practice to treat a wide variety of psychological and behavioral difficulties that can interfere with leading a happy life, including anxiety, depression, stress-related medical disorders, and addictions. You will learn how different techniques, including exercises that develop compassion and self-compassion, can help us work effectively with these conditions.

The course will also address how to use mindfulness to engage with inevitable existential challenges, such as loneliness, alienation, aging, trauma, illness, and death, and how these difficulties can become pathways to greater psychological freedom. In addition, the course will address the role of wisdom and ethics in psychological well-being, from both ancient and modern scientific perspectives.

Throughout the course, you will explore recent neurobiological and clinical discoveries, what they can teach us about finding well-being, and how this enriches what we can learn from ancient wisdom traditions. The course concludes with a look at the relatively new field of positive psychology and what it can add to discoveries from studying and practicing mindfulness for finding a path to well-being. ■

Why Mindfulness Matters

Lecture 1

Throughout this course, you will learn what mindfulness is—and isn't—and what modern science is revealing about how it can resolve both everyday and more serious problems while helping to make people's lives richer and happier. Recently, there has been an explosion in scientific research about how mindfulness practices change both the structure and functioning of our brains as well as how they can improve all sorts of outcomes. You are encouraged to regularly engage in mindfulness practices to help you develop mindfulness.

What Is Mindfulness?

- In Western psychotherapy and neuroscience, mindfulness is a translation of the term *sati*, from the ancient language Pali, in which the teachings of the historical Buddha were first written down.

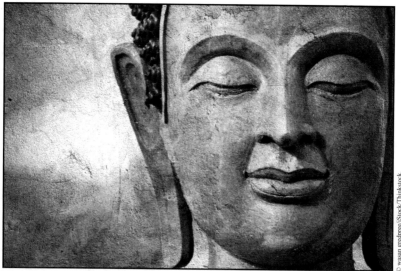

The founder of Buddhism, the Buddha was a teacher who lived in northern India between the 6th and 4th centuries B.C.E.

Sati connotes awareness, attention, and remembering. In addition, there is a sense of nonjudgment and deep acceptance, a kindness or friendliness, to the enterprise.

- There are three components of mindfulness: awareness of present experience with acceptance. Now that mindfulness practices have become part of mainstream psychotherapy, people are trying to construct scales to measure this.

- The Dunning-Kruger effect, discovered in social psychology by David Dunning and Justin Kruger, says that our actual competence at a whole host of different life endeavors is inversely proportional to our perceived competence. When we don't have that much mindfulness developed, we think of ourselves as pretty mindful. But when we develop more mindfulness, then we actually notice how often the mind wanders.

- The way in which one develops a sense of mindfulness is by studying mindlessness. You've probably had life experiences in which they simply unfolded on automatic—where the mind was one place and the body was somewhere else. For example, when you drive a common route, you aren't thinking about the directions you're taking.

- Most of the time, our minds are not in the present moment. And yet the moments that matter to us are all situations in which our mind shows up. We spend an inordinate amount of time lost in memories of the past and fantasies of the future.

How Mindfulness Practice Can Help

- Life is difficult for everybody. Everything changes, and loss is inevitable. Psychoanalytic writer Judith Viorst wrote a book in the 1980s called *Necessary Losses*. Her basic premise was that you could understand a great deal about human unhappiness by looking at our difficulties dealing with loss.

- Self-esteem is our remarkably robust habit of comparing ourselves to others. In fact, in the Buddhist tradition, this is said to be the last neurotic tendency to fall away before highest perfect enlightenment.

- Different people get caught on different domains or dimensions. In other words, we compare ourselves in different ways. For one person, it's about who is wealthier. For someone else, it's about who is smarter, or who is more physically fit, or who has more artistic talent. The concern for rank in the primate troop manifests itself in we humans with these constant preoccupations for how we compare to others.

- Mindfulness practices can help us with all of this. They can help us to see and accept things as they are, rather than as we wish them to be. For example, they can help us with dealing with the inevitability of illness or even death. It can also help us loosen our preoccupation with self—with the concern with where we rank in the baboon troop.

- In fact, it's been shown to quiet parts of the brain that are associated with self-referential thinking. It can even help us to experience the richness of the moment more fully. And this promotes savoring, which research shows to be a very important component of most paths to well-being.

- Finally, it helps to connect us to a world outside of ourselves, to something larger. And this is particularly important given our ultimate prognosis. And it's another reason why mindfulness practices figure prominently in so many spiritual traditions.

- Mindfulness can also help us get along with one another better. It helps us to see the other person more clearly and not believe so much in our judgments. So, we don't get caught as much in condemning the other person who has upset us today. It also helps us to not take things so personally. So, we can realize that much of the time, the other person's behavior, even if it's disturbing to us, isn't really about us. Rather, it reflects their own struggles at the moment.

- And it can help us to be present in relationships. And this is essential to being able to provide empathy for others and to support others, which is quite important if we're going to get along, particularly during difficult times. It also helps us learn not to act on urges compulsively. So, then, we can respond thoughtfully, rather than reacting automatically out of our hurt or anger.

Mindfulness Practices and Scientific Findings
- Mindfulness practices are moving into the mainstream of psychology, neuroscience, and medicine as their positive effects on the mind, the brain, and the whole body are being studied. Mindfulness practices keep important parts of our brain from withering with age. They also activate brain circuits associated with being happy, energized, and enthusiastically engaged in life. They even lengthen telomeres, the ends of chromosomes that get worn down with stress, resulting in cell death associated with aging.

- To experienced mindfulness students, it can seem strange that a millimeter of change in brain tissue shown on an MRI, or a shift in EEG activity, is more convincing in our modern age than the reports of living people or thousands of years of testimony from monks and nuns who have successfully used these practices to find peace, fulfillment, and wellness.

- But for people relatively new to the practice, the scientific findings are important, especially given the tenacity of competing—and often questionable—religious, philosophic, and medical claims over the ages. After all, how do we know that proponents of miracle cures and all sorts of solutions to life's problems aren't just fooling us or themselves?

- It's encouraging for people who have found mindfulness practices to be personally transforming, or have taught these practices to others, to know that science is now validating time-honored observations about their power.

- Mindfulness practice is also itself a form of empirical inquiry, an investigative tool for a sort of inner science. It enables us to carefully observe the processes that create distress, and then alleviate it, in our own minds and bodies. Mindfulness practices can be remarkably transformative.

- There has been a recent explosion of research into how mindfulness practices can help us with a remarkable variety of psychological difficulties. It turns out that everything from anxiety and depression to the challenges of intimate relationships, aging, and raising children can be helped with mindfulness practices.

How to Become More Mindful
- The way that we become more mindful is through mindfulness practices. Many people assume that mindfulness practice is about developing a blank mind, or getting the thought stream to shut up. That only happens during very intensive retreat practice. It is, however, about developing a different relationship to our thoughts—so that we can observe them coming and going and not believe in or identify them so very much.

- Most people enter these practices when they're having a rough time. And they secretly hope that this will get rid of the negative emotions and help them escape pain. The practices don't actually work that way. We actually feel our emotions, and even our pain, more vividly. But because we don't resist that pain or emotion, we end up suffering much less.

- Even though these practices were refined by monks and nuns and other enunciates, they're not actually about withdrawing from life. We might take a little time to step back to develop these capacities. But they are for the purpose of engaging so much more richly and fully in life. And even though, occasionally, we run up against wonderful experiences of bliss or peace, they're not really about seeking bliss or peace. They're about learning to be with whatever might arise.

- Finally, even though we call these "mindfulness practices," they're really mind and body practices, because they're very much about noticing that all of our experience in consciousness occurs from the mind-body more broadly.

- Under the umbrella of mindfulness practices, there are three skills that we're going to try to develop. The first skill is focused attention, which is traditionally called concentration. And that helps us observe things clearly. The second skill is what neurobiologists now call open monitoring, which is used to see how the mind creates suffering for itself. Finally, the last skill is acceptance and loving-kindness, which is used to soothe and comfort.

- Neurobiological evidence shows that the mental skills cultivated by these three different meditation types represent overlapping yet distinct brain processes. Most mindfulness practices develop one or another of these three skills.

Suggested Reading

Germer, "Mindfulness."

Gunaratana, *Mindfulness in Plain English*.

Hanh, *Peace Is Every Step*.

Kabat-Zinn, *Wherever You Go, There You Are*.

Siegel, *The Mindfulness Solution*, chapter 2.

Questions to Consider

1. During which moments of your day do you find yourself being most mindful? When are you most mindless?

2. Reflect on moments in which your mind makes comparisons between yourself and others. What are the criteria it uses? Which domains matter most to you in judging yourself and others (e.g., wealth, intelligence, fitness, social status, generosity, popularity, spiritual attainment, etc.)?

Why Mindfulness Matters

Lecture 1—Transcript

Welcome to our course on the science of mindfulness. Now, most people don't start a course like this because they've just fallen in love, won the lottery, and gotten a promotion. Rather, we get interested in these things when we want to better understand the cause of our psychological or physical suffering and how to find a path to greater well-being.

Luckily, mindfulness practices can provide just such a path. They did it for an accountant I work with who once loved sports but was disabled by back pain for years until he learned, through mindfulness practices, that he could work with the pain in a new way and return to a full athletic life. And they did it for an artist, who had become so afraid of her panic attacks that she no longer went out with friends. But she was able to return to a full life by learning to be with her fear in a new way. And they even did it for a high-powered executive who came to see me because he was so accustomed to relieving his stress with alcohol, that it was now affecting his health. But he was able to use mindfulness practices to transform the emotions and impulses that were driving him to drink.

So what is this mindfulness that was so helpful to these folks? Well, mindfulness, as we're using it in Western psychotherapy and in Western neuroscience, is actually a translation of an ancient Pali term. And Pali was the vernacular language in which the teachings of the historical Buddha were first written down. And the word in Pali is *sati*, S-A-T-I. And it connotes awareness, attention, and remembering. Now, the awareness and attention part are pretty much the way we use them in English, to be aware and to pay attention. But the remembering is different. It's not about remembering what we had for breakfast or, for that matter, even remembering some childhood trauma. It's about remembering to be aware and to pay attention. So it's about developing the intention to pay attention throughout the course of the day.

Now, I was attending a conference at the University of Massachusetts Medical School, where scholars and researchers and clinicians were gathering to discuss the use of mindfulness practices in psychotherapy. And there was a Buddhist scholar there named John Donne from Emory

University. And John had a criticism. He said, you know, I think as you're talking about *sati*, you're missing something. And here was his illustration. He said, imagine a sniper, poised on top of a building, getting ready to take out an innocent victim. Now, that sniper would be very aware and very attentive. And every time his mind wandered from the task at hand, he'd be returning it. And John said, I don't think that's exactly the attitude you're trying to cultivate in yourselves as psychotherapists, nor the attitude you want to have in your patients or your clients. Something's missing. I like to think of what's missing as the Rogers—Carl Rogers and Mr. Rogers.

Now, Carl Rogers was a pioneering psychotherapist who developed the idea of unconditional positive regard and reflective listening. To be able to be with the other person with a kind of presence in which they accept whatever comes to the person's mind and whatever the person says. And Mr. Rogers, as we all know, was a television character who taught young children and who just exuded a sense that, you're OK, sweetheart, no matter what happens and whoever you are.

So together, this adds a sense of non-judgment and deep acceptance, a kind of kindness or friendliness to the enterprise. So putting these together, my colleagues and I, when starting to write about mindfulness practices in the context of psychotherapy, identified three components: It's awareness of present experience with acceptance. And now that mindfulness practices have become part of mainstream psychotherapy, people are trying to construct scales to measure this.

And what they discover is, if you could try to construct such a scale, and you basically ask people, "Are you aware of present experience with acceptance?" Almost everybody endorses that. They say, oh, sure. That's me. It's actually an example of something known as the Dunning-Kruger effect, which is an effect discovered in social psychology by David Dunning and Justin Kruger at Cornell University. The Dunning-Kruger effect says that our actual competence at a whole host of different life endeavors is actually inversely proportional to our perceived competence.

You could think of this as the Homer Simpson effect. When Homer goes out on one of his misadventures, he's supremely confident that he knows what he's doing. It's just us in the audience who have some doubts. So what happens with mindfulness is when we actually don't have that much mindfulness developed, we think of ourselves as pretty mindful. But when we develop more mindfulness, then we actually notice how often the mind wanders.

Lucky for you, it turns out that the way in which one developed a sense of mindfulness is by studying mindlessness. And I happen to be a lifelong expert at mindless behavior. Let me give you a few examples. I remember once I was driving in the Boston area to give a talk on a topic related to this at one of the universities in town. And I live west of town. And I was hassled and harried and a little bit distracted. And somehow, when it came time to get onto the Massachusetts Turnpike, I found that the automobile was going west rather than east.

Now, the Mass Pike is a toll road. And it was built a long time ago. So the toll stations were built rather far apart from one another because they're expensive to construct. And I can tell you that if you've just headed west rather than east, subjectively, they're about 100 miles apart from one another. There was plenty of time to think, what had happened here. I had no conscious recollection of any—we'll call it a volitional entity named Ron that had decided to go west rather than east. Simply, the body was sitting in the car, and the car headed off in that direction.

Curious. Who did that? How did that occur? Even if you've never gone the wrong way on the Massachusetts Turnpike, I bet you've had other life experiences in which they simply unfolded on automatic—where the mind was one place and the body somewhere else entirely. We also notice that we spend an inordinate amount of time lost in fantasies of the past and fantasies of the future. The past we call memories. For example, has the thought crossed your mind since this lecture started, I wonder if this lecture is going to be any good. It would cross many of our minds. And if we think about that, it's actually about projecting into the future and thinking, am I going to feel gratified that I took the time to listen to it? Am I going to feel good about having purchased the course? Or for that matter, any time we go into a restaurant, and we look at the menu, and we think, is this meal going to feel more gratifying, or that meal feel more gratifying? Will I enjoy this more?

Will that one make me feel guilty? These all have to do with thoughts about the future.

I happen to know the answer to this as a native New Yorker. I think we all learn it through genetic transmission or some kind of epigenetic phenomena. But have you ever wondered what the leading cause of admissions is on Sunday mornings in Manhattan to emergency rooms? When I ask audiences about this, people will say, gunshot wounds, the effects of drinking too much the night before. Actually, it's none of those. It's bagel cutting incidents.

What's happening is people are at home, perhaps with family or with friends, and they get into some kind of a discussion and, sure enough, one hand cuts right through the flesh of the other. In fact, I was talking about this topic to an audience in Texas. And a fellow said to me, "You know it happened to me. I was in Manhattan. I was with my sister. We started to talk about our mother, again. One hand sliced right through the other. I went to the emergency room. And the first thing the triage nurse said to me was, 'Do you know, the leading cause of admissions here every Sunday morning are people like you?' " So apparently it's true.

Now, on top of this, we have a remarkable tendency to always try to get to the good stuff. This is things like, washing the dishes and thinking, I can't wait to be done with this so that I can have my cup of tea or go call my friend. Or perhaps the thought, let me finish my paperwork so I can get home. Or let me get through this traffic so I can get to the park where I want to go. We're constantly trying to get to the good stuff. And this is really interesting when we ponder, what are the moments in our lives that really matter?

So take a moment to consider that. Think of some experience you've had that do you think, that's precious. I'm so glad I was there for that. When I ask audiences about this, it's usually things like the birth of a child or perhaps a wedding or perhaps an intimate conversation with a friend or maybe watching a sunset. The next question is, where was your mind during that activity that you felt was very meaningful? Was it thinking about the past or the future? Or did it actually show up, was it actually present for the experience at hand? The correct answer is, I think, it was present for the experience at hand. So we have this really odd juxtaposition. Most of the time, our minds are actually not in the present moment. And yet the moments that matter to us are all situations in which our mind shows up.

I'm sorry to say, it gets worse. It turns out that life is difficult for everybody. There are lots of reasons for this. I just want to address a couple of them. First, you may have noticed that everything changes, and loss is inevitable. There's a psychoanalytic writer named Judith Viorst who wrote a book in the 1980s called *Necessary Losses*. And it was on the bookshelf of virtually every psychotherapist. I don't know how many actually read it, but it was on a lot of bookshelves. And her basic premise was, you could understand a great deal about human unhappiness by looking at our difficulties dealing with loss.

Now, this starts very early. I don't want to give up my diapers and start using the potty. The current arrangement suits me just fine. School, with all those strange people and weird teacher? No, thank you. I will stay home with you, Mom. And even though some of these changes may have some excitement connected to them, they also, typically, have a lot of fear and a lot of concern. I remember when it was time to give up my Toyota Corolla and get a minivan because we had given birth, or my wife had given birth to twin daughters. And I wasn't so pleased about it. It didn't seem like such a cool idea.

And then, when they had grown up 18 years later, and they were ready to go to college, I thought, this is how it works? I spend 18 years trying to forge a good relationship with them, trying to prepare them for life, trying to feel connected, and now they're going to abandon me like a lot of girls did when I was 18 myself? Who designed this system? Now, luckily, my wife has little bit more wisdom about these matters than I do. And she pointed out that, had they been so impaired that they couldn't go off to college, I'd be even more upset. And I'll grant her that—but the change wasn't very easy.

And as I project forward and think, someday, perhaps, entering assisted living or a nursing home, even if they're playing The Stones for my whole generation, I don't think I'm going to be so pleased about the change. Perhaps you yourself have noticed changes. Have you noticed any changes in your body since you were 20? Have you welcomed and embraced them all? Change is hard.

And we have other problems. I was once listening to an interview on National Public Radio that Terry Gross is conducting with Robert Sapolsky, who's a wonderful stress physiologist. He's an excellent teacher. And she's asking him about his life's work. And he was describing that his colleagues essentially spent years hiding behind blinds of vegetation in the African Savannah, watching baboon troops. And what they would do is they would wait for a particularly juicy soap opera-like interaction among the baboons. They go in. They'd anaesthetize all the baboons. Draw blood. And try to come up with some conclusions about stress physiology.

So Terry Gross said, well, that's an interesting way to have spent a career. What did you learn? Dr. Sapolsky said, well, the first thing we learned was, it's really hard to anaesthetize a whole group of baboons without screwing up their stress hormones. But apparently, he found some way to get over that hurdle. So Terry said, did you learn anything else? He said, yes. Another thing we learned was that stress physiology is far more complex than we had ever anticipated. We thought that there were going to be a few hormonal systems interacting. And it turns out that there are hundreds.

Now, Terry Gross is a good interviewer and she was looking for take-home point. So she said, well, is there anything that has really stood out? He said, well, yes, there is one particularly robust finding. What's that? It's quite bad for your health to be a low-ranking male in a baboon troop. Now, we may think of ourselves as the smart monkeys, as somehow above this, that this doesn't apply to us. But the way in which it shows up in humans is concern about what we call self-esteem.

It's our remarkably robust habit of comparing ourselves to others. In fact, this is said in the Buddhist tradition to be the last neurotic tendency to fall away before highest perfect enlightenment. So how does this work? Well, different people get caught on different domains or dimensions. We compare ourselves in different ways. For one person, it's about who's wealthier. For someone else, it's who's smarter or who's more physically fit, who has more artistic talent, who has more sense of style, better-behaved kids, the better-behaved spouse.

This becomes particularly humorous when we get into the context of meditators or people involved in spiritual practices. Then it's who makes fewer comparisons? Who's less competitive? Who's more selfless? It doesn't matter. The concern for rank in the primate troop manifests itself in we humans with these constant preoccupations for how we compare to others.

Now, assuming that you're like me and you also make these comparisons, do you always win? I once asked that question to a group of psychotherapists. And I said, who here always wins? A guy raised his hand. And I thought, avoid him at lunch. Bad sign, right? And on top of this, we have another problem. I'll often ask those same groups of psychotherapists, who here is going to die. Usually at tops, 20 percent of the hands go up. But of course, we know our prognosis for all of us is quite poor in this regard. No wonder happiness is so elusive.

Now, mindfulness practices can help us with all of this. They can help us to see and accept things as they are, rather than as we wish them to be—like, for example, being better able to deal with the inevitability of illness or even death. It's not an accident that so many hospice workers practice mindfulness meditation so that they can be with folks who are at the end of life. It can also help to loosen our preoccupation with self, with the concern with where we rank in the baboon troop.

In fact, it's been shown to quiet parts of the brain that are associated with self-referential thinking. It can even help us to experience the richness of the moment more fully. And this promotes savoring which research shows to be a very important component of most paths to well-being. And finally, it helps to connect us to a world outside of ourselves, to something larger. And this is particularly important, given our ultimate prognosis. And it's another reason why mindfulness practices figure prominently in so many spiritual traditions.

Now, mindfulness can also help us to get along with one another better. It helps us to see the other person more clearly and not believe so much in our judgments. So we don't get caught as much in condemning the other person who has upset us today. It also helps us to not take things so personally. So we can realize that much of the time, the other person's behavior, even if it's disturbing to us, isn't really about us. It rather reflects their own struggles at the moment.

And it can help us to actually be present in relationships. And this is essential to be able to provide empathy for others and to support others, which is quite important if we're going to get along, particularly during difficult times. It also helps us to learn not to act on urges compulsively, so that we can respond thoughtfully rather than react automatically out of our hurt or anger.

Over the coming lectures, we'll be looking much more at what mindfulness is and isn't, and what modern science is revealing about how it can resolve both everyday and more serious problems while helping to make our lives richer and happier. Now is a great time to be studying this. Since we're in the midst of an explosion in scientific research about how mindfulness practices change both the structure and functioning of our brains as well as how they can improve all sorts of health outcomes.

For over 30 years, I've been privileged to be part of a group of clinicians and researchers in and around Harvard Medical School, all of whom have had personal long-term meditation practices. It's been exciting for all of us to see these practices moving into the mainstream of psychology, neuroscience, and medicine, as their positive effects on the mind, the brain, and the whole body are being studied. We're seeing that mindfulness practices actually keep important parts of our brain from withering with age. And they also activate brain circuits associated with being happy, energized, and enthusiastically engaged in life. They even lengthen telomeres, the ends of chromosomes that get worn down with stress, resulting in cell death that's associated with aging.

Now, to experienced mindfulness students, it can seem strange that a millimeter change in brain tissue, as shown on magnetic resonance imaging or a shift in EEG activity, is more convincing in our modern age than reports of living people who are meditating, or thousands of years of testimony from monks and nuns who have successfully used these practices to find peace, fulfillment, and wellness. But for people relatively new to the practices, the scientific findings are really important, especially given the tenacity of competing and often questionable religious, philosophic, and medical claims about cures. After all, how do we know that the proponents of various miracle solutions and cures for medical problems and cures for other sorts of life problems aren't just fooling themselves or trying to fool us? It's encouraging for those of us who have found mindfulness practices to be personally transforming, and have taught them with positive results to others, to know that science is now validating time-honored observations about their power.

Mindfulness practice is also, itself, a form of empirical inquiry, an investigative tool for a sort of inner science. It enables us to carefully observe the processes that create distress and that alleviate it in our own minds and bodies. And I think you'll agree, once you've seen the results in the laboratory of your own mind, that mindfulness practices simply feel remarkably transformative. This is also a great time to be studying mindfulness practices, given the recent explosion of research into how they can help us with a remarkable variety of psychological difficulties.

It turns out that everything from anxiety and depression to the challenges of intimate relationships, aging, and even raising children can be helped with mindfulness practices. In fact, over the last few years at the meetings of the ABCT, that's the American Association of Behavioral and Cognitive Therapies—and this is the convention where clinical psychology professors and their students come to present the latest research on empirically-validated new psychotherapies—it turns out that the majority of presentations are now on mindfulness- and acceptance-based treatments. This has indeed become the mainstream of scientifically-based modern psychotherapy.

Sound good? Want to become more mindful? Let's take look at how to do just that. The way that we become more mindful is through mindfulness practices. And we can look at this through an analogy with physical fitness. Physical fitness is strength, endurance, and flexibility. But the way we develop physical fitness is through things like calisthenics, working out at the gym, going for a bike ride, that sort of thing.

So mindfulness is awareness of present experience with acceptance. But the way we develop mindfulness is through mindfulness practices.

Now, since many of these practices are borrowed from Asian traditions, they can seem a little strange to us initially. And I'd like to clear up a few misconceptions about them. Many people assume that mindfulness practice is about developing a blank mind. There is a story of Jon Kabat-Zinn, who has done a lot to introduce mindfulness practices to Western audiences and into medical practice. And he's leading a meditation retreat. And a fellow brings him a comic. And it's one of these comics that comes from bubble gum, a Bazooka Joe comic. And in the comic, there's Joe sitting in full Lotus meditation posture, looking very serene and very serious. And next to him is his sidekick, Mort. And Joe was saying, since I've discovered meditation, my mind is a complete blank. And Mort's saying, gee, Joe. I thought you were born that way.

This is not about developing a blank mind or getting the thought stream to shut up. That only happens during very intensive retreat practice. It is, however, about developing a different relationship to our thoughts, so that we can observe them coming and going and not believe in or identify them so very much.

As I mentioned, most people enter these practices when they're having a rough time. And they secretly hope that this will get rid of the negative emotions, will help us to escape pain. The practices don't actually work that way. We actually feel our emotions more vividly, and even feel our pain more vividly. But because we don't resist that pain and don't resist that emotion, we wind up suffering much less.

Even though these practices were refined by monks and nuns and other enunciates, they're not actually about withdrawing from life. We might take a little time to step back to develop these capacities. But they are for the purpose of engaging so much more richly and so much more fully in life. And even though, occasionally, we run up against wonderful experiences of bliss or peace, they're not really about seeking bliss or peace. They're about learning to be with whatever might arise. And finally, even though we call these mindfulness practices, they're really mind and body practices because they're very much about noticing that all of our experience in consciousness occurs from the mind-body more broadly.

So under the umbrella of mindfulness practices, there are actually three skills that we're going to try to develop. And the neurobiologists are helping us to clarify them. The first skill is focused attention, traditionally called concentration. And that helps us to observe things clearly.

The second skill the neurobiologists now call *open monitoring*. It used to be called, or it's called in the Zen tradition, *choice-less awareness*, or even *mindfulness*, per se. And I know that can be a little confusing. It's when people started introducing mindfulness practices into the West, they used the umbrella term mindfulness to actually cover a number of different sub-practices. And open monitoring is used to see how the mind creates suffering for itself.

Finally, the last skill is acceptance and loving kindness, which is used to soothe and comfort. Now, the neurobiological evidence is that the mental skills cultivated by these three different meditation types actually represent overlapping yet distinct brain processes. Let's talk a little bit more about focused attention and open monitoring. Focused attention involves choosing an object and following it closely, like the breath or a sound. Whereas open monitoring involves opening the field of awareness to whatever arises in consciousness. Actually, focused attention and open monitoring develop the first two aspects of mindfulness. They develop awareness of present experience. And we can think of the relationship between those two as kind of like the old days when we had cameras with a manual focus lens. In those days, if you wanted to be a photographer, first you had to get the skill down of how to focus the lens. If you didn't have that skill down, you were going to be pretty much limited to Impressionism. But once you got that skill down, you could take a picture of anything at all. In the same way, we use focused attention to be able to refine the attention of the mind to be able to see what's happening in each moment. And then, we can open it to whatever arises in awareness, to see how the mind creates suffering for itself.

Now, the third skill is acceptance. And here's one way to understand that. What would you feel inside if you saw a very cute little puppy just barely able to stand, looking at you with big brown eyes, wagging its tail? Would you likely feel a sense of harsh, critical judgment? Probably not. You would feel something that goes like, ah. You know what that feeling's like. Now, even if that puppy were to pee and poop at the wrong time, in the wrong place, even if it weren't to listen to instructions, you would think, well, he's young. He just needs training.

You'll likely find when you take up mindfulness practices that your mind does pee and poop at the wrong time, in the wrong place. And it doesn't listen to instructions. And we want to have the same attitude toward it. It's OK. It just needs training. This third component, acceptance, is often just as hard as paying attention. We need to constantly let go to develop what the meditation teacher, Joseph Goldstein, calls a "soft and spacious mind." Now, most mindfulness practices develop one or the other of these three skills.

We can understand the development of different religious and philosophical schools throughout history as responses to our evolutionarily-determined and neurobiologically-hardwired predisposition toward psychological distress. They're all ways of finding happiness or well-being in the face of our shared biological and existential predicaments. Often independently, many different religions and philosophical schools have either developed forms of mindfulness practice themselves, or they've hit on insights similar those that we encounter when we practice mindfulness. It just happens that of all the world's religious traditions and philosophical traditions and wisdom traditions, mindfulness practices have been developed and refined the most in Buddhist monasteries. This doesn't mean, though, that you have to become a Buddhist to benefit from them.

The original teachings of the historical Buddha were remarkably pragmatic and avoided many questions we usually think of as religious. He eschewed metaphysical speculation about things like the origins of the universe, what exactly happens after death, or even the existence of God or gods. He called himself a "physician of the mind." And said, I teach the origins of psychological suffering and its alleviation. This is one reason why practices drawn from Buddhist teachings are such a natural fit with mental health professionals. After all, we're trying to be effective physicians of the mind ourselves.

Because of their practical nature, most people find that Buddhist techniques and teachings needn't interfere with their cultural identifications or their personal philosophic and religious beliefs. And this has made them good candidates for study neurobiologically and to integrate into medical and psychological treatments. So it's primarily mindfulness practices drawn from Buddhist traditions, that we're learning change brain structure and function, and move ourselves in desirable directions to help alleviate psychological distress. But as we'll also see, mindfulness practices drawn from other Western and Eastern religious, philosophic, and psychological traditions can also be part of a scientifically-supported path to well-being.

Also, the practices themselves are taking new form as they are being used in modern scientific psychotherapy with its emphasis on the nuance of interpersonal relationships of all kinds. So while religious and philosophical systems are providing tools for scientifically-informed paths to well-being, insights from science are prompting these ancient traditions to evolve as they are being practiced in the modern world.

Throughout the course, I'll encourage you to regularly engage in mindfulness practices yourself. Like swimming, making love, or eating a gourmet meal, you can read or hear about it, but that won't give you the understanding or the benefits that you will get from actually doing it. And it appears that mindfulness development is dose-related. Do a little practice, develop a little mindfulness—do a lot of practice, develop a lot of mindfulness.

So I'll introduce some practices to you during the lectures. But also encourage you to practice them on your own. Most people find it helpful to follow recorded instructions at least for the first several times they try a practice. Whether I'm teaching these to mental health professionals or to my patients, I find that without either a live teacher or recorded instructions, it's hard for most beginners not to get lost in daydreaming, to stay focused on the practice.

And that's why we've provided longer audio recordings of mindfulness practices in this course to guide you. Now, in the next lecture, we'll look at how our brains evolved for survival rather than for happiness, and how this sets us up for countless difficulties. Difficulties that mindfulness practices were developed to help us resolve. And we'll also learn how to start practicing mindfulness ourselves so that we can train our brains not only to thrive, but also to flourish.

Our Troublesome Brains
Lecture 2

I
n this lecture, you will learn how our brains evolved for survival rather than for happiness and how this sets us up for countless difficulties—difficulties that mindfulness practices were developed to help us resolve. In addition, you will learn how to start practicing mindfulness so that you can train your brain not only to thrive, but also to flourish. Understanding what science is revealing about why various problems plague us is important for being able to use the practices effectively.

Stress-Related Disorders

- By some estimates, over 80 percent of visits to the doctor's office in the developed world are for stress-related disorders. After upper respiratory diseases (which we actually catch more easily when stressed because of our weakened immune system), the most common ailments are all either caused or exacerbated by stress, including chronic back and neck pain, gastrointestinal distress, headaches, insomnia, and problems with sexual functioning.

- Then, there are many medical problems that are the result of habit disorders like eating or drinking too much or eating unhealthy foods. And, of course, many people seek medical help for anxiety and depression.

- These problems don't just exist because of the difficulties living in today's fast-paced world. Hardwired, evolutionarily determined tendencies that cause our stress are active even during the best of times. From what science is uncovering about the evolution of our brains, we have learned that most of us have minds that are predisposed to making ourselves unhappy.

- And these predispositions set us up for so many psychological and physical difficulties and disorders. Of course, there are exceptions—

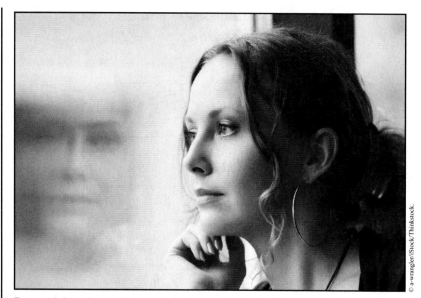

Research has shown that people who engage in mindfulness practices experience fewer stress-related problems than those who do not.

there are a few individuals with minds that are naturally at peace, who are easily contented. And these people have far fewer stress-related problems than others.

The Evolution of the Human Brain

- Research is showing that our propensity to psychological distress is universal. That's good news—it means that it's not necessarily our fault or failure. In addition, we humans have developed mindfulness practices that can help counteract our propensities for distress.

- Science suggests that we didn't actually evolve to be happy. The cortex of the brain mostly evolved to analyze the past and imagine the future—and to remember past moments of pleasure and pain and to figure out how to maximize future pleasure and avoid future pain. So, the cortex doesn't just think any thoughts; it thinks thoughts tailored to the demands of our environment.

- Our ancestors lived in small bands. It was uncommon for them to meet unknown people, and it was dangerous when they did. In addition, they were faced with starvation, parasites, illness, injury, and the hazards of childbirth and didn't have painkillers or police departments.

- Our ancestors could make two possible mistakes: Thinking that there was a lion behind the bushes when it was actually a beige rock and thinking that there was a beige rock behind the bushes when it was actually a lion. The cost of the first mistake was needless anxiety, while the cost of the second was death. So, we evolved to make the first mistake a thousand times to avoid making the second mistake even once.

- Our ancestors remembered every bad thing that happened and spent much of their lives anticipating more trouble. And this is the mind they bequeathed to us.

Negativity Bias

- Cognitive scientists say that we have developed what's called a negativity bias. For example, notice what comes to your mind when you see the words "Bill Clinton." In an informal sampling, about 80 percent of people immediately think about either Monica Lewinsky or a blue dress.

- One reason for this is the existence of the amygdala, which is an almond-sized part of the brain that reacts more to negative than positive stimuli. The negative contaminates the positive more easily than the positive contaminates the negative. This is why we remember Monica Lewinsky and why negative ads dominate political campaigns.

- Other animals, which presumably don't think as much as humans do, also have a negativity bias. If you run a rat through a maze and at the end of a given pathway give the rat an electric shock, one trial learning will work, and the rat won't go down that pathway again. But if you run the rat through a maze and at the end they get food, they need several different trials before they actually learn it. But rats are much less likely than we are to spend their time, when not confronted by danger or pursuing food, thinking about the electric shock or thinking about the food.

- Negativity bias emerged in harsh settings very different from our own, but it continues to operate today. For example, on a daily basis you might drive in traffic, try to diet, watch the news, juggle housework, pay bills, or go on a date. Even in relatively safe situations, we react as though they're life-or-death situations and often expect the worst.

Survival Systems
- On top of our hardwiring, learning changes the brain. So, the negative expectations and outlooks that develop from our negativity bias become new pathways in the brain. Scientists used to think that the brain reaches maturity at age 25 and deteriorates after that. We now know that it's more like a muscle. While it ultimately weakens, throughout our life, areas of the brain we use become stronger. Scientists call this experience-dependent neuroplasticity.

- Other tendencies that predispose us to unhappiness include difficulties accepting change, because everything we enjoy or love eventually leaves or changes, and preoccupation with self, which is difficult given our changing fortunes and poor prognosis.

- All of this interacts regularly with another important survival system that we share with many other animals: our emergency response, or fight-freeze-flight, system. Basically, it's the arousal, which can feel like desperation, we experience when we're threatened.

- This emergency arousal system is activated by every one of our negative thoughts. While our bodies evolved to be able to handle these emergency responses from time to time, they don't do very well when this system is activated all day long. It's this constant activation that sets us up for so many ailments.

- In addition, there's another survival system that occupies a lot of our attention. While we evolved to expect the worst, we're also hardwired to pursue pleasure and try to avoid pain. This makes a lot of sense evolutionarily, because pursuing pleasure and avoiding pain motivates us to do things that help perpetuate our DNA.

- Generally, activities that perpetuate our DNA are experienced as pleasurable, including returning to homeostasis, having sex, eating, sleeping, alleviating (most) pain, and enhancing social rank. So, we get hooked on seeking these things. And when we don't have the conditions that help perpetuate our DNA, or fear that we'll lose them, we become distressed.

- Our fear-response system is activated not only by threats, but also by fear that we won't get what we evolved to want. These motivational systems—that drive us to seek pleasure and fear threats—are continuously interacting with our propensity to recall the past and imagine the future. They drive us to do things in the pursuit of happiness that don't actually sustain our feelings of well-being for long.

- Many of the things we do to pursue good feeling, such as shopping, are subject to the hedonic treadmill—you need more and more to keep the same level of well-being. And then there are all of our pursuits that feel good in the short run but leave us feeling bad in the long run, such as eating too many donuts.

- It makes perfect sense that we would've evolved to be drawn to sweets and fats given that getting enough calories used to be a challenge, but it wreaks havoc for our modern lives in the developed world, where sufficient calories are all too readily available. With all of these evolutionarily hardwired systems operating, it's no wonder that we so often find life to be difficult.

The Effects of Mindfulness Practices
- Mindfulness practices were developed in response to our complex evolutionary predicament. They're systematic methods for gaining

insight into how the mind instinctually creates suffering for itself. Mindfulness practices include techniques designed to interrupt these natural processes of mind.

- Of course mindfulness practices are not the only tools we humans have developed to deal with our hardwired tendencies toward psychological distress. For example, people have developed programs of positive thinking—affirmations of various sorts—to counteract our negativity bias. And there are all sorts of psychotherapy designed to replace negative thoughts with positive ones.

- Historically, diverse cultures have developed a wide variety of religious beliefs and rituals that help us feel safer in an uncertain world. Studies have shown that all of these approaches—positive thinking, religious faith, and conventional psychotherapy—can enhance our sense of well-being.

- Mindfulness practices are another set of tools. They may be particularly far-reaching in their effect on well-being because they address two challenges simultaneously: They can provide profound insight into the patterns of mind that create suffering, radically changing our views of ourselves and others, and they retrain the brain to not automatically respond in its instinctual patterns.

- What are some of the insights into distress-generating patterns we get from mindfulness practice? We notice that we relate to all experience as either pleasant, unpleasant, or neutral. We see that we habitually try to hold on to the pleasant, push away the unpleasant, and lose interest in the neutral. This causes an inordinate amount of distress when paired with our negativity bias.

- We evolved to both expect unpleasant experiences and to constantly work to try to avoid them. Having these tendencies coexist sets up a continuous tension for many of us that we experience as feeling stressed much of the time.

- We also see that trying to grasp, or hold on to, changing phenomena causes suffering. We see that our thoughts are not reality; in fact, they constantly change with our changing feeling states. And we see that all that actually exists is the present moment—despite the fact that we're hardwired to be constantly seeking pleasure and avoiding pain, which means living in memories of the past and fantasies of the future.

- Reading, hearing, or talking about mindfulness isn't the same as practicing it. In fact, it's very difficult to understand what these practices are like unless you try them. It's very important to practice regularly. And keep in mind that different variations have different effects.

Suggested Reading

Gilbert, *Stumbling on Happiness*.

Hanson, *Hardwiring Happiness*.

Hanson and Mendius, *Buddha's Brain*.

Siegel, *The Mindfulness Solution*, chapter 1.

Questions to Consider

1. In what situations do you notice the negativity bias operating most strongly in your experience?

2. What did you find most challenging about trying breath awareness practice? When you reflect on that challenge, does it illustrate anything about the everyday functioning of your mind and what might cause you psychological distress generally?

Mindfulness Practice

breath awareness: A brief version of a foundational formal meditation practice.

Our Troublesome Brains
Lecture 2—Transcript

Did you know that by some estimates, over 80 percent of visits to doctor's offices in the developed world are for stress-related disorders? After upper respiratory diseases, which we actually catch more easily when stressed because of our weakened immune system, the most common ailments all are either caused by or exacerbated by stress. Chronic back and neck pain, gastrointestinal distress—both lower GI and upper GI—headaches, insomnia, problems with sexual functioning. Then there are lots of medical problems that are the result of habit disorders, like eating or drinking too much, or eating unhealthful foods. And of course, many people seek medical help for anxiety and depression.

How did this possibly come about? Well, we'll be talking later in the course about how to use mindfulness practices to address these sorts of problems. Understanding what science is revealing about why they plague us is important for being able to use the practices effectively. And as it turns out, these problems don't just exist because of the difficulties living in today's fast-paced world, or because of stressful moments. If we pay careful attention, we can see that hardwired evolutionarily-determined tendencies that cause us stress are active even during the best of times.

Let me give you an example. I love vacations. Of course, relaxing and enjoying central pleasures is nice. But the really great part about vacations is how they illuminate the workings of my mind. I might be on a beautiful Caribbean beach with perfect temperature, glistening white sand, and clear waters, but still, my mind can create trouble. I can spy a dark cloud on the horizon and start worrying that it might rain. Or my wife and I can start talking about our kids, and soon I'm worrying about them. Or in those rare moments when everything's really perfect, I'll start thinking that it won't last, before long I'll have to return home, and eventually I'll be too old or infirm to enjoy the beach.

I used to think that it was just me that was so crazy. But as I've learned what science is uncovering about the evolution of our minds and our brains, I've come to realize that most of us have minds and brains that are predisposed in this way to making ourselves unhappy, and these predispositions set us up for all sorts of psychological and physical disorders.

Of course, there are exceptions. There are few individuals with minds that are naturally at peace, who are easily contented, and these folks have far fewer stress-related problems than the rest of us. My friend, the meditation teacher and psychologist Jack Cornfield, has studied how these remarkably happy and healthy individuals function. Here's what he's learned.

If you can sit quietly after difficult news, if in financial downturns you remain perfectly calm, if you can see your neighbors travel to fantastic places without a twinge of jealousy, if you can happily eat whatever's put on your plate and fall asleep after a day of running around without a drink or a pill, if you can always find contentment just where you are, you are probably a dog. For those of us who happen to be human, it's not so easy. Research is showing that our propensity of psychological distress is quite universal. That's good news! It means it's not our own fault or failure. And there's other good news too. We humans have developed mindfulness practices that can help to counteract our predispositions to distress.

You know, the American Declaration of Independence guarantees the right to life, liberty, and the pursuit of happiness. But why do we have to pursue it like it's some sort of fugitive? For centuries the world's religions and philosophic traditions have sought answers to this question. Only relatively recently has science suggested an answer. We didn't actually evolve to be happy.

Let me illustrate what I mean. Imagine for moment the existence of Lucy. She was *Australopithecus* and she lived some 3.2 million years ago. It could be that she's our great-great-great-great-great-great-great-great-, etc., grandmother. Scientists think that either she or a hominid somewhat like her was likely our common ancestor.

Imagine what it was like for her out there on the African Savannah competing with the other wildlife. Imagine, for example, that she came face to face with a lion. What might she do? Well, she could bare her teeth or show her claws, but that probably wouldn't be too effective. She could rely on her hide for protection, but that, too, wouldn't help much; her fur was really quite silly. She wasn't really all that fast.

If you've ever had the opportunity to go on a walking safari in Africa— and I'm delighted to say I have had such an opportunity—the standard setup looks like this: There's a group of tourists, usually in a line, and usually one or two guys (the guides) with big guns. And they give an orientation talk at the beginning. And that talk always features one important admonition. They say, whatever happens, don't run. Why? See that lumbering hippopotamus over there in the mud puddle?—42 miles an hour when he gets going. See those half dead rhinos hardly even moving behind the trees?—48 miles an hour when they get going. Everything out there is faster than you are. And if you start to run, they're going to just think you're prey.

So we couldn't outrun the predators. Our sense of sight was OK, not as good as a giraffe or a hawk, perhaps, but better than those rhinos. Our sense of hearing was also mid-range. And our sense of smell didn't help us out very much at all; it was pretty weak. Just ask your dog for comparisons. And yet, we know that we survived. We know our ancestors survived. How did they do it? Well, they had a few things going for them. Lucy had a prehensile or opposable thumb so she could pick things up. And she had exquisite fingers. Just take a moment to examine your fingers right now—if you're not driving or in some other indisposed circumstance—and notice how exquisitely sensitive they are and how much dexterity we have. And think: Do you know any other animals that have anything like this ability to manipulate objects? Probably not. And of course, we also had an usually sophisticated brain. Now the thumb and fingers didn't cause much trouble. I'm afraid I can't say the same for the brain.

By two million years ago our hominid ancestors, *Homo habilis*, was intelligent enough to start making stone tools. And our own species, *Homo sapiens*, the clever ape, emerged about 200,000 years ago. And over the course of evolution, our cortex grew three times larger. It grew to deal pretty much with the same environment that Lucy faced. The situation didn't change much until humans had started building cities much later.

So this bigger cortex had a great value for survival. The problem is it also set us up for an awful lot of psychological suffering. As we'll soon see, this was in part because it had to coexist with another important survival mechanism, and the two together are recipe for misery. But let's first look at what the cortex spends a lot of its time doing.

It mostly evolved to analyze past and imagine the future, and to remember past moments of pleasure and pain, and figure out how to maximize future pleasure and avoid future pain. So as the cortex thinks, it doesn't just think any thoughts, it thinks thoughts tailored to the demands of our environment.

Let's look more closely at the environment our ancestors lived in. They were grouped in small bands, and it was very uncommon to meet unknown people, and dangerous when they did. Also starvation, parasites, illness, injury, and the hazards of childbirth were all commonplace, and there were no painkillers and no police departments. This world was the womb of the human brain and it was a rough place.

Now, our ancestors could make two possible mistakes. Let's imagine it was Lucy and that she was looking at some bushes and she spied a beige shape behind the bushes. The first mistake would be thinking, eh, I think it's a lion, when it's actually a beige rock. The second mistake would be saying, eh, it's probably a beige rock, when it was really a lion. The cost of the first mistake: needless anxiety; the cost of the second mistake: death. So we evolved to make the first mistake a thousand times to avoid making the second mistake even once.

Now, we can imagine that there might have been some happy hominids around singing "Kumbaya," thinking about dynamite sexual experiences or luscious pieces of fruit that they had experienced. Those folks generally weren't our ancestors, because statistically they died before reproducing. Our ancestors were the ones who spent each day remembering every bad thing that had happened, and spent much of their lives anticipating more trouble. And this is the mind they bequeathed to us. It's quite easy to see it in operation when we do some mindfulness practice.

Now, cognitive scientists say we develop what's called a *negativity bias*. I'll give you an example of how this works. I'm going to say two words, and simply notice whatever comes to your mind when you hear them. Ready? Bill Clinton. In my informal sampling, about 80 percent of people immediately think either Monica Lewinsky or a blue dress. And the negativity bias is why it's so easy to ruin a reputation.

My friend, Rick Hansen, who wrote a wonderful book called *The Buddhist Brain* said, "Our minds evolve to be Velcro for bad experiences and Teflon for good." Bad experiences stick, good ones slide off. If you got 20 things done today but made one mistake, what do you think you'll think about at night when you go to bed? If your boss gives you a generally positive review, but there's one area for improvement, which one sticks in the mind? From a survival standpoint, sticks have much more urgency and impact than carrots.

There are many other examples. There's a part of the brain called the amygdala. It's an almond shaped little area, and it's designed to evaluate our environmental circumstances and decide whether something's a threat or not. It turns out the amygdala reacts far more rapidly and more thoroughly to negative than to positives stimuli.

In relationships, trust is easy to lose and hard to regain. The negative contaminates the positive more easily than the positive contaminates the negative. This is why we remember Monica Lewinsky and negative ads dominate political campaigns.

There's a couple of researchers, they're a married couple themselves, the Gottmans in Seattle, and they've been spending decades studying the interactions between members of romantic couples and seeing which kinds of interactions lead to lasting and wholesome relationships and which ones lead to dysfunctional ones. And they've determined that there's a basic ratio. It basically takes five positive interactions between members of a couple to undo the effects of only one fight.

Now, other animals who presumably don't think so much also have a negativity bias. If you run rats through a maze and at the end of a given pathway give the rat an electric shock, one-trial learning will work; the rat won't go down that pathway again. But if you run the rat through a maze and at the end they get food, they need several different trials before they actually learn it. But rats are much less likely than we are to spend their time, when not confronted by danger or pursuing food, thinking about the electric shock or thinking about the food. I'm afraid I can't say the same for us.

The negativity bias emerged in harsh settings very different from our own, but it continues to operate today. If we drive in traffic, try to settle a squabble between siblings, try to diet, try to deal with housework, paying bills, or even go on a date, we have our negativity bias operating. Even in relatively safe situations, we react as though they're life or death challenges, and very often we expect the worst.

On top of our hard wiring, learning also changes the brain. So the negative expectations and outlooks actually start to deepen the more we experience them. When I trained as a psychologist, scientists thought that the brain reaches maturity around the age of 25 and then deteriorates after that. We now know that it's much more like a muscle. While ultimately it weakens, throughout our life, if we use parts of our brain, they become stronger; if we don't use them, they become weaker. Scientists call this *experience-dependent neuroplasticity*, and it's like a riverbed that deepens over time. And we already discussed other tendencies that predispose us to unhappiness. Our difficulties accepting change, the fact that everything we enjoy or love eventually leaves or changes, and our preoccupation with self and self esteem, which is so difficult given our changing fortunes and poor prognosis.

Now, all of this interacts regularly with another important survival system that we share with many other animals: It's our emergency response or fight, freeze, flight system. Basically, it's the arousal—which can feel like desperation—that we experience when we're threatened. This emergency arousal system is activated by every one of our negative thoughts. While our bodies evolved to be able to handle these emergency responses from time to time, they don't do very well when the system is activated all day long. And it's this constant activation that sets us up for so many of the ailments I mentioned earlier.

And as if this weren't enough, there's another survival system that occupies a lot of our attention. While we evolved to expect the worst, we also evolved to be hardwired to pursue pleasure and try to avoid pain. This makes a lot of sense evolutionarily since pursuing pleasure and avoiding pain motivates us to do things that help to perpetuate our DNA.

Generally, activities that perpetuate our DNA are pleasurable experiences. So returning to homeostasis—if I'm cold, getting warmer, if I'm warm, getting cooler. Having sex, obviously, typically feels good and helps perpetuate DNA. Eating when we're hungry, sleeping when we're tired, alleviating pain, generally, and even enhancing social rank all helps our DNA to get propagated. So we get hooked on seeking these things.

And when we don't have the conditions that help to perpetuate our DNA, or fear that we'll lose them, we become distressed. Or fear response system is activated, not only by threats, but by fear that we won't get what we evolve to want. These motivational systems, the desire to seek pleasure and fear threats, are continuously interacting with our propensity to recall the past and imagine the future. And they drive us to do all sorts of things in the pursuit of happiness that don't actually sustain our feelings of well being for very long.

Take for example what it's like to buy a car or go shopping for a new outfit. It starts with just thinking about making the purchase. We'll use the car as an example. We start to see cars out on the road that look attractive to us and think, oh, it might be nice to have that one. Oh, this other one could be cool. Then we actually go to the showroom and check them out, and might get quite excited about how it feels to drive them. At a certain point, we decide to take the leap and we buy the car. And there may be some fear, but there's a lot of excitement that goes in with that. And after a few days, we kind of start to get used to owning it. And it's different for different people, but it doesn't take that long before we start to habituate to having the car. And instead of it being the new source of joy, the new source of pleasure, it starts to become a means of transportation. But luckily, our minds can start thinking about buying something else, which is exactly what they do.

Now, many of the things we do to pursue positive or good feelings are like shopping: They're subject to the hedonic treadmill. We need more and more to keep the same level of well being. Hedonic comes from the same root as hedonism, having to do with pleasure. And then they're all of our pursuits that feel good in the short run but leave us feeling really badly in the long run, like eating too many doughnuts or too many well-marbled steaks.

It makes perfect sense that we would have evolved to be drawn to sweets, in fact, given that getting enough calories used to be a challenge. But it wreaks havoc on our modern lives in which, in the developed world at least, there are sufficient calories all too readily available. And with all of these evolutionary hardwired systems operating, no wonder so often we find life to be difficult.

Mindfulness practices were developed in response to this complex evolutionary predicament. They're systematic methods for gaining insight into how the mind instinctually creates suffering for itself. Mindfulness practices include techniques designed to interrupt these natural processes of the mind.

Of course, mindfulness practices aren't the only tools we humans have developed to deal with our hardwired tendencies towards psychological distress. For example, people have developed programs of positive thinking, affirmations of various sorts to counteract our negativity bias. And there are all sorts of psychotherapy designed to replace negative thoughts with positive ones. And historically, virtually every culture has developed some kind of religious belief or ritual to help its members feel safer in an uncertain world.

Now, studies have shown that all of these approaches—positive thinking, religious faith, conventional psychotherapy—can enhance our sense of well being. Mindfulness practices are simply another set of tools. Now, they may be particularly far reaching in their effect because they address two challenges simultaneously. First, they can provide profound insight into the patterns of mind that create suffering, and that can radically change our views of ourselves and others. They can also retrain the brain to not automatically respond in its instinctual patterns.

So what are some of the insights into the workings of the mind that we get from mindfulness practice? Well, one of the first things we observe is that we relate to all experiences either pleasant, unpleasant, or neutral. And we see that we habitually try to hold on to the pleasant, push away the unpleasant, and we kind of lose interest in the neutral. And this causes an inordinate amount of distress when paired with our negativity bias, because we evolve to both expect unpleasant experiences and to constantly work to try to avoid them. Having these tendencies co-exist sets up a continuous tension for many of us that we experience as feeling stressed much of the time.

We also see that trying to grasp or hold on to changing phenomena causes suffering. We see that our thoughts aren't reality. In fact, they constantly change with our changing feeling states. And we see that all that actually exists is the present moment, despite the fact that we're hardwired to be constantly seeking pleasure and avoiding pain, which means living in memories of the past or the future.

Do these sound like worthwhile insights? Want to experience them more often? As I mentioned in the last lecture, talking about mindfulness isn't the same as practicing it. In fact, it's very hard to really understand what these practices are like unless we try them. It's really important to practice regularly. And different variations, different sorts of practices, have different effects. So let's try a few minutes of mindfulness practice together to get started with the actual experience of doing this.

It helps in doing breath awareness practice to start with an alert and dignified posture, with the spine more or less straight up and down. It also usually helps to begin with the eyes closed. Even though this can be done with the eyes open, when the eyes are closed it's usually easier, particularly as a beginner, to focus. So sit with your eyes closed.

To find the alert and dignified posture, it may help to imagine a string tied just to the top of your head pulling up toward the sky, gently elongating the spine. Then notice your breathing. If all is going well, the breath is already there and it's happening quite naturally.

Now there are two places where the breathing is normally observed. One is in the rising and falling sensations in the belly: the way in which as we breathe in, the belly expands a little bit, and as we breathe out it contracts a little bit. The other traditional place is at the tip of the nose, where we notice that the air enters kind of cool and leaves a little bit warmer. Just notice wherever you feel your breath most clearly, and start to feel it. See if you can feel the breath through its full cycles, from the beginning of an inhalation all the way to the end of an exhalation, and then onto the next cycle. It doesn't matter what form you find the breath in. If it's slow and deep, that's fine. If it's shallow and rapid, that's fine too. We're just using it as an object of awareness, a way to expand our awareness of present experience with acceptance.

Just feel each in-breath and each out-breath. See if you can develop an attitude of interest or curiosity in the moment-to-moment sensations of each breath. Notice that each is unique. Now, it would not be unusual as you begin to follow the breath for thoughts to enter the mind. That's OK; they're our friends. We're simply going to allow them to come and go, like clouds passing through a vast sky. Should you notice that your attention becomes hijacked by a train of narrative thought, such that it leaves the breath behind entirely, just congratulate yourself—that's a moment of mindfulness, of seeing what the mind is doing. Then gently and lovingly bring your attention back to the moment-to-moment sensations of the breath.

In this way, the breath helps to anchor our attention in the present moment. And we practice feeling the breath as if there were nowhere else to go, nothing else to do, just this moment of our lives. We're not trying to make anything special happen; we're just practicing bringing our attention back to moment-to-moment sensory experience.

And to bring this brief period of practice to a close, I'm going to ring a bell. And I want you to listen to the sound of the bell from the beginning of the ring until it trails off into space and you can no longer hear it.

Before going on to the next lecture, you'll want to try practicing for a longer period. I recommend you try following the recorded breath awareness meditation that's included as an audio file with the course. You'll need a quiet space where you can listen to it on a computer, or copy it to a phone, an iPod, or a similar device. It takes about 25 minutes.

When you do the longer meditation, I'd like you to watch out for a few challenges. The challenges that arise in meditation practice are usually the same sorts of difficulties our minds present during the rest of daily life. And, in fact, when they occur during meditation it gives us insights into how the mind creates trouble. They reflect the fact that our brains evolved to seek opportunity and avoid threat.

But what do I mean by this? Most of us have two common states, we're either involved in anxious goal-seeking activity trying to get something, acquire something, or we're avoiding threats, or we're spacing out, sometimes slipping into sleep. Mindfulness practice trains the brain for a third possibility, awake, alert, relaxed attention. Sometimes this doesn't come easily. Instead, we run into various kinds of difficulties. Here are a few of the most common.

We can find that our minds are quite restless. Living in the modern world is a lot like having bees inside of your head. There's constant, constant activity. And sometimes the activity stings us. In the Buddhist traditions, this is often called having a monkey mind. That the mind is as though it's a monkey inside the house, going from one window to the next, just rapidly jumping around from place to place.

The other thing we find is that there's something called the *default mode network* at work. And this is what happens when we're not involved in goal-oriented activity, there's a self-referential system that's constantly involved in reviewing who we are and how we're doing.

We see restless mind most in the experience of boredom. What makes one situation boring and not another? Many of us are happy to go off and watch a sunset where not much is happening, and think of it as a rich and fulfilling opportunity. In fact, we spend a lot of money to do it sometimes to see a sunset on a Caribbean beach or at a lakeside. And yet, sometimes, we could just be following the breath and say, this is boring, I need something more. So it becomes very interesting to examine what's making the difference for us. And then there's the danger of sleepiness. When we're not frenetically pursuing some kind of pleasure or avoiding some kind of pain, often we just fall asleep.

Now the typical instruction in mindfulness practice is, whatever happens, you can simply bring your attention to that. But it's tricky when what's happening is sleep, because when we enter into REM, when dreams start happening, it's as though the volitional entity is gone. There's nobody running the show. We're simply being carried down the stream of dreams unfolding. So there're traditional remedies for this. In Zen practice they suggest, try meditating at the edge of a particularly deep well. A high cliff will work, also. It kind of livens things up and helps us to pay attention.

And then there's anxiety. And this is one of the hardest states to just be with. We feel compelled to take action, to either medicate it, or move, or do something. And this probably developed because it was so important evolutionarily to take action in response to danger. Anxiety is a danger response.

Post-suicide inquiries, it turns out, that many people, when they attempt to take their life, it's not because they feel sad or even depressed, it's because they felt so anxious and they just wanted it to stop. So neurobiologically, what's happening is it's the activation of the amygdala and our host fight or flight system resulting in adrenaline flying through the system. And the solution, while we're doing mindfulness practice, is to simply attend to the component parts and observe them in detail. The tightness in the body, the heart racing, the urge to get up and distract ourselves, we simply allowed these to be the objects of our meditative attention.

And then there are all the unwanted feelings that arise. It's said that in psychoanalysis, if you spend enough time on the couch, sooner or later everything you've ever wanted to not think or feel will come into awareness. Well the same, I'm afraid, is true with mindfulness practice—everything comes up. In the long run, that's going to be helpful because it's going to allow us to integrate these contents. And then there's physical discomfort: the desire to scratch or adjust posture. And here, we try a different approach, which is simply to bring our full attention to the physical sensations when they occur.

So now that you know some of what may come up, you'll be armed with the knowledge you need to try some longer periods of practice. And after trying the longer breath practice, you can go on to the next lecture, when we'll explore some other ways to cultivate mindfulness, including how to do this without taking extra time out of a busy day.

Informal, Formal, and Intensive Practices
Lecture 3

In this lecture, you will learn about the options for meditation practice: informal mindfulness practice, formal meditation practice, and intensive retreat practice. Throughout this course, you can practice all of the forms of informal and formal practice that you learn about in this lecture. You want to create rituals so that you do them regularly. It's often best if you try to do formal practice at the same time of each day. And if you do a longer dose of mindfulness practice, it's actually easier to get into it—because you'll notice the effects that your practice is having on your life.

Being versus Doing
- Like learning a musical instrument, learning mindfulness is a dose-related activity. If we do a little bit of practice, we develop a little bit of mindfulness. If we do more, we develop more mindfulness.

- Experience-dependent neuroplasticity is the way in which parts of our brain bulk up when we use them over and over. Neurobiologist Donald Tabb says that neurons that fire together wire together.

- All mindfulness practices involve "being." And this is a little unfamiliar for most of us, because we have a constant focus on "doing." Many of us have worries about falling behind. We're constantly involved in making sure we stay on top of the things we need to do.

- It can be very difficult for most of us to be in the now, because being in the now opens the door to all sorts of unwanted thoughts, images, and feelings. In fact, our constant activity is one way that we defend against, or push unpleasant things out of, our awareness.

- Mindfulness means cultivating awareness of present experience with acceptance. And to do this, typically, we need to slow down a bit and pay attention. Slowing down can be really difficult in our information age, because it's so speedy.

- We could think of mindfulness as single-tasking. Some people think that it is actually possible to multitask, but cognitive scientists say, instead, that attention is like a pie. If you try to do two things at once, each gets 50 percent of your attention. If you try to do four things, each gets 25 percent of your attention.

Options for Meditation Practice

- In practicing mindfulness, there are options for meditation practice: informal mindfulness practice, formal meditation practice, and intensive retreat practice. Informal mindfulness practices are things we do during the course of our busy day that develop some mindfulness. Formal meditation practice is when we take time out of the day to actually set aside resources to just develop mindfulness. And intensive retreat practice is when we decide to go away somewhere and practice mindfulness in a continuous way over the course of many days.

- We don't have experimental data on the neurobiological and behavioral effects of informal practice. Experienced meditators report that doing these informal practices help to sustain and deepen the effect of formal practices during the day.

- For example, telephone meditation is a practice suggested by the Vietnamese Zen teacher Thich Nhat Hanh. Next time your phone rings, first you have to set it so that it doesn't pick up immediately and go to an automatic answering system. Give yourself enough rings so that you can actually listen to it. And just stay with the sound of the phone, and let your attention on what's going on in the present moment be something to bring you back to awareness of present experience with acceptance.

- Nowadays, virtually all phones have some kind of caller ID, and this allows for another opportunity. So, first, we listen to the sound of the phone. Then, we notice the number, and we see what emotional response comes up with each number. We have associations to different numbers. Interestingly, when a different number shows up, very different emotions arise in the body.

- An alternative is called taillight meditation. Next time you're in traffic, use the color and the texture of the form of the taillights on the vehicle in front of you as an object of meditation. Instead of our usual reaction, which is thinking about how the traffic is going to make you late, simply take in the texture and the experience of the visual field.

- Because mindfulness practices are becoming so mainstream, it appears that vehicle manufacturers are designing taillights that are especially conducive to mindfulness practice. Many of them look like mandalas. They're concentric circles of light emitting diodes that kind of evoke some Tibetan sand painting or perhaps Navajo spiritual art. Some, in fact, are two interlocking mandalas, to give you a sense of the interconnectedness of all beings in the universe and a real sense of the oneness of the present moment.

- In addition, there are many other mindful driving practices you can do. Simply try turning off the radio and focus on the sights and sounds of the other traffic, nature, and the environment. Try to not drive on automatic—not thinking about the break and the accelerator but, rather, bringing attention out to the environment of the moment.

- We can engage in mindfulness practice while walking the dog, walking to and from the car, waiting in line, or waiting for the bus. All that is required is that we resist the temptation to check our smartphones every 30 seconds, turn on some media, or do something to bring us out of the moment. Any activity in which we can single-task and be present becomes an opportunity for informal mindfulness practice.

- If we want to take our mindfulness practice the next level, we have to do some formal meditation. And this is what we have a wealth of data coming out supporting the efficacy for. It turns out that formal meditation practice changes both brain structure and brain function.

- Research has found that people who do a lot of meditation practice develop more robust brain structures in certain areas. The cerebral cortex thins as we get older. Sara Lazar at Mass General Hospital in Boston studied the cerebral cortices of older meditators, people who have been doing it for years, and matched controls, who were the same age and had similar life circumstances but hadn't been meditating. Several areas of the brain don't deteriorate in the meditators in the way that they normally do in a non-meditators.

- Scientists have known for a long time that when people are happy, relaxed, or engaged in life, there's a lot of left prefrontal activation. But when they're anxious, stressed, or hyper-vigilant (in survival mode), there's a lot of right prefrontal activation.

- Richard Davidson at the Laboratory for Affective Neuroscience at the University of Wisconsin–Madison conducted a study involving the activation of the prefrontal cortex. He wired up a Tibetan monk who had thousands and thousands of hours of meditation practice and found that he was off the charts in terms of the degree to which he leaned left, in the favorable direction, versus leaning right.

- Mindfulness practices involve restraint. They're not about becoming an ascetic, or trying to wipe out desire; rather, they're about not just doing what comes naturally, but taking some time to focus on what's going on in the current moment.

- If you have had the opportunity to do some breath awareness training, you might notice the experience of an itch or an ache coming up and not act on it. Perhaps you saw that the itch or the ache would transform by itself.

- This happens with other things, too. We can see anger arising and not just act on it, but notice that it transforms by itself. Mindfulness practices help us to realize that we have choices about whether or not to act on our impulses. And this restraint turns out to be an essential ingredient in using mindfulness practices to work with a host of psychological and behavioral difficulties, including anxiety, addictions, interpersonal conflicts, and stress-related medical disorders.

- If you want to take your mindfulness practice to the next higher level, you might consider an intensive retreat, which is where you would go off and spend several days all day in mindfulness practice. The typical setting of an instructor retreat is out in nature, and people don't talk or check their cell phones. They don't even make eye contact with one another after the opening of the retreat but, rather, keep their eyes cast downward in what's often called noble silence.

- The idea is to develop sufficient concentration and sufficient open-monitoring skills to really notice what the mind is doing in each moment. And what emerges is really amazing. There's a concept in psychoanalysis called transference, which means that we don't actually see other people as they are but, rather, as reflections of other people that they remind us of.

- The mind makes up stories about other people we see doing things, even though we have minimal data about them. Most of the time when our minds present these kinds of stories, we think we're describing reality. The mind picks up on little tidbits and endlessly weaves whole stories.

Walking and Eating Meditation

- During a retreat, one of the kinds of practice that we do a lot of, so as not to get too stiff, is walking meditation. Walking meditation is a wonderful practice, because it can be done both as an informal practice as well as a formal meditation practice.

- Walking meditation has a number of different benefits. First, it easily transforms from a formal meditation to an informal practice. And it's an opportunity to be mindful whenever we're walking.

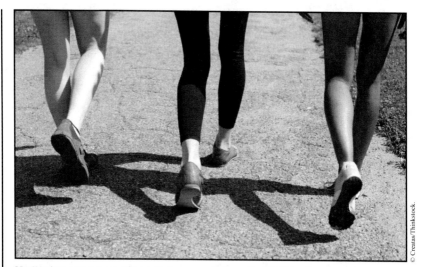

Meditation can be practiced during a routine walk with friends or anytime you are walking in your daily life.

We tend to walk a lot in our lives, and when we're feeling more agitated, restless, or sleepy, it's easier than following the breath. Simply, it brings more wakefulness. And when were agitated, it's difficult to sit still—it's easier to be in motion. So, it's quite helpful when we're dealing with anxiety or depression.

- Another practice that also works quite well as both an informal practice and a formal practice is eating meditation. Like walking meditation, eating meditation easily becomes an informal practice or a formal practice. And it's an opportunity to be mindful whenever we're eating. After all, there are a lot of opportunities for that, because you have to eat. It's also very helpful when we're distracted, because eating is a very vivid object of awareness, or stimulus, so that if the mind is jumpy and is easily distracted, it's easier to focus often on food.

- In addition, eating meditation is very useful if you ever struggle with eating appropriate amounts of food. When we eat mindfully— instead of scarfing down to self-soothe or to distract ourselves—

we tend to notice when we're full. We notice the sensations of distension in the stomach, and we also have time for a natural feedback loop to occur.

• Normally, when we eat, if we would eat slowly enough and attentively, as the food reaches the duodenum, a signal is fed back to the hypothalamus that says that there's satiation happening, meaning that you have eaten enough. And we find when we eat mindfully that most of us eat far less than we normally would. In addition, interestingly, even though we're eating less, we feel a lot more satisfied.

Suggested Reading

Hanh, *Peace Is Every Step*.

Kabat-Zinn, *Full Catastrophe Living*.

Pollak, Pedulla, and Siegel, *Sitting Together*.

Siegel, *The Mindfulness Solution*, chapter 3.

Questions to Consider

1. Choose three activities that you do most days that could be used as informal mindfulness practices (e.g., walking the dog, showering, eating breakfast, driving to work, listening to the phone ring, etc.).

2. Try a few periods of walking and eating meditation. How does your mind respond to these practices, compared to how it responds to the breath awareness practice?

Mindfulness Practice

eating meditation: A foundational practice that can be done either as a formal meditation (using a raisin or larger quantity of food) or as an informal practice (just paying attention to the process of eating during daily life).

walking meditation: A foundational formal meditation practice that can be done initially as a concentration, or focused-attention, practice. Once some concentration develops, it can be expanded to be an open-monitoring, or choiceless-awareness, practice. After spending some time doing formal walking meditation, we naturally find it easy to use walking as an informal practice whenever walking in daily life.

Informal, Formal, and Intensive Practices
Lecture 3—Transcript

There's an old story about a tourist who's lost in New York and late for a performance, and he spies a guy with a violin case in a tuxedo. And he rushes up to the musician and says, "Help me. Help me. How do I get to Carnegie Hall?" And the musician pauses, and looks at the tourist, and seems to be scoping him out, looking up and down. And the tourist is getting more and more frantic, expecting an answer. And finally, pensively, the musician says, "Practice, practice."

Now, like learning a musical instrument, learning mindfulness is a dose-related kind of activity. If we do a little bit of practice, we develop a little bit of mindfulness. If we do more, we develop more mindfulness. I mentioned earlier, experience-dependent neuroplasticity, the way in which, when we use parts of our brain over and over, they actually bulk up. Donald Hebb, the neurobiologist says, "Neurons that fire together wire together."

All mindfulness practices involve being. And this is a little unfamiliar for most of us, because we have a constant focus on doing. Many of us have worries about falling behind. Some time ago, I received a phone call from a woman in the United Kingdom and she said, "I'd like to interview you." She was a journalist. She said, "I'm doing a report on FOMO, would you agree to be interviewed?" I say, "Sure. What's FOMO?" She said, "Oh, you don't know? It's Fear of Missing Out." It's apparently a thing. We're constantly, constantly involved in making sure we stay on top of the things we need to do. You know, if we we were to update René Descartes' famous maxim for the modern era, we would probably say, "I have a to-do list, therefore I am." Or these days maybe, "I have Facebook friends, or text messages to return, therefore, I am."

It can be very hard for most of us to be here now, because being here now opens the door to all sorts of unwanted thoughts, images, and feelings. In fact, our constant activity is one way that we defend against or push unpleasant things out of our awareness. So mindfulness means cultivating something different. Mindfulness means cultivating awareness of present experience with acceptance. And to do this, typically, we have to suspend our urgency to do stuff. We need to slow down a bit and pay attention. The intention is key here. Slowing down can be really hard in our information age, because it's so speedy. Most of us nowadays are drinking from the fire hose of information that's coming in so quickly and in such volume.

Historians say that a person with a smartphone in his or her pocket today has access to more information more rapidly than an American president did before the internet. Think Bill Clinton. It wasn't that long ago. So slowing down helps to increase our awareness.

We could think of mindfulness as single-tasking. I found it quite horrifying that in my state, Massachusetts, they had to pass a law saying no texting while driving, as though that might seem like a reasonable idea to some people. Of course, some folks, and you see this more among younger people, think it is actually possible to multitask. Cognitive scientists say it's not so. Attention is like a pie. If you try to do two things at once, each gets 50 percent of your attention. If you try to do four things, each guess gets 25 percent of your attention.

In practicing mindfulness, there are different ways to go about this. And they're similar to the different ways we might go about developing physical fitness. If I wanted to develop a little bit of physical fitness, but I was busy, and I didn't have a lot of time or resources to devote to it, I could make simple adjustments and get more physically fit. I could take the stairs instead of the elevator; I might walk somewhere, rather than moving my car; I might even bicycle someplace, rather than taking the bus. And if I do those things, I would develop a little bit of physical fitness.

But if I want to take my physical fitness to the next level, and really become strong and have strength and endurance, I would have to take some time out of my day to do things devoted to developing physical fitness. I would need to go to the gym, go on a long bicycle ride, perhaps go hiking. Similarly, we have options for meditation practice, which we'll talk about shortly. If I really, really want to jump start my physical fitness, and get super fit, I might decide to devote my next vacation to it and go off to some place where I'm either hiking day after day, or going to a place where I could work out in the gym quite regularly.

So for mindfulness, the equivalent of these things are what we called informal mindfulness practice, formal meditation practice, and intensive retreat practice. Informal mindfulness practices are things we do during the course of our busy day that develop some mindfulness. Formal meditation practice is when we take time out of the day to actually set aside resources to just develop mindfulness. And intensive retreat practice is when we decide to actually go away somewhere and practice mindfulness in a continuous way over the course of many days.

And let me give you an example of what these are like. Well, we don't have experimental data on the neurobiological and behavioral effects of informal practice. Experienced meditators report that doing these informal practices help to sustain and deepen the effect of formal practices during the day. Take for example telephone meditation. This is a practice suggested by the Vietnamese Zen teacher, Thích Nhất Hạnh. He says to try this: Next time your phone rings or chirps or plays old Beatles songs, first you have to set it so it doesn't pick up immediately and go to an automatic answering system. Give yourself enough rings so you can actually listen to it. And just stay with the sound of the phone, and let your attention to what's going on in the present moment be something to bring you back to awareness of present experience with acceptance.

Nowadays, virtually all phones have some kind of caller ID, and this allows for another opportunity. So first, we listen to the sound of the phone. And then we notice the number, and we see what emotional response comes up with each number. I don't think it's exotic numerology, I think we have associations to different numbers. But interestingly, when a different number shows up, very different emotions arise in the body.

An alternative, actually one of my favorites that I practice all the time, is called "tail light meditation." This means next time you're in traffic, use the color and the texture of the form of the tail lights on the vehicle in front of you as an object of meditation. Instead of our usual reaction, which is, oh, damn. Now there's traffic, I'll be late. Simply take in the texture and the experience of the visual field.

I'm happy to announce that because mindfulness practices are now becoming so mainstream, it appears that the vehicle manufacturers are designing taillights especially conducive to mindfulness practice. Many of them look like mandalas. They're concentric circles of light emitting diodes that kind of evoke some Tibetan sand painting, or perhaps Navajo spiritual art. And some, in fact, are two interlocking mandalas to give you a sense of the interconnectedness of all beings in the universe, and a real sense of the oneness of the present moment.

There are many other mindful driving practices you can do. Simply try turning off the radio, or turning off the scores, and focus on the sights and sounds of the other traffic, of nature, of the environment. We're trying to not drive on automatic. Not to be like a 16-year-old driver who's anxiously thinking about the break and the accelerator, but rather as a driver who brings attention out to the environment of the moment.

Yet another option is shower meditation. Think back to your last shower, this morning, or last night, or a week ago Tuesday—I'm not going to judge. Unless you're particularly shy, you were probably naked. And if you live in the developed world, there would be thousands of droplets of water caressing your naked body, and you were able to adjust them for a Goldilocks kind of moment. Oh, no. That's a little too cold. Oh, no. That's a little too warm. Ah, just right.

Now this is, potentially, a very rich sensual experience. You're using soap and probably massaging everywhere on your body, including your private parts. (I travel a lot, talking about these kinds of things, and I like reading the names of soaps. The last hotel called it Jasmine Zen, which I thought was perfect for shower meditation.) So this can be a very rich sensual experience. And yet, I find that if I don't approach a shower as a kind of mindfulness practice, I'm perfectly capable of spending the entire shower lost in the thought stream, thinking about my to-do list, or what happened this morning. In fact, I can get to the end of a shower and think, did I wash my hair? Or was that yesterday? Shower meditation transforms the experience.

So you see, it can really be anything. It can be walking the dog, walking to and from the car, walking anywhere. It can be waiting. Waiting in line, or waiting for the bus. All that is required is that we resist this temptation to check our smartphone every 30 seconds, turn on some media, do something to bring us out of the moment. Any activity in which we can single-task and be present becomes an opportunity for informal mindfulness practice.

Now if we want to take on mindfulness practice the next level, we have to do some formal meditation. And this is what we have wealth of data coming out supporting the efficacy for. It turns out that formal meditation practice changes both brain structure and brain function. I'll give you a few examples, just to whet your appetite.

It's found that people who do a lot of meditation practice develop more robust brain structures in certain areas. Many of us worry about our hair thinning when we get older. Well, that's not nearly so serious as the fact that the cerebral cortex thins as we get older. And my friend and colleague Sara Lazar at Mass General Hospital in Boston studied the cerebral cortices of older meditators, people who have been at it for years, and matched controls, who were the same age and similar life circumstances, but hadn't been meditating. And it turned out that several areas, such as the insula—which involves proprioception, noticing what's going on in the body in each moment—and areas of the brain that are involved in integration between affect or emotions and cognitions don't deteriorate in the meditators in the way that they normally do in the non-meditators.

Or another interesting study, done by Richard Davidson at the Center for Affective Neurobiology at the University of Wisconsin Madison—and this study involved the activation of the prefrontal cortex. It turns out that when people are happy, relaxed, engaged in life, there's a lot of left prefrontal activation. But when they're anxious, stressed, or hyper-vigilant, when they're in survival mode, there's a lot of right prefrontal activation. This has been known for a long time. Dr. Davidson wired up a Tibetan monk who had had thousands and thousands of hours of meditation practice, and found he was off the charts, in terms of the degree to which he leaned left, in the favorable direction, versus leaning right. And we'll talk much more about other neurobiological studies later in the course.

All of these practices involve restraint. They're not about becoming an ascetic, or trying to wipe out desire, but rather, to not just do what comes naturally, but take some time to focus on what's going on in the current moment. Hopefully, you've had the opportunity to do some breath awareness training and notice the experience of an itch or an ache coming up, and not acting on it. And perhaps you saw that the itch or the ache would transform by itself. And this happens with other things, too. We can see anger arising and not just act on it, but notice it transforms by itself. The same with sadness. The same with all sorts of things. Mindfulness practices help us to realize that we have choices about whether or not to act on our impulses. And this restraint turns out to be an essential ingredient in using mindfulness practices to work with a host of psychological and behavioral difficulties, including anxiety, addictions, interpersonal conflicts, and stress-related medical disorders.

If you want to take your mindfulness practice to yet the next higher level, you might consider an intensive retreat. And that's where you would go off and spend several days, basically spending all day in mindfulness practice. The typical setting in structured retreat is out in nature, and we don't talk, we don't check our cell phones, we don't even make eye contact with one another after the opening of the retreat, but rather keep the eyes cast downward in what's often called *noble silence*. And the idea is to develop sufficient concentration and sufficient open monitoring skills to really notice what the mind is doing in each moment. And what emerges is really amazing. There's a concept in psychoanalysis called *transference*, which means, we don't actually see other people as they are, but rather we see them as reflections of other people that they remind us of. Let me give you an example of how this shows up on a retreat.

I could be there, and, perhaps, on the third morning, or so, and it's breakfast time. And I'm looking across the room, spying somebody serving herself oatmeal. And I just notice these feelings arising in the heart. What grace, what beauty. Oh, I feel so in love. Or I might turn to another person in another part of the room and say—silently in my mind, of course—four prunes. I can't believe he took four prunes. Don't you just hate people who are so narcissistic, so involved with themselves that they don't care about the community, they just care about themselves?

And the mind continues making up these stories, even though we have minimal data about the other people we're with. Now most of the time when our minds invent these kinds of stories, we think we're describing reality. What we see in an intensive meditation retreat is, oh, no. The mind picks up on little tidbits, and weaves whole stories, endlessly.

There was a journalist who was attending a silent retreat, and he was cheating because one of the rules is you're not supposed to write or read so as to develop more concentration and more mindfulness. But he was taking notes because he was going to write an article. And it was the second night of the retreat. And in his notebook he wrote, "Sitting a silent meditation retreat is a lot like being trapped in a phone booth with a lunatic."

Now during a retreat, one of the sorts of practice that we do a lot of, so as not to get too stiff, is walking meditation. And walking meditation is a wonderful practice, because it can be done both as an informal practice, as well as a formal meditation practice.

In walking meditation, we're going to use the sensations of the legs walking through space and the feet touching the ground as our object of awareness. There are a number of different ways to do this. I'll show you a couple of variations. If you can join me now that would be great, otherwise you can try this a little bit later.

Simply start by standing still—and you may wish to close your eyes for a few moments—and feel what it feels like to have the feet planted on the ground and the legs aligned beneath the hips and just what it feels like to stand and take a breath or two. Just arriving in the present moment. One way to do this is to then pick an area where you can walk—and it doesn't have to be very long. Ten feet is sufficient, longer if you've got space outside to do this. Just very slowly and deliberately, begin walking. And you're feeling the sensations of lifting the leg, moving forward in space, stepping. Lifting, forward, stepping. Some people find it helpful to actually note the movements, to silently say in the mind "lifting, forward, stepping." Or else just to feel the sensations.

When you get to the end of whatever your path is, take a moment to stand, feel the feet on the ground again, maybe feel the breath, then slowly turn around again and head back in the other direction. This is decidedly a journey to nowhere. Lifting, forward, stepping. Lifting, forward, stepping. Just as with the breath meditation, if the mind tends to wander, to get lost in thought, that's fine—it's just once you've noticed that the mind has left the sensations of the legs and feet entirely, just gently bring it back to the sensations of walking. Again, when you get to the end, just breathe and feel the body. Mindfully change positions.

If you find that walking very slowly and deliberately like I'm doing here makes you unsteady—because sometimes that happens at first—you can quicken the pace a little bit. Still bringing your attention to the sensations. And at the end of the path, stopping and breathing. Mindfully changing direction. Here, too, you can do the noting, so it can be "lifting, placing, lifting, placing, lifting, placing," the idea being that most of the attention goes to the sensations of the body moving through space and the noting is only used to bring our attention back to what's going on.

We just continue in this way and you'll find that as with the breath awareness, after awhile some more attention and concentration begins to develop, and we start to notice subtler and subtler changes in the body, the sensations of moving. And that's all there is to it. You can do that any time you like when you have a few minutes free. It's an easy way to practice some mindfulness in motion.

Walking meditation has a number of different benefits. For one thing, it easily transforms from a formal meditation to an informal practice. And it's an opportunity be mindful whenever we're walking. We tend to walk a lot in our lives. And when we're feeling more agitated, or restless, or sleepy, it's easier than following the breath. Simply it brings more wakefulness. And when were agitated, it's hard to sit still. It's easier to be in motion. So it's quite helpful when we're dealing with anxiety or depression.

Another practice that also works quite well, both as an informal practice and as a formal practice, is eating meditation.

Now we're going to do some eating meditation. And we're simply going to use what we're eating as an object of awareness. It helps to do this with either a raisin, or I have a Craisin right now (a dried cranberry), or some other little piece of dried fruit that's small and simple. Once you gather that up, allow your eyes to close and just come back into the present a little, take a breath or two. Then open your eyes and begin looking at your morsel. Look at it as though you've never seen it before—which actually, you haven't. Notice its hills and valleys, where it's shiny, where it's smooth. Perhaps, if it's something like a raisin, you can see where in its former life as a grape it once attached to the vine. Take it in as though you are a visitor from a foreign culture or even another planet and have never seen one of these things before. Really notice what it's like visually.

Then allow your eyes to close and continue exploring it, but this time tactilely. Feel it between your thumb and your forefinger. Notice the hills and the valleys, and the smoothness and the roughness. Take in the morsel through the sense of touch. Notice how different this is in consciousness than taking it in through the visual channel.

Now this next step may feel a little peculiar, but gradually and slowly—mindfully, if you will—take the morsel and lift it up until it's just outside your ear canal. Roll it between your thumb and forefinger and see if you can hear the faint crackling sound it makes, and notice how radically different this is than the other sensations. Just listen.

Then gradually lower the morsel until it's below one nostril. Breathe in predominantly through that nostril—you'll find that we can kind of do this; we can favor one nostril or the other. Notice the aroma that comes from it. It could be very faint. Then try putting it under the other nostril and then notice the aroma. See if it's the same or different.

Next, moving to a moment that maybe you're anxiously anticipating with pleasure—or with dread, depending on how you feel about what you're about to eat—bring the morsel until it's just outside your lips. Notice any feelings of anticipation that arise. Then allow your tongue to reach out and capture the morsel as only it knows how to do. Just hold it between your tongue and the roof of your mouth. See what happens. Notice how the mouth responds to the morsel. How the morsel responds to the mouth. Notice too how the mind responds the whole drama with a sense of liking it or disliking it, pleasant or unpleasant. Just take in the full experience. Notice how the morsel tends to change as you hold it there between your tongue and the roof of your mouth.

Now use your tongue to begin to explore it. Once again, take in the hills and the valleys, the smooth parts and the rough parts. Notice how different they are perceived through the perception of the tongue. Then use your tongue to maneuver your morsel so that it's being cradled between your upper and lower molars. Just hold it there and see what that feels like, again noticing the sensations in the mouth and the mind's response to the sensations—like it, don't like it.

Now, once, and only once, bring your molars together and see what happens. Notice all of the sensations that appear in the mouth, and again notice the mind's response to those sensations. Then use your tongue to examine your handiwork. Explore all the feelings that come up and all of the sensations of your newly transformed morsel. At each moment, we're noticing the symphony of sensations that unfold, and how complex the whole operation is.

And then very slowly and deliberately, continue chewing so that you feel each time that your teeth come together. Notice all the sensations that arise with each chew—again, the propensity to like some and dislike others. When the swallow reflex starts to kick in, let that happen naturally. Continue chewing until you get to the point where the morsel is gone or mostly gone. And then notice the sensations of the mouth now that the morsel is largely headed down the alimentary canal.

Take a breath or two to feel this, and notice particularly if any desires or urges come up—perhaps the desire for another piece of the dried fruit, perhaps the urge to floss. Whatever arises, just feel it for a moment. When you're done, open your eyes and decide whether to have another.

Like walking meditation, eating meditation easily becomes an informal practice or a formal practice. And it's an opportunity to be mindful whenever we're eating. And after all, there are a lot of opportunities for that because you've got to eat. It's also very helpful when we're distracted, because eating is a very vivid object of awareness. It's a very vivid stimulus, so that if the mind is jumpy and is easily distracted, it's easier to focus often on food.

And, as we'll see, it's very useful if you ever struggle with eating appropriate amounts. When we eat mindfully, instead of snarfing down to self-soothe or to distract ourselves, we tend to notice when we're full. We notice the sensations of distension in the stomach. And we also have time for a natural feedback loop to occur. Normally, when we eat, if we eat slowly enough and attentively, as the food reaches the duodenum, a signal is fed back to the hypothalamus that says, there's satiation happening. I've had enough. And we find when we mindfully that most of us eat far less than we normally would. And interestingly, even though we're eating less, we feel a lot more satisfied.

So you can practice all of these forms of informal practice and formal practice throughout the course. Remember Carnegie Hall and experience-dependent neuroplasticity. You want to create rituals for this so that you can do them regularly. It's often best with formal practice to try to do it the same time of each day, like when I get up in the morning, or when I get home from work, or perhaps before bed.

There's a program called Mindfulness Based Stress Reduction, which is basically a standardized eight-week course for teaching mindfulness practice. And they found, in designing the program, that if you do a longer dose, it's actually easier to get into this. And they asked people to do 45 minutes to an hour a day, six days a week of practice. And one of the reasons for asking folks to do that is people who do that notice that, this is really transforming my life. My consciousness is different.

So try to pick a few practices and stick to them. There's a Zen metaphor about that that says, a finger pointing to the moon isn't the moon. To reap the benefits of these practices, we have to actually do them. So in the next lecture, we're going to focus on one of the most challenging but important insights that come from mindfulness practice. It's the key insight by which mindfulness practices can lead us to greater happiness, fulfillment, and well-being, and it's how mindfulness practices can change our sense of who we are.

Who Am I? The Perils of Self
Lecture 4

During your meditation, have you discovered a "self"? Or have you found an ever-changing kaleidoscope of changing sensations, thoughts, and images? This question hasn't been discussed extensively yet among clinicians as mindfulness practices are being adapted into Western psychotherapeutic interventions. But advances in neurobiology are beginning to bring the question to the forefront among biological researchers. This lecture focuses on the self—the key insight by which mindfulness practices can lead us to great happiness, fulfillment, and well-being. And it's how mindfulness practices can change our sense of who we are.

The Sense of Self

- In their original context of Buddhist psychology, mindfulness practices were designed to help us see more clearly into the nature of the self—or, to be more precise, how we construct a sense of self moment to moment.

- Buddhist tradition, and Western cognitive science, suggest that try as we may, all we find if we examine our experience carefully are sensations and images, accompanied by a remarkably persistent narrative. The "I" or "me" can't actually be found.

- It's said that if we practice intensively enough, we'll see that we're actually not who we usually think we are. Instead, we'll see ourselves as a modern physicist, biologist, or cognitive scientist might describe us.

- How do we develop a separate sense of self that divides the world into objects and doesn't notice the fluid interconnections of things—doesn't notice that two people are part of the superorganism? Buddhist psychology outlined the process about 2,500 years ago.

And this formulation aligns remarkably well with how a cognitive scientist would describe it today.

Sense Contact and Perception

- In the Buddhist psychological formulation, our sense of ourselves starts with the coming together of a sense organ with a sense object, and then we have awareness of that object. So, this involves six senses: seeing, hearing, smelling, tasting, touching—and the sixth sense is everything else. The sixth sense is not direct sensory contact; it's an experience happening in the mind.

- What we start to see is that we are psychophysiological organisms that don't exactly exist. But we occur moment by moment. And the first occurrence of this involves sense contact. We don't stay at the level of sense contact for very long. We organize sensory experience into perceptions.

- Consider looking at the word "perception." Can you visualize the letters? Are you able to see simply the shapes of letters, basically fluid forms against a contrasting background, or do sounds arise in the mind?

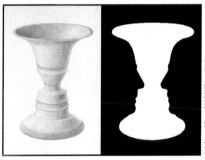

Rubin's goblet looks like either two faces looking at each other or a goblet, depending on how you look at it.

- Another example is an image that looks like two things simultaneously: two faces facing one another, and the faces themselves define a goblet. As we look at it, we can see it as one or the other. And if you can picture that, are you actually able to see both the faces and the goblet simultaneously, or do they actually appear in rapid oscillation?

- Most of us find that they appear in rapid oscillation—that it constellates itself as a goblet, and then as two faces. In fact, the mind kind of struggles to make it into one or another. This makes perfect sense evolutionarily, because deciding between a beige rock and a lion mattered a lot to us.

- There's a well-known video of students playing basketball, and they're wearing black shirts and white shirts. The task that people are assigned is to watch how many times the students in the white shirts pass the basketball on the video. In the middle of the video, a big black gorilla comes in, beats his chest, and exits the stage.

- When people are asked to count the number of times the students with the white shirts pass the basketball, about two-thirds of the audience simply doesn't see the gorilla. This is called inattentional blindness. Perception—what we see—is terribly conditioned by culture, language, and desire. What happens in the video is that we're trying to get the number right, so we don't see the gorilla at all.

- Perception constructs and categorizes, and omits details, and fills in all sorts of missing information. Have you ever been in a situation where you were ostensibly in the same place as someone else and saw the same thing, but you ended up perceiving it very differently?

- A study was done in which they took X-rays of the lungs, and they asked 24 radiologists to perform a familiar lung nodule detection task. They placed a gorilla 48 times larger than the average lung nodule in the last slide, and 83 percent of the radiologists didn't see it. And they did eye tracking, which revealed that the majority of the radiologists who missed the gorilla looked directly at it.

- Our perception is radically influenced by what's going on with our desires. And we fill in things, too. Consider a large, round circle with two small circles placed about two-thirds of the way up the middle of it. Can you visualize that? What might it be? Virtually everybody sees a face, or a few people tend to see bowling balls. We fill in details like this all the time, even though the nose (and even the thumb hole from the bowling ball) is missing.

Emotional Tone

- We don't stay at the level of perception for very long. We add an affective, or emotional, tone to the experience. Everything that happens, we see it and feel it to be pleasant, unpleasant, or neutral. We love some things, and we hate others.

- Then, we develop what are called intentions and dispositions. We try to hold on to pleasant experience, push away unpleasant experience, and ignore neutral experience. When we do this over time, we develop habits of intention. We can also call them dispositions. Behavioral scientists call them learned behaviors or conditioned responses. Many of us actually refer to these dispositions—these habits of holding on to some things and pushing away others—as our personality.

- Sense organs connect with sense objects, and that's experienced in consciousness. There are feelings, intentions, and perceptions happening. It's all happening at once. What mindfulness practice reveals is that it's all impersonal—there's nobody home. There's simply a continuous flow of moment-to-moment experience, with a new self being born and dying in each moment. There isn't even a stable witness; there's just impersonal experience unfolding.

- Our normal sense of self creates all sorts of trouble. Instead of thinking of having a self, we might more accurately think that selfing occurs—because in each moment, we're responding out of this sense of agency, or the sense of "I." And we respond very differently when the experiences belong to "me." It creates all sorts of further distortions, and endless suffering comes from this. These are the self-evaluative thoughts, including "I'm better than you" or "I'm not talented" that happen.

- Whenever experiences arise, we tend to not just take them as they are, or see them clearly; instead, we reflect on what they mean about ourselves. When we identify with the self, it makes pleasure and pain personal. It creates this fantasy of being able to control your experience, your insecurities, your competitive feelings, and all of these kinds of defensive things follow.

Identifying with the Self

- Karma is associated with the teachings of many Indian cultures and also Eastern cultures generally. Karma is traditionally understood in terms of reincarnation. The idea is that how we perform in this life determines how we will be reborn in the next.

- But karma can also be seen in moment-to-moment intentions. What becomes reborn is a certain constellation or attitude in consciousness. So, your intention in one moment tends to shape the perceptions and feelings in the next moment, which creates the reality of the next moment.

- The Buddha said that our identity is being recreated moment by moment and that the continuity of self simply can't be found—it's illusory. All we have are frames in a movie and the mind's tendency to string these frames together into a narrative, starring you, that makes you feel that you exist. And all sorts of suffering, preoccupation with what's going to happen to you, result from this.

- Carl Jung, the student and colleague of Freud, had a similar observation. He talked about what happens when we identify with some mental contents and reject others. He said that when we do this, it creates a kind of split-off shadow. It's almost a form of dissociation, a kind of splitting caused by trying to avoid pain.

- So, if you think of yourself—because you have a self-concept—as being generous, hardworking and intelligent, then your greedy, lazy, and dumb side is going to be your shadow. And you're going to have trouble every time you have a life circumstance that highlights the fact that you're greedy, lazy, or dumb, to some degree. And you'll go through the world seeking affirmation of who you want yourself to be, or who you think of yourself as being.

- The very construction of the self sets us up for many difficulties. Indeed, the sense of self is a universal category of experience. But it really is experienced differently in different cultures. And one of the things we see through mindfulness practice is how the self is actually constructed not only by our moment-to-moment experience, but by the culture in which we live.

- We all get hooked on different dimensions or domains that define ourselves. For one person, it's about physical beauty, while for another, it's athletic talent that gets the focus. This causes all sorts of difficulties.

- The other thing that we discover is that there is no single self to be found. And we see this all the time in meditation practice. In fact, it can be very useful in dealing with emotional difficulties to notice if there's no single, coherent self—to notice if there's a committee.

- Often, when we're in distress, there are conflicts among different parts. There's a part of you that wants to achieve more and be successful in your career. But there's a part of you that wants love and connection and wants to spend more time with friends and family. Seeing what each part wants and needs can really help us.

- There's a popular form of psychotherapy called internal family systems, which invites us to take time to recognize, honor, and draw out the fears and needs of each of these different parts. When each part is recognized in this way, the part itself feels safer, calms down, and doesn't need so much to run the show.

- When we're not identified with a single sense of self, this can facilitate a tremendous amount of flexibility—because then we don't have to be one way or the other. And we can be much more accepting of our diverse, and often complex, experiences.

- This also has tremendous implications for our development. Mindfulness practices, like forms of psychotherapy, become a sort of loosening process, where the goal becomes not to be more one way or more of the other way—in the sense of becoming more perfect—but to develop a sense of psychological flexibility.

- In fact, there are some mindfulness-based psychotherapies like acceptance and commitment therapy, where the explicit goal is not feeling good about yourself—not even being successful in your endeavors—but simply having psychological flexibility. The goal is being able to be whomever or whatever you are in each moment.

- And this provides enormous relief from worrying so much about ourselves, about how we compare to others, or about our pleasure or pain. It helps us to identify with something larger than ourselves. And this identification with something more than oneself becomes particularly important in any path to well-being.

Suggested Reading

Fulton and Engler, "Self and No-Self in Psychotherapy."

Olendzki, "The Roots of Buddhist Psychology."

Siegel, *The Mindfulness Solution*, chapter 8.

Questions to Consider

1. In your meditation practice, when and how does your sense of self arise? Is it found in bodily sensations, visual images, or thoughts passing through the mind?

2. Imagine that you had a day in which you had no concerns about how others see you. How would it be different from a typical day?

Who Am I? The Perils of Self
Lecture 4—Transcript

I hope you've had some opportunities by now to do some breath awareness meditation and to do some formal and informal walking and eating practice. And you're beginning to see how these practices can bring insight into how the mind creates suffering for itself.

I wonder during your meditation, did you discover a little homunculus inside? Did you find a self? Or did you find an ever-changing kaleidoscope of different sensations, thoughts, and images? This question hasn't been discussed extensively yet among clinicians as mindfulness practices are being adapted into Western psycho-therapeutic interventions, but it's becoming a hot topic with advances in neurobiology that are bringing the question into the forefront of biological research.

In the original context of Buddhist psychology, these practices were designed to help us see more clearly the nature of the self—or to be more precise, how we construct a sense of self, moment to moment. Buddhist tradition and Western cognitive science suggests that try as we might, all we find if we examine our experience carefully are sensations and images, accompanied by a remarkably persistent narrative about our desires, about our fears, about who we think we are. The I, or the me, can't actually be found. It's said that if we practice intensively enough, we'll see that we're actually not who we usually think we are. Instead, we'll see ourselves as a modern physicist, biologist, or cognitive scientist might describe us.

Let's do a little thought experiment to illustrate how this works. Consider the experience of a little girl eating an apple. And let's say she bites into that apple and looks at the remaining apple, and sees half a worm. She's a smart little girl. She realizes what's going on, and she's about to spit out the chewed material in her mouth. Now I ask you to consider, what is that chewed material? Would you say that the chewed material is still essentially the apple? Or has it already become the little girl? If I asked you to vote on that, what would you select?

Now let's assume that there's no half of a worm, and she continues eating the apple. But if she were having a bad day, it could still come up. So that stuff that's now in her stomach, how would you vote about that? Would you say that that's still essentially the apple? Would you say, nah, now it's the little girl? How would you vote? Or imagine taking it a little further. Imagine she's having a good day. She continues to digest it, and that material gets into her intestines. And in the process, the fructose of the apple is broken down into glucose. It gets absorbed into her bloodstream, and it's now her blood sugar. What's that? They're certainly atoms of the apple; would you say they're still the apple? Or would you say no, now they're the little girl?

And we might take this even further. Imagine that the glucose molecules of the blood are being picked up by the cells. And through the magic of the Krebs cycle, and ATP, and all the things you might have learned about in high school biology, her cells are using the energy in that glucose in order to recombine amino acids and create new cellular structures. Those new cellular structures, since they're fueled by the apple, are they still the apple? Or have they now become the little girl? Most people at this point vote, I think they're the little girl.

But there is of course, part of the apple that we don't digest. We call this "fiber" or "cellulose." And let's imagine that that's continued down the alimentary canal, and is now being aggregated, preparing to go into a familiar white porcelain receptacle. Now that stuff, how would you vote? And here, I'll give you three options to make it easier. That stuff, we could say, it's still the apple—after all, it's cellulose from the apple. It's the little girl—it's been in there for a little while. Or I'll give you a third option: It's something else. Most people vote for it's something else. It's interesting—we don't like to identify with our feces as either us, or to think of our feces as what we eat. We like to think that's something else.

So, have you noticed the problem here? There isn't a sharp line of demarcation between where the apple ends and where the girl begins. In fact, we might say that it's an apple-girl system that's unfolding in each moment. And there are countless other examples of this.

Consider looking at a picture, if you would, of just the tops of the fingers of a hand. Can you imagine that? Where the palm is hidden—can't see the palm. Now if you just looked at the tops of the fingers, you'd say, well, these four entities or objects, they clearly have a familial connection. They're similar to one another, but they certainly also look quite separate. That is indeed how we usually see objects in the world.

What's revealed in mindfulness practice is the whole hand. We actually notice that the separate, individual things of the world are part of larger organisms. We see the interconnections.

Consider an ant colony for a moment. All of the different elements in the ant colony have separate roles. There's the queen, the worker, the drone. Biologists, starting actually in the late 1700s, defined organisms like ant colonies as superorganisms. They're any organisms in which the different so-called individuals have differentiated roles, and the whole system collapses if they're not all present.

One could consider human beings as a sort of superorganism. Do you happen to be a subsistence farmer? I'm not either. That means we're quite dependent on one another to provide energy, to provide food, to provide shelter, and all of the things we need for our survival. Yet most of the time, at least I, don't recognize this.

If I'm running late to see a patient, and I'm running into a convenience store because I have several hours back-to-back this afternoon and I'm afraid that I'm going to be hungry, I just want to quickly buy a sandwich before my first appointment. And there's a fellow in front of me who's decided that this is his red letter day. And he has carefully chosen 23 scientifically selected lottery numbers that he's playing. And I'm waiting and waiting, worried that I'm going to be late. I don't see him as part of me. I don't see us as part of the same superorganism. Rather, I see him as a problem. And in fact, when there are laser beams coming out of my eyes burning holes in the back of his skull, screaming why don't you just set the money on fire? It'll be so much quicker and have the same result. He doesn't sense this, but I don't feel connected with him.

What I notice when I do mindfulness practice is—and this is a little horrifying to see—is that basically, I see other things in the world in terms of how they might fulfill or thwart my desires. So other people, for example, are friends, others who might support me, or perhaps enemies in some way, they might threaten me. Or perhaps servants, they might do something or give me something. Or when I'm not being vegetarian, which for me is much of the time, I might see other beings as meat, something that I might actually eat.

So how do we develop this separate sense of self, which divides the world into objects and doesn't notice the fluid interconnections of things, doesn't notice that you and I are part of the superorganism? Well, Buddhist psychology outlined the process some 2,500 years ago. And this formulation aligns remarkably well with how a cognitive scientist would describe it today.

In the Buddhist psychological formulation, our sense of ourselves starts with the coming together of a sense organ with a sense object, and then we have awareness of that object. So this involves six senses. Seeing involves the eyes coming into contact with the visual field, hearing, the ears coming into contact with the audio field, and going on with smelling, tasting, and touching.

The sixth sense is interesting. The sixth sense isn't some woo-woo kind of sixth sense. It's everything else. So if I asked you right now, if you're not driving, to close your eyes for a second and conjure up an image of your mother, whether she's alive or no longer, you can probably do that. That would be an example of the sixth sense. It's not direct sensory contact; it's an experience happening in the mind. Or if I were to ask you to count silently to three—do this right now—that would be an example of the sixth sense. Collectively, they're typically called "thinking."

So what we start to see here is we are psychophysiological organisms that don't exactly exist, but we occur moment by moment. And the first occurrence of this involves sense contact. Now we don't stay at the level of sense contact for very long. We organize sensory experience into perceptions.

I'm going to create some sounds and I want you to just listen and see if you can hear these sounds as just sense sensations. Ready? Here they come. Elephant. Elephant. Are you able to just experience those as sensations? Or did an image of a certain animal with a trunk come to mind? It's probably the latter.

Or for example, consider looking at an English written word, typed out, let's say. Let's say you see the following letters, P E R C E P T I O N. Can you visualize those? Are you able to see simply the shapes of letters, basically fluid forms against a contrasting background? Or do sounds arise in the mind? For me when I do this, I cannot *not* read it. The best I can do is break it up into PER, and CEP, and TION. But I can't not read it. Now were they written in something other than English, I'd have no trouble not reading them.

I remember when I was traveling around Thailand with my wife a number of years ago, and she was navigating in the back of the motorbike, and I was driving. And we would get to an intersection. And the sign would say long squiggle, long squiggle, medium squiggle to the left, short squiggle, long squiggle, short squiggle to the right. And luckily, the Lonely Planet had things written out in Thai. And I could say, "Sweetheart, which way do we go?" And she could usually figure it out. So if things are written in Thai, I'm fine with staying at the sensory level and not organizing them into perception. But when things are written in English, I don't have that option.

Now finally, when you see the image that most of us have seen in introductory psych classes that looks like two things simultaneously—you could see two faces facing one another, and the faces themselves define a goblet. And as we look at it, we can see it as one or the other. And if you can picture that, are you actually able to see both the faces and the goblet simultaneously? Or do they actually appear in rapid oscillation?

Most of us find that they appear in rapid oscillation. That it constellates itself as a goblet, then as two faces. And in fact, the mind kind of struggles to make it into one or another. Now this makes perfect sense evolutionarily. Because deciding, beige rock? Nah, lion. Nah, probably beige—nah, maybe lion. It mattered a lot to us.

You know there's this well-known video of students playing basketball and they're wearing black shirts and white shirts. And the task that people are assigned is to watch how many times the kids in the white shirts pass the basketball. And what happens is in the middle of the video, a big, black, gorilla comes in, beats his chest, and exits the stage. And when people are asked to count the number of times the white shirts pass the basketball, about two-thirds of the audience simply doesn't see the gorilla. It's really quite remarkable.

This is called *inattentional blindness*. And we see that perception, what we see, is terribly conditioned by culture, by language, and by desire. What happens in the video is, we're trying to get the number right, so we don't see the gorilla at all.

And what happens is perception constructs and categorizes, and it omits details, and it fills in all sorts of missing information. Now have you ever been in a situation, let's say, with a spouse, or a boyfriend, or girlfriend, some loved one, maybe a parent or a child, where you both were ostensibly in the same place, but you wound up perceiving it very differently? Have those differences in perception ever caused trouble? For most of us, they have.

So a particularly wonderful recent study was done in which they took X-rays of the lungs. They asked 24 radiologists to perform a familiar lung nodule–detection task. And they were playing with the theme from the video I just described, and they placed a gorilla 48 times larger than the average lung nodule in the last case, the last slide. And 83 percent of the radiologists didn't see it. And they did eye tracking and it revealed that the majority of them, who missed the gorilla, looked directly at it. So our perception is radically influenced by what's going on with our desires.

And we fill in things too. Consider a large, round circle with two small circles placed about two-thirds of the way up the middle of it. Can you visualize that? What might it be? Virtually everybody sees either a face, or a few people who probably are into this tend to see bowling balls more. We fill in details like this all the time, even though the nose and even the thumb hole from the bowling ball are quite missing.

I'm sorry to say it gets worse because we don't stay at the level of perception for very long. We add an affective, or emotional or hedonic tone to all the experience. Everything that happens, we see it, feel it to be pleasant, unpleasant, or neutral. We love some things, and we hate others. And then, we develop what are called *intentions* and *dispositions*. I talked about this earlier. We try to hold on to pleasant experience, push away unpleasant experience, and we tend to ignore the neutral.

When we do this over time, we develop habits of intention. We have different words for these. We can call them dispositions; behavioral folks call them *learned behaviors*, or *conditioned responses*; and many of us actually refer to these dispositions, these habits of holding on to some things and pushing away others, as our personality. Now how does that work?

Now, we see this most clearly in adolescence. When you're talking to a teenager and you're asking them about themselves, they'll say well, I'm this kind of person. I'm into this kind of music; I'm not into that kind of music. I like reading, or I hate school. Or I'm big on this kind of sport.

I remember when I went college shopping with my twin daughters. Where I live in the Boston area, there's a lot of emphasis on education, and there are a lot of institutions of higher education nearby. So we were doing one of these tours of going to various liberal arts campuses in New England, and each one was more lovely than the last. They would have ivy covered walls. They would have wonderful athletic facilities, rivaling the things you'd find in Olympic stadiums these days. They would have diverse cafeterias. They had the meat and potatoes crowd, they had something for vegans, they had something for the sushi and Asian fusion group.

These are practically designed as adolescent theme parks, with everything a kid might want. So we finished touring one of these colleges and it was wonderful—great curricular offerings on top of all of that. And I asked my daughter what she thought. And she said, "Well, it's a great school. But I don't think I'm going to apply." And I said, "Why not?" And she said, "Well, did you see what the kids were wearing?" And I said, "Clothes. Jeans and flip-flops, like you, your sister, and all your friends wear." And then I got the eye roll. "Oh, Dad, you are so out of it. Didn't you get it? Didn't you see it in the cafeteria? All the kids are totally emo."

Now if you don't happen to have had a child of the same age as mine, you might have missed this. Adolescents have these complex ways of differentiating and categorizing the different social groups. When I was a kid, we basically had three. We had the kids who were intellectual and academic, and I don't even remember if we quite called them "nerds" yet. And then we had the athletes, who were called "jocks" at the time. And then we had a third group that went by different names. But they're basically the kids who were on the pre-penitentiary track. It was simple back then.

Well now, there are a lot more possibilities, and emo is one of those categories. Emo apparently refers to emotional, and these are kids who are artistically inclined. They feel a lot of angst, and they like to express it in creative work. So they may write novels, they may perform in plays, they may paint pictures. They're not quite as dark as the goth kids. The goth kids are basically, frankly, suicidal. The emo kids, they're OK. But they feel a lot. And somehow, my daughter was able to see what these kids were wearing, identify that they're emo. She's not emo, so she would never go to that school.

Now as grown-ups, we may think this doesn't affect us. But I think it does. I often ask audiences of mental health professionals, and I'll say, "How many of you listen to National Public Radio?" which in the US is our kind of educational radio channel, and the vast majority of them raise their hands. And then I ask, "How many you either currently drive, or aspire to drive some day, a Hummer?" And none of the hands go up. What is it? Do I have great clinical insight? Sociological acumen? No. It turns out that virtually nobody who listens to National Public Radio ever drives a Hummer. In fact, the Hummer may not even have stations on that part of the dial, because it would be no use for them.

So it's a mad house in there. There're sense organs connecting with sense objects, that's being experienced in consciousness. There's feeling happening, intentions happening, perception happening. It's all happening at once. What mindfulness practice reveals is that it's all impersonal. There's nobody home.

As the neurobiologist Wolf Singer put it famously, "[The brain and the mind] are like an orchestra without a conductor." There's simply a continuous flow of moment-to-moment experience, with a new self being born and dying in each moment. There isn't even a stable witness. There's just impersonal experience unfolding.

Now our normal sense of self creates all sorts of trouble. We might more accurately think of—instead of thinking of having a self, think that "selfing" occurs, because in each moment, we're responding out of this sense of agency, or the sense of I. And we respond very differently when the experiences belong to me. It creates all sorts of further distortions. And endless suffering comes from this. These are the thoughts of, I'm better than you, or I'm worse than you; I'm a moral person, I'm an immoral person; I'm talented, I'm not talented—and all of these other self-evaluative thoughts that happen. So whenever experiences arise, we tend to not just take them as they are, or see them clearly, but we reflect on what do they mean about me?

There's a famous quote about this that's attributed to Wei Wu Wei, who masquerades as though he's an ancient Taoist scholar. He's actually a British guy from the modern era. And his quote is this, "Why are you unhappy? Because 99.9 percent of everything you think, and everything you do, is for yourself. And there isn't one."

When we identify with the self, it makes pleasure and pain personal. It creates this fantasy of being able to control my experience, and my insecurities, my competitive feelings, my aggression, jealousy, and all of these kinds of defensive things follow.

Einstein put it beautifully. Here's what he said. He said,

> A human being is part of the whole called by us universe. … We experience ourselves, our thoughts and feelings as something separate from the rest. A kind of optical delusion of consciousness. This delusion is a kind of prison for us, restricting us to our personal desires and to affection for a few persons nearest to us. Our task must be to free ourselves from the prison by widening our circle of compassion to embrace all living creatures and the whole of nature

in its beauty. The true value of a human being is determined by the measure and the sense in which they have obtained liberation from the self.

Now this has very interesting implications. And it touches on the idea of karma, which many of you probably know is associated with the teachings of many Indian, but also eastern cultures generally. And karma is traditionally understood in terms of reincarnation. The idea is that how we perform in this life determines how we will be reborn in the next.

But karma can also be seen in moment-to-moment intentions. What becomes reborn is a certain constellation or attitude in consciousness. So my intention in one moment, whether I'm grasping onto something, pushing it away, acting out of anger, acting out of love, my intention at this moment tends to shape the perceptions and the feelings in the next moment, which creates the reality of the next moment.

Now the Buddha has been described as being like Copernicus of the mind because he said that our identity is being recreated moment by moment, and that the continuity of self simply can't be found—it's illusory. All we have are frames in a movie and the mind's tendency to string these frames together into a narrative, starring me, that makes me feel that I exist. And all sorts of suffering, preoccupation with what's going to happen to me, result from this.

The Copernican shift he made was a figure ground shift, like the one Copernicus did when he said, you know, we can understand the solar system more clearly if instead of seeing the earth as the center, we see the earth as part of this larger set of entities.

And Carl Jung in a certain way—the student and colleague of Freud's—had a similar observation. He talked about what happens when we identify with some mental contents and reject others. He said that when we do this, it creates a kind of split-off shadow. It's almost a form of dissociation, a kind of splitting caused by trying to avoid pain. So if I think of myself—because I have a self-concept—as being generous, hardworking, and intelligent, then my greedy, lazy, and dumb side is going to be my shadow. And I'm going to have trouble every time I have a life circumstance that highlights the fact that I'm greedy, lazy, or dumb, to some degree. And I'll go through the world seeking affirmation of who I want myself to be, or who I think of myself as being. And if I'm in a relationship with somebody who does something that illuminates my greediness, my laziness, or my lack of being very smart, I'm going to get very uncomfortable and I will probably react to them in some kind of negative way. So we start to see how the very construction of the self sets us up for lots, and lots of difficulties.

As you're listening to this though, you may be thinking, but wait a minute. Of course I exist. And indeed, the sense of self is a universal category of experience. Every language has words for you, and for me. But it really is experienced differently in different cultures. And one of the things we see through mindfulness practice, is we see how it is actually constructed not only by our moment to moment experience, but by the culture in which we live.

As I mentioned earlier, we all get hooked on different dimensions or domains that define ourselves. For one person, it's physical beauty—am I attractive enough? For another, it's athletic content, athletic talent. For somebody else, it's financial status—am I rich or poor? For yet another, it would be artistic creativity—you know, am I better able to express myself and create new works this way? For someone else, it's academic degree, or even whether they're wearing the correct designer outfit.

A patient came in to see me and she was really in distress. She had been a former model, and clothing mattered to her, and appearance mattered to her, not surprisingly. And she had apparently gone to a Bar Mitzvah on Long Island and felt that she wasn't wearing the right level of designer dress. I didn't even know that designer dresses come in different levels, but she certainly did, and she had felt out of place. That had been a very painful experience for her because she was afraid about other people and how they would look at her.

So this causes all sorts of difficulties. The other thing that we discover is that there is no single self to be found. And we see this all the time in meditation practice. If I were to ask you, how was your last meditation session? You might report, if you're being accurate, well, there was part of me that was trying to attend to the breath. There was part of me that was fantasizing about the future. There was part of me that was judging myself for fantasize about the future. We should really ask the committee how it went.

You know, in fact, it can be very useful in dealing with emotional difficulties to notice if there's no single coherent self, to notice if there's a committee. Often, when we're in distress, there are conflicts among different parts. Well there's a part of me wants to achieve more, and be successful in my career, but there's a part of me that wants love and connection, and wants to spend more time with my friends and family. There's a part of me that thinks it's very important to be social, and yet there's another part of me that completely craves and hungers for solitude. Seeing what each part wants and needs can really help us.

There's a popular form of psychotherapy called Internal Family Systems. It's practiced a lot in the Boston area. And this invites us to take time to recognize, honor, and draw out the fears and needs of each of these different parts. When each part is recognized in this way, the part itself feels safer, calms down, and doesn't need so much to run the show. When we're not identified with a single sense of self, this can facilitate a tremendous amount of flexibility because then we don't have to be one way or the other, and we can be much more accepting of our diverse, and often complex, experiences.

This also has tremendous implications for our development. Mindfulness practices, like forms of psychotherapy, become a sort of loosening practice, and loosening process, where the goal becomes not to be more one way or more of the other way in the sense of more perfect, but to develop a sense of psychological flexibility. In fact, there are some mindfulness-based psychotherapies like Acceptance and Commitment Therapy, also called ACT, where the explicit goal is not feeling good about yourself, not even being successful in your endeavors, but simply having psychological flexibility—being able to be whoever, or whatever you are, in each moment. And this provides enormous relief from worrying so much about ourselves, from how we compare to others, about our pleasure or pain. It helps us to identify with something larger than ourselves. And this identification with something more than me becomes particularly important in any path to well-being.

Now both philosophers and scientists have described the interdependence that's revealed through mindfulness practice, the sense of being part of the superorganism. Here's how Thích Nhất Hạnh, the Zen teacher, describes this insight.

> Looking deeply into a flower we see that the flower is made of non-flower elements. We can describe the flower as being full of everything. There's nothing that is not present in the flower. We see sunshine, we see the rain, we see clouds, we see the earth, and we also see time and space in the flower. ... A flower, like everything else, is made entirely of non-flower elements. The whole cosmos has come together in order to [make] the flower manifest herself. The flowers is full of everything except one thing: a separate self or a separate identity.

Or as the astronomer Carl Sagan once famously said, "If you want to make an apple pie from scratch, you must first create the universe."

So I invite you to try a little exercise. Imagine what a day would be like if you no longer thought about yourself as a separate individual. And as a result, you had no concerns about how you or others saw yourself. This is a day in which you actually get it, that what you are is simply part of this larger, constantly changing, fluid collection of atoms and molecules that we call the universe. How might you dress if your sense of self didn't matter? How might you act with other people? What would you do during the day? What would matter to you? And in particular, how might you feel if it wasn't about me anymore, but it was simply about whatever you were engaged with? Most people find when they make the shift that all sorts of wonderful opportunities open up.

In our next lecture, we're going to look at the implications of these insights into the nature of the self for psychological well-being, and we'll see how we may be able to go beyond—as Freud once put it, as the goal of psychoanalysis—changing "neurotic misery into common unhappiness."

Mindfulness or Psychotherapy?
Lecture 5

In this lecture, you will learn that there are many parallels between Western psychotherapies and the traditions from which many mindfulness practices come. But they diverge in the understanding of the self—the ultimate goal. However, the practical differences may not really be so profound, because traditional students of mindfulness may have full enlightenment of their ultimate goal. But that ultimate goal is rarely attained. Instead, in ways that would be quite recognizable to Western health professionals, students of mindfulness become more mature and balanced.

The Eightfold Path

- Many mindfulness practices that are used in Western psychotherapy come from Buddhist psychology. One reason is that Buddhist psychology has much in common with Western psychotherapy. Like modern scientific psychology, Buddhist psychology is nontheistic. It doesn't discuss God or gods in any way.

- Rather, it has a fundamental principle—the Pali term for which is *ehipassiko*, which translates roughly as "come and see for yourself." The way we understand mindfulness practices is by doing them and making them real in our own experience and discovering what we discover. It is not based on doctrine. It's also a systemic approach, and it uses empirical methodology and questions authority.

- Mindfulness supports open-mindedness by helping us to take our thoughts more lightly. In this regard, it's very similar to the scientific posture that we see in Western psychology and psychotherapy. Also like Western psychotherapy, the goal of mindfulness is the alleviation of suffering. And it actually has a system similar to Western medical practices that includes identification of symptoms, etiology, prognosis, and treatment.

- The symptom is the unsatisfactoriness of all experience—the fact that the mind creates suffering no matter what's happening. The etiology is seen as our distorted views, our misunderstandings about reality. And the prognosis is surprisingly good. As we've taken up these practices in Western psychological circles, we've primarily focused on concentration, or focused attention; open monitoring, or mindfulness; and acceptance practices, such as loving-kindness meditation.

- Actually, these were part of a much larger treatment plan in Buddhist traditions called the Eightfold Path, which is about "right" concentration, mindfulness, effort, livelihood, action, speech, intentions, and view. The word "right" doesn't mean "right" in a moral sense as opposed to wrong. It means optimal, wholesome, or that which is most likely to alleviate suffering.

- We've already discussed concentration and mindfulness. Right effort involves having the right degree of control versus letting go. Right livelihood, in the modern context, means doing work in the world in which we're not causing more harm than good. Right action is about thinking about everything we do in terms of whether it is going to be helpful to others or hurtful to others. Right speech involves honesty, but it also involves not speaking in ways that create divisions or derision and not being abusive or hurtful in our speech. Right intentions is about orienting ourselves always toward our own sanity and alleviation of suffering. Finally, right view is about seeing the world clearly.

Similarities between Mindfulness Practices and Psychotherapies
- There are many overlaps and parallels among different psychotherapies and between mindfulness practices and psychotherapies. They're certainly all designed to move us in a similar direction, toward greater well-being. Recently, many mental health professionals have come to believe that mindfulness might actually be a central curative element in most other forms of psychotherapy because it accomplishes several nearly universal therapeutic goals.

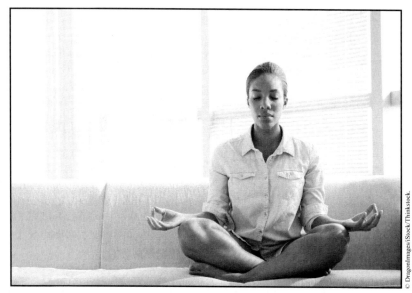

Mindfulness practices are designed to move you toward greater well-being.

- Mindfulness, like many forms of therapy, loosens the repression barrier. When we start practicing mindfulness, the previously unnoticed thoughts and feelings—the things we've pushed out of our awareness—start to become evident. We become more sensitized to what's happening in the mind and less distracted by our constant activity. Also, our impulses become clearer. Finally, our defensive strategies become apparent, which ultimately allows us to reintegrate these contents.

- The second way that mindfulness helps to accomplish a task that's pretty universal in psychotherapy is that it treats the thinking disease. The basic idea with cognitive behavior therapy is to develop metacognitive awareness, which means to notice what thoughts are rising and passing in the mind. And it focuses, in particular, on identifying rational thoughts and differentiating them from irrational thoughts.

- Dynamic psychotherapy, which is the vast array of psychotherapies that have come out of psychoanalysis, is more interested in understanding the origins of our personal narrative. How did we come to believe we are who we are? How did we to construct our world? The idea is to loosen the identification with the story. And we also look to see how it plays out in relationships, and the idea of this is to create a new personal narrative.

- In Buddhist psychology, the idea is that distorted beliefs lead to suffering. This is not unlike what we're seeing in the other traditions, but in Buddhist psychology, the problem is not embracing reality in a very radical sense; instead, the problem is seen as not realizing that everything is always changing. We can hold on to nothing, not realizing that the mind creates distress, regardless of external circumstances, and that our conventional sense of self is illusory.

- Buddhist psychology is very skeptical of thought generally. This is, in part, because it sees thought as supporting essentialism, meaning that it is our thoughts about things that make things real. And thought also creates self. Descartes commented on this when he said, "I think; therefore, I am."

- First, in mindfulness practice, unlike psychotherapies, there's no need to replace one thought with another. Rather, we start to see thoughts as just mental objects, like any other, including an itch or an ache. If we notice an itch while engaging in mindfulness practice, turn our attention to the itch and watch it dissipate.

- In the same way, in mindfulness practice, we start to simply watch thoughts coming and going. As a result, they become less serious to us, which means that we don't need to suppress or repress them so much. Nothing is unthinkable, and our identifications with roles start to loosen. When we take this attitude, we develop a kind of freedom.

- The third way that mindfulness practice performs something that psychotherapies also are designed to do is by being a form of exposure treatment. Exposure is perhaps the most universal element in all of our diverse psychotherapies. It's simply facing our fears, longings, or aggressive impulses. One way we could understand mindfulness practice is its exposure to everything.

- Finally, both mindfulness practice and psychotherapy provide holding, which is a term that was introduced by pediatrician and psychotherapist D. W. Winnicott, who discovered that simply holding a baby provides so much comfort to the child. One way in which mindfulness practices and psychotherapy provide holding is simply the relationship with the therapist—having another human being who is accepting and nonjudgmental and keeps confidentiality.

- With both mindfulness practice and psychotherapy, it tends to get worse before it gets better. In psychotherapy, usually people notice that they have so many difficult thoughts and feelings and might start to think that they are crazy. In behavioral treatment, there's often self-monitoring, and people notice that they're having irrational thoughts all the time. And in mindfulness practice, we see just how unruly the mind is.

Differences between Mindfulness Practices and Psychotherapies

- There are also ways in which mindfulness practices and psychotherapies are different—where mindfulness practice veers off from conventional treatments. In behavior therapy, as well as psychodynamic treatment, we're typically seeking normalcy.

- Mindfulness traditions have a much more radical goal. They're looking for insight leading to complete psychological, emotional, moral, and spiritual emancipation—what's been called enlightenment. Traditionally, the starting point is actually common unhappiness or normalcy. It's only recently, as mental health professionals are adopting it, that we start also seeing that we can use mindfulness practice to move us from states of particular distress to normal unhappiness.

- Another important difference is a different view of the self. In the Western view, there's this emphasis on separateness rather than connection to family, tribe, or nature. In fact, our models of healthy Western development have included being well individuated, being aware of boundaries, knowing one's needs, having a clear identity and sense of self, and having good self-esteem. Buddhist psychology says that we suffer when we don't know who we really are, and it's the attempt to buttress the self that's the central cause of our suffering.

- One of the goals of Western psychotherapy—to improve self-esteem and have a cohesive sense of self—is actually seen as a form of pathology from the Buddhist perspective. One way we could conceptualize the goal of Buddhist psychology is to shift our universe from a world that is mostly about "me" to a world that is mostly not about "me." It's a subtle shift, and it occurs over time.

- Buddhist psychology actually has a very radical psychological goal as well. We erect defenses against pain, ways in which we shut down, pull back, and turn off to others. And we think that they're going to keep us safe, but they leave us very isolated in a kind of anxiety of the separate self. The alternative is to try to develop a kind of spacious tender awareness—to stay with whatever is and not to leave these feelings in order to feel better.

- In psychotherapeutic circles, we talk about having adaptive and healthy defenses, not be radically open and aware. The Buddhist psychological approach is not a path to perfection, but it's a path to wholeness. It's about transforming our view to be able to allow everything in and to not judge them as better and worse.

Suggested Reading

Epstein, *Psychotherapy without the Self.*

Fulton and Siegel, "Buddhist and Western Psychology."

Shapiro and Carlson, *The Art and Science of Mindfulness.*

Siegel, "East Meets West."

1. In what ways are the goals of Buddhist psychology and conventional Western psychotherapies similar and different?

2. How is the self conventionally viewed in Western cultures, and how does this compare to how it is viewed in Buddhist psychology?

Mindfulness or Psychotherapy?
Lecture 5—Transcript

There's a famous Zen teaching story that points to the power of mindfulness practice to fortify us to work with life's inevitable challenges. It's said that in medieval Japan, there was this marauding general who came to a town, and he was very sadistic. He and his men were raping women. They were committing horrible acts of vandalism, burning down farms. They were killing the able-bodied boys and men. It was really a horrible, horrible scene. And this general really wanted to vanquish the town. And he caught wind that they respected and revered their Zen master.

So he took his horse and he galloped up the hillside into the main hall of Zen temple. And there, sitting on his *zafu*—his meditation cushion—was this little old man. And the general raised up his bloody sword over the head of Zen master and he said, "Don't you realize I could run you through with this sword without blinking an eye?" And the Zen master looked up, and he said, "Yes. And I, sir, can be run through with a sword without blinking at eye." And it's said that at that moment, the general became flustered and left town.

Now, it's not always going to work as a military intervention, but it does say something about the power of these practices to build the kind of courage inside of us. So how did the Zen master become so courageous? He did it by following a detailed treatment plan with mindfulness practice at its core, that's designed to cultivate well-being as well as courage. The ancient treatment plan has much in common with what we know to be effective in modern psychotherapy.

I mentioned earlier that many mindfulness practices that are used in Western psychotherapy come from Buddhist psychology. One reason is that Buddhist psychology has much in common, actually, with Western psychotherapy. Like modern scientific psychology, Buddhist psychology is non-theistic—it doesn't posit God or discuss God or gods in any way. It's not based on doctrine. Rather, it has a fundamental principle, the Pali term for which is *ehipassiko*. And *ehipassiko* translates roughly as "come and see for yourself." Take nothing on doctrine. Try these things out. Try these practices we're suggesting. And see in the laboratory of your own mind and body what you find to be true. It's also a systemic approach and systematic approach. And it uses empirical methodology and questions authority.

The Dalai Lama frequently meets these days with large convocations of neuroscientists and clinicians and researchers into psychotherapeutic change. And what he says at virtually every meeting is, "If you Western scientists discover some principal or some finding that contradicts a basic doctrine or tenant of Buddhism, that will be OK. We'll just have to change Buddhism, won't we?" And there's a venerable history of this. You see it particularly in the Zen tradition. There's a famous line by the Zen master Linji, who's the founder of the Rinzai sect in the 9th century. And he said, "If you meet the Buddha on the road, kill him!" And that may seem a little odd when we first hear about this. And the scholars have spent much time discussing what that's really about.

And what it's about is, if you feel that the teaching comes from the outside, if you feel that you can understand these principles by reading some text or passing down what your teacher said, kill that. That's not how we understand these practices. The way we understand them is by doing them and making them real in our own experience and discovering what we discover.

There's a Zen saying that goes along with this that says, "Great questioning, great awakening; little questioning, little awakening; no questioning, no awakening." And mindfulness supports this open-mindedness by helping us to take our thoughts more likely. And in this regard, it's very similar to the scientific posture that we see in Western psychology and Western psychotherapy. Also like Western psychotherapy, the goal of mindfulness is the alleviation of suffering. And it actually has a system the same way we do in Western medical practices that includes identification of systems, symptoms, noticing with the etiology is, having a prognosis, and a treatment plan.

The symptom is the unsatisfactoriness of all experience, the fact that the mind creates suffering no matter what's happening. The etiology is seen as our distorted views, our misunderstandings about reality. And the prognosis is surprisingly good. As we've taken up these practices in Western psychological circles, we've primarily focused on concentration or focused attention, open monitoring—or mindfulness, per se, or choice-less awareness—and acceptance practices, such as the loving-kindness meditation that we've discussed.

Actually, these were originally part of a much larger treatment plan. You may have heard of it. The treatment plan is called, in Buddhist traditions, the Eightfold Path. And it's about right concentration, mindfulness, effort, livelihood, action, speech, intentions, and view. When we use the word "right" here, though, it doesn't mean right in a moral sense as opposed to wrong, it means optimal, wholesome, or that which is most likely to alleviate suffering.

We've already discussed concentration and mindfulness. Let's look at the other factors. Right effort involves having the right degree of control versus letting go. We don't want to be so lax in our approach to mindfulness practices that we just sit there and daydream, but we don't want to be so tight that we're trying to get every thought to stop or stay rigidly on the breath.

Right livelihood, traditionally, meant not selling or buying slaves, selling or buying weapons, or selling or buying poisons. In the modern context, it means doing work in the world in which we're not causing more harm than good. Right action is broader than that. It's about thinking about everything we do in terms of whether it is going to be helpful to others or hurtful to others.

Right speech, as you might imagine, involves honesty, but it also involves not speaking in ways that create divisions or derision. And also involves not being abusive or hurtful in our speech. Right intentions is about orienting ourselves always toward our own sanity and alleviation of suffering. Finally, right view is about seeing the world clearly, and we'll talk more about that in a bit.

There are many overlaps and parallels among different psychotherapies and between mindfulness practices and psychotherapies. They're certainly all designed to move us in a similar direction, toward greater well-being. Recently, many mental health professionals have come to believe that mindfulness might actually be a central curative element in most other forms of psychotherapy because it accomplishes several nearly universal therapeutic goals.

Let's look at a few of them. First, mindfulness, like many forms of therapy, loosens the repression barrier. What do I mean by that? Well, it turns out that all of us, when we experience difficulty in life—and it could be a small sadness or significant trauma—tend to push feelings out of awareness. When things are painful and difficult to take in in the moment, our minds have a mechanism by which we can either ignore them or forget them.

What happens when we start practicing mindfulness is that previously unnoticed thoughts and feelings, the things we've pushed out of our awareness, start to become evident. We become more sensitized to what's happening in the mind, less distracted by our constant activity. Also, our impulses become clearer. So that if I have an angry feeling and an impulse to harm, that shows up. If I have a warm feeling and an impulse to bring somebody closer to me, that shows up. We start to notice all these things.

And then finally, our defensive strategies become apparent. We start to notice when we're rationalizing. We start to notice when we're creating thought streams in order to make ourselves feel better or to block things out of awareness. So whether we're on the psychoanalytic couch or sitting on the meditation cushion, sooner or later, everything we've ever wanted to not think, feel, or remember tends to come into awareness.

And this is a good thing because this ultimately allows us to reintegrate these contents. Because what happens is, when we're pushing contents out of awareness, that requires a certain amount of effort. And that effort, actually, is experienced as a kind of constant stress as we're threatened by the fact that these thoughts and feelings might come back into our awareness.

The second way that mindfulness helps to accomplish a task that's pretty universal in psychotherapy is it treats the thinking disease. You've probably heard of cognitive behavior therapy or CBT. It's the most widely-studied, empirically-supported method. Or it has been, historically, until the mindfulness and acceptance-based treatments have recently come onto the scene. And the basic idea in cognitive behavior therapy is to develop what's called *metacognitive awareness*.

It's to notice what thoughts are rising and passing in the mind. And it focuses, in particular, on identifying rational thoughts and differentiating them from irrational thoughts. And when we see irrational thoughts, the idea is to refute them as well as to label them and categorized them. There are many different forms of irrational thought. There's overgeneralization. In other words, somebody rejects me and I think, oh, everybody hates me. There's catastrophizing. I think something might go wrong and I imagine horrible things are going to happen. It'll be the end of my life as I know it.

There's all sorts of magical thinking. When we have adversity in our life, thinking that it's our fault, for example, because we didn't do this, or we didn't do that. And other things, such as disqualifying the positive—these are the actions of the negativity bias at work, in which we might notice the one negative thing that happened during the day and disqualify the 20 positive things that happened. There's even, in CBT, the idea of thought stopping, which is when there're particularly troublesome thoughts, people might even wear a rubber band on their wrist. And every time one of those thoughts comes up, they will just snap the rubber band to bring their attention away from it.

Psychodynamic psychotherapy, which is really the vast array of psychotherapies that have descended or come out of psychoanalysis, that's more interested in understanding the origins of our personal narrative. How did we come to believe we are who we are, believe the things that are important that we think are important? How did we come to construct our world? And the idea is to loosen the identification with the story. If we see how we came upon it during our childhood experience, we're much more likely to be able to take it lightly. And say, oh, OK. That's a constructed story. It's not necessarily reality with a capital R.

And we also look in psychodynamic psychotherapy about how it plays out in relationships, including in the relationship with the therapist in this moment when thoughts and feelings come up in treatment. And the idea of this is to create a new personal narrative. In Buddhist psychology, the idea is that it's distorted beliefs that lead to suffering—not unlike what we're seeing in the other traditions. However, here, the problem is not embracing reality in a very radical sense. The problem is seen as not realizing that everything is always changing—we can hold on to nothing; not realizing that the mind creates distress, regardless of external circumstances—whether things are going well or poorly, it nonetheless generates senses of dissatisfaction; and that our conventional sense of self is illusory—what we spoke about earlier. Buddhist psychology is very skeptical of thought generally. And this is, in part, because it sees thought as supporting essentialism. By that, I mean, it is our thoughts about things that make things real.

So if I look at a chair, and I think, chair. It's actually the thought of chair that makes me see the chair as a separate object. Or I look at a person, and I think, criminal. It's the thought of them as a criminal that makes them a separate object and makes it so I don't see them and me as part of the same superorganism. And thought also creates self. Descartes commented on this years ago when he said, "I think, therefore I am." And we know that constant judgments create alienation because we wind up living in a world of good people and bad people, good things and bad things.

In mindfulness practice, unlike psychotherapies, there's no need to replace one thought with another. Rather, we start to see thoughts as just mental objects, like any other, like an itch or an ache. So we're sitting there in our meditation practice—and I hope, by the way, that you are sitting there in your meditation practice between the lectures, not all the time but taking some time out to practice—and an itch or an ache might arise. Right? So what do we do with that? We simply watch the itch, turn our attention to it, and watch it dissipate. In the same way, what we start to do in mindfulness practice is simply to watch thoughts coming and going. They become less serious to us. When they're less serious to us, when we don't believe in them in the same way, then we don't need to suppress or repress them so much. And on the other side, our attachment pleasant fantasies diminish as we think, if I have a fantasy that I'm the greatest thing on Earth and I think, ah, there we go again with another narcissistically-inflated fantasy. And I can go on to looking at the tree.

Nothing is unthinkable. And our identifications with roles start to loosen. So how do we actually put this into practice? Well, when we're sitting and doing our meditation practice, we simply are with an object of attention, such as the breath, and a thought arises. And we simply allow the thought to arise and to pass, like a cloud passing through the sky. We might observe our bodily responses to the thoughts. And we might even observe how cognition follows affect and affect follows cognition, by which I mean a feeling arises, like there's a wave of sadness for example, and it's followed by a sad thought. Or wave of anger arises, and it's followed by an angry thought. They work hand-in-hand, mutually creating one another. And we can also watch our impulse to cling to the pleasant thoughts and reject the unpleasant ones. There's even a practice called "noting" that I invite you to try when you do your meditation, which is simply sitting—and, again, being with an object of awareness, such as the breath—and every time a thought comes in, just gently and sub-vocally saying, "thinking, thinking."

A modification of this involves labeling the type of thought—judging, planning, remembering. Whatever it is, we simply see them as objects. And we use the labeling so as not to get caught in the narrative because it's very easy—and I'm sure you've noticed this if you're doing the practice—it's very easy to simply get swept into the thought stream, to leave the breath entirely and get lost in a daydream or a plan or to-do list check. And when we take this attitude, when we allow everything to rise and pass, and we simply notice them like clouds going through the sky, we develop a kind of freedom. Suzuki Roshi, the Zen master, once asked this question. He said, "If you had a cow or sheep who was quite agitated, and you wanted to help the animal to calm down, what do you think the best thing to do would be? Would it be to shackle it or tie it up in ropes? Or do you think giving it a wide pasture would help?" The natural answer is the wide pasture. And one of the ways of mindfulness practice is really modifying traditional Western psychotherapeutic practices is by emphasizing much more the need to give the mind this wide pasture.

Now the third way that mindfulness practice performs something that psychotherapies also are designed to do is by being a form of exposure treatment. Now, exposure is perhaps the most universal element in all of our diverse psychotherapies. It's basically, simply facing our fears, facing our longings, facing our aggressive impulses. In the behavioral tradition, we literally set up exposure circumstances. You're afraid of bridges? We'll go over bridges with you. In psychodynamic psychotherapy, it occurs much more by simply allowing whatever comes to mind to come to mind and then exploring the things that are difficult. But exposure is a central component of not only psychodynamic and behavior therapies but virtually all other the forms of treatment. And one way we could understand mindfulness practice is it is exposure to everything. We're developing the muscle of bearing experience, of being able to be with whatever arises. Because if we're allowing the mind to be this open space, the ache arises, the itch arises, the pain arises, and thoughts arise and feelings arise.

That's how the Zen master evolved to the point where he could be run through with a sword without blinking an eye. He did it by simply sitting moment after moment—in his case probably hour after hour—allowing pleasant and unpleasant experiences to arise and pass and not taking action to fix them, by repeatedly being with experience and noticing its impersonal nature.

Finally, both mindfulness practice and psychotherapy provide holding. What do I mean by holding? Holding is a term that was introduced by a very well-known pediatrician and psychotherapist named D. W. Winnicott. And he had watched a lot of moms holding their kids, and saw the way that simply holding a baby provides so much comfort to the child. And there's a way in which mindfulness practices and psychotherapy provide holding. One way is simply the relationship with the therapist, having another human being who's accepting. And the therapist is nonjudgmental and keeps confidentiality and the like.

Behavioral treatments, they provide holding by giving people homework. It's a way of taking the treatment home with you. Holding in mindfulness practice happens by taking refuge in the present moment because no matter what's happening, we can always return to right now, knowing that there are these traditional teachings, not as doctrine but as a rough map, a guide that we might follow. Knowing that we're in the community of so many other people who are doing these practices with the same intention of finding sanity and finding a way to live in the world that doesn't promote more suffering—we have their reports to give us some support. And simply having a physical posture in which we sit in a kind of dignified and relaxed way and having an object of concentration provides some support and holding.

Now in both mindfulness practice and psychotherapy—and maybe you've seen this already, maybe you haven't—it tends to get worse before it gets better. And this is like what we see in medicine. If you have a wound that's infected and you go to the doctor, well, the doctor's going to have to open the wound up to clean it out. And it's going feel worse to open it up than it did to leave it be. But the chances of it healing are quite slim if we don't open it up. So in the same way, in mindfulness practice as well psychotherapy, initially it gets worse. In psychotherapy, usually people notice, oh my god, I've got so many difficult thoughts and feelings. I start realizing, I'm really nuts. Or in behavioral treatment, for example, often there's self-monitoring done. And people notice, god, I'm having irrational thoughts every minute. And in mindfulness practice, we see just how unruly the mind is, how, like the puppy we were talking about, it tends not to follow instructions very well and it does pee and poop in the wrong place in the wrong time quite a bit.

Now, there are ways in which these practices are different also, where mindfulness practice veers off from conventional treatments. In behavior therapy as well as psychodynamic treatment, typically, we're seeking normalcy. In behavior therapy, we're seeking rational and adaptive behavior. And in psychodynamic psychotherapy, as Freud famously said, the goal was to transform "hysterical misery into common unhappiness [so that his patients could be] better armed against the unhappiness."

Mindfulness traditions have a much more radical goal. They're looking for insight leading to complete psychological, emotional, moral, and spiritual emancipation—what's been called "enlightenment." Traditionally, the starting point is actually common unhappiness or normalcy. It's only recently, as mental health professionals are adopting this, that we start also seeing that we can use mindfulness practice to move us from states a particular distress to normal unhappiness.

Another really important difference, as we've discussed in the last lecture, is a different view of the self. In the Western view, there's this emphasis on separateness rather than connection to family, tribe, or nature. In fact, our models of healthy Western development have been things like being well individuated, being aware of boundaries, knowing one's needs, having a clear identity and sense of self, and having good self-esteem.

The problem with good self-esteem is we can't all live in Lake Wobegon, where all the women are beautiful, and all the children are above average. Rather, what happens is, we wind up feeling better or worse about ourselves, comparing ourselves to others, and obviously half of the time, at least half of us are going to come up short.

Buddhist psychology says, we suffer when we don't know who we really are, and it's the attempt to buttress the self that's the central cause of our suffering. And that's because our concept itself is based on the fundamental misunderstanding that we discussed before. One of the goals of Western psychotherapy, to improve self-esteem and have a cohesive sense of self, is actually seen as a form of pathology from the Buddhist perspective. Now, why, you might ask? What's wrong with developing a stronger, more positive sense of self? Well, as the Beatles said, there's a lot of pain in "I, me, me, mine. I, me, me, mine."

I had a patient who taught this to me in stunning relief very early in my practice. It was my first year of private practice. And he came to see me and he had just sold his oil trading business for $30 million cash. And he kept using that expression, $30 million cash. And I kept imagining the wheelbarrow. You know, what does that look like? And he was really quite adrift and quite despondent. And I was eager. I was thinking, this is going to be one of these meaning-of-life treatments. It's not just, well, my baby done left me, or I lost my job, or I failed the test at school. This is going to be what really matters because he had enough money. He'd been successful. Now what matters? And I had a longstanding interest in Buddhist psychology, a longstanding interest in other philosophic forms of inquiry, so I was very, very eager to work with this fellow. And as often happens when a psychotherapist has a clear idea of where they want the treatment to go, I wasn't connecting very well with him at all because he actually had no interest in the meaning of life. He just wanted to these feelings to go away.

Nonetheless, he came back for a few sessions. And it was probably in maybe the third or the fourth session when he looked transformed. He was beaming. He was animated. And I commented. I said, "What happened?" And he said, "I've just come up with a business plan by which I think I could parlay my $30 million into a $50 million enterprise. And I think that if I could establish a $50 million company, then I'd feel like I had been successful." And there was no irony in his voice. He was completely serious about it.

It was a great teaching to me, because I had my own narcissistic concerns having just come from working in a teaching hospital and all sorts of other difficulties. And I realized, it doesn't matter how successful we are. I want to give you of little exercise that may illustrate this for you. I want you to think of the goals that you had when you were younger. And we've had so many of them—it starts early. It could be when I get to ride a bicycle, then I'll really feel like I've made it and I'll be happy. When I can walk to the store alone because I'm a big enough boy, then that'll do it. Oh, if only I could have a girlfriend or a boyfriend, that would certainly do it for me. And then, there's looking forward to graduating from high school, perhaps, or college and maybe getting a professional or graduate degree. Or perhaps getting married or having kids or a house. Think of your own life. You've probably had some milestones like this that you looked forward to. And you thought, when I get there, that's going to feel really good.

When I'm talking to groups of psychotherapists, we all share the moment in which we got a professional degree. And it took a lot of work and a lot of effort. And I ask folks, when you awoke this morning, did you say, wow, I'm so happy I have my professional degree? And the whole group cracks up. Because usually nobody—sometimes there's one person—but rarely more than one person who felt that way. And I ask you, when you woke up this morning, did you think, this is so great. I can go to the store alone, or ride a bicycle, or I graduated from college. Probably not.

What happens to us is what happened to the fellow in the oil trading business which is we simply habituate to the new level. And then, it becomes the new normal and it no longer works for us anymore. My friend and colleague, the meditation teacher Tara Brach, talks about the trance of unworthiness. And this comes from a finding—it was quite surprising. When Eastern meditation teachers first came to the West and started teaching Western students, they were amazed at our self-criticism. They said, every Westerner thinks they're terrible meditator. What's this all about?

Asian cultures clearly have their own problems but this, apparently, is not one of them. And it seems to be related to the Western cultural emphasis on a separate itself. Everything is like a test to see, how am I doing? How am I doing? How do I compare to others? And my friend, Tara, says, "Anxiety is kind of the primal the mood of the separate itself. If we feel separate from others and isolated from the larger world, we're always feeling in danger. And we're always giving ourselves these sorts of report cards."

Now, one way we could conceptualize the goal of Buddhist psychology is to shift our universe from a world that's mostly about me to a world that's mostly not about me. It's a subtle shift and it occurs over time, but we can start to see how many of my thoughts are basically evaluative thoughts about me or thoughts about me getting what I want or avoiding what I don't want, versus thoughts about the bigger picture. How many of you, when you've been anxious recently, have been mostly anxious about global climate change? The science says we should be anxious about global climate change, but it's not what grips most of us most personally.

Now, Buddhist psychology actually has a very radical psychological goal as well. All of us have had our hearts broken. Think back, perhaps, to the last time that happened to you. Maybe it was recently. Maybe it was back when you were a teenager. And when your heart was broken, let's say in a love relationship, was your first impulse, oh, let me be vulnerable again? I would love to have the possibility of intimacy again. You might have longed for contact with somebody, but the idea of this kind of vulnerability again— probably, no. In fact, when it has happened to me, I'm thinking particularly earlier in my life, I kind of adopted the Simon and Garfunkel, "I am a rock" posture. Like, I think I'll take a break from this.

So we erect these defenses against pain, these ways in which we kind of shut down and pull back and turn off to others. And we think that they're going to keep us safe. But the problem is they leave us very alone and they leave us very isolated in this kind of anxiety of the separate self which doesn't work out so well. The alternative is to try to develop a kind of spacious tender awareness, to stay with whatever is, and not to leave these feelings in order to feel better.

There is a mythological kingdom that existed in Tibet before Buddhism came there, called Shambhala. You may have heard of it if you're interested in such matters as Shambhala Press—they publish a lot of wisdom literature. And the highest attainment in the Shambhala kingdom was to be a Shambhala warrior. But these warriors are not like warriors in the conventional sense. They didn't have weapons and shields and that kind of thing. They were warriors of the heart. And the idea was to be so open to our felt moment-to-moment experience that we defend it against nothing. And the image they use for this is to go through life like a cow without its skin. All of the nerve endings exposed. Wow. We don't see that very much as an ideal in Western psychotherapeutic circles. In psychotherapeutic circles, we talk about having adaptive and healthy defenses, not be this radically open and aware.

So this Buddhist psychological approach is not a path to perfection. But it's a path to wholeness. It's about allowing everything in. You may have heard of Tantra, Tantric yoga, or Tantric Buddhism. Many of us—at least I heard of it as an adolescent, and I thought, that sounds good. It sounds like it's basically an excuse for having sex and calling it spiritual awakening because there is a sexual element to it. But that's not the main point of Tantric practices. The main point is using all of the everyday, intense, nitty-gritty feelings of longing, of love, of loss, of anger, all of our instinctual life, and, rather than trying to block it out, rather than trying to defend against it, using it as energy for awakening—embracing it all.

As one of the Zen patriarchs said, "The boundary of what we can accept in ourselves is the boundary of our freedom." So ultimately here, it's about embracing all these contents and embracing ordinariness, noticing we're all Bozos on this bus. We're all like dandelions in a field. When you look at a field of dandelions, it looks lovely. Do you think, "Oh, well, that's a nice field of dandelions, but the real celebrity wonderful dandelion is in the 234th row from the front, the 89th in from the left"? No. That seems absurd.

This is about transforming our view of things to be able to allow all these contents in and not be judging them as better and worse. So there are many parallels between Western psychotherapies and the traditions from which many of our mindfulness practices come. But they diverge in the understanding of the self, in the ultimate goal. Yet, the practical differences may not really be so profound because traditional students of mindfulness may have full enlightenment of their ultimate goal, but that ultimate goal is rarely attained. Instead, in ways that would be quite recognizable to Western health professionals, students of mindfulness become more mature and balanced, embodying more of what a currently popular Zen saying goes, like this, they say, "You're perfect just as you are, and there's room for improvement."

In our next lecture, we're going to explore the area where mindfulness practices are evolving most rapidly and are going furthest beyond their roots in Buddhist psychology. And this is as they're being taken up by Westerners and applying them to our interpersonal relationships.

Attention and Empathy in Relationships
Lecture 6

In this lecture, you are going to explore the area where mindfulness practices are evolving most rapidly and are going furthest beyond their roots in Buddhist psychology, as they're being taken up by Westerners and applying them to interpersonal relationships. Specifically, you will learn how mindfulness practices can help you develop attention, empathy, open-mindedness, and acceptance—all of which are critical when you're trying to cultivate and maintain relationships with other people.

Attention

- Mindfulness is a kind of training in being present. Our normal state—especially in an era of smartphones, computers, and constant connectivity—is a kind of partial attention. Multitasking distracts us from uncomfortable feelings, and it makes us feel like we can achieve more, but it leaves us more disconnected. Of course, we do have moments of full attention.

- Sometimes danger can help. For example, when we reach to get a tomato from a bin, we might do so with partial attention. When we slice it, we use full attention. Danger can highlight our level of attention. But, often, just the intention to pay attention works, such as deciding to turn our full attention to a friend or loved one.

- Concentration practices help to increase attention, simply by repeatedly practicing paying attention to an object. Every time the mind wanders, bring it back home to the object. Insignificant events can become vivid or rich. We see this in our informal practice—brushing our teeth, showering, or driving. If we bring full attention to these, they become very rich, rewarding, full experiences in themselves, instead of obstacles or difficulties on the way to other things.

- The Dalai Lama says that it takes him about four hours a day of meditation practice to have this form of attention. But even if we do less than that, we can develop some of this ourselves. In addition, Sigmund Freud suggested that a psychoanalyst should practice what he called evenly hovering attention, which he defined as to listen without the trouble of keeping in mind anything in particular.

- Mindfulness practice helps us to cultivate this by practicing presence independent of context. Most of the time, we're interested in the context—and labeling it and thinking about it. Mindfulness, instead, helps us to simply do open monitoring, to be present to whatever arises.

- This develops a rare gift of wholehearted attention. Usually, in order to pay more attention, we turn up the volume in some way. We go for a much more interesting or more entertaining stimulus. With mindfulness practice, we can turn up our attention instead.

- By helping us to simply be present, mindfulness practice also helps us to stay with discomfort. One way the mental muscle gets strong is simply by "being with" the itch or the ache or whatever happens in our life and just feeling it and not moving.

- The other way it helps is by seeing emotional events as impersonal uprisings or phenomena. This helps us to develop affect tolerance, the ability to really be with feelings. When we start to notice feelings simply as neurobiological events, they are transformed, and we're able to tolerate them at much higher levels.

Empathy
- In psychotherapy, we find that other people can only really be close with us if we can tolerate both our feeling and their feeling simultaneously. In the Buddhist tradition, one of the ways that we learn to tolerate these feelings is by noticing not only their impersonality—not just building up the muscle of tolerating discomfort—but also noticing that everything changes.

- Evenly hovering attention is undefended, unconflicted, tolerant, and open attention. In mindfulness practice, much of the time, we're defending against unpleasant experiences. We're trying to hold on to the good ones and push away the bad ones. Instead, what we're trying to develop in our relationships is a kind of radical acceptance of all contents, and being able to tolerate emotions in this way is necessary for developing empathy.

- Empathy is a particular kind of attention. As far as neurobiologists now understand it, empathy works through the action of mirror neurons. For example, when we watch a scary movie, we're not involved in the action, yet our bodies react very much as though we are in the midst of it.

- The way in which we sense what another might be experiencing is actually by sensing events in our own body. And the greater our inner attunement and our tolerance of this, the greater our capacity is to be empathic.

- Sara Lazar researches changes in brain structure that happen with meditation practice. One of these is in the insula. There are parts of the insula that don't shrink with age. The insula is very much involved in proprioception, which means feeling inner sensations in the body.

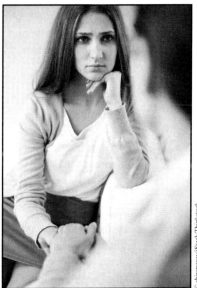

- When we can feel what's happening inside of us, we can understand others. It helps us develop what modern psychologist call theory of mind, which is simply the awareness that other people don't

Mindfulness practice cultivates empathy, which is a specific kind of attention.

live in your head—that they actually have different experiences from you. But you can get a resonating feeling about their experience by tuning into some of your own. This is critical for relationships generally.

- Acceptance is also critical for empathy. Mindfulness practice helps cultivate acceptance by simply seeing the judgments about ourselves and others like other thoughts—like itches or aches simply coming and going. And this helps us to see ourselves and others more clearly. When we can accept our own imperfections, difficulties, joy, and sorrows, we become more accepting of others, and they feel our trust and acceptance.

Open-Mindedness

- Mindfulness practice also helps us to stay open-minded. There is a Greek myth about Procrustes, who was the son of Poseidon. Procrustes lived in a fortress that was along a major thoroughfare in ancient Greece, and every once in awhile when a passerby would come, he would invite him or her in to spend the night. And if it was evening, and the passenger was tired, he or she often took him up on his offer.

- What the travelers didn't realize was that Procrustes had a bed of a fixed length, and in the middle of the night, if Procrustes felt that the traveler was too long for the bed, he'd make an adjustment. He'd come in and cut off the feet. If he felt that the passenger was too short, he'd come in and stretch him or her out. This became known, metaphorically, as the Procrustean bed.

- This myth propagated, and we still know it today, because it has a certain resonance with a very basic psychological experience. This is what Jean Piaget, the pioneering cognitive scientist, called assimilation and accommodation. He pointed out that when young children are developing, they develop what he called schemas for the world. These are understandings of how the world works. It can be basic, such as one thing is a chair while another is a bed, or it can be more complicated, such as a good person is like this while a bad person is like that.

- As we develop, we do one of two things: As we get new information or data, we either assimilate it into our existing schemas, or we accommodate, changing those schemas to account for the new information. As we get older, we become better and better at assimilation and not as good with accommodation.

- That attitude doesn't work very well in relationships, because in relationships, if we think we know what the other person is thinking or feeling, that can cause trouble. We do much better if we have a kind of radical uncertainty. And mindfulness helps us to have this uncertainty because we see all of our thoughts as simply coming and going. We don't trust them as much.

Acceptance

- Early in the history of mindfulness practices, when they came to the West and were being taught in meditation centers, there was a lot of emphasis on concentration and open monitoring. Now, the skill of acceptance is gaining a lot more attention. This is critical for relationships. One way to develop the skill of acceptance is to do acceptance practices. And one of those is called loving-kindness practice.

- In Buddhist traditions, loving-kindness practices are designed to cultivate an open, quivering heart. And the image they often use is of a mother with a child. Whether the experience is joyous or painful, they say, it's as a mother would feel toward her child leaving home to marry or pursue a profession, or as a mother would respond to her sick or injured child. This is the attitude of heart that we're trying to cultivate.

- But, of course, the mind can be a little ornery, and sometimes when we try to cultivate one thing, other things come up. In fact, ambivalence is pretty universal. So, what we want to do is realize that negative emotions may arise when we start to try to generate these loving-kindness feelings. Cynicism, anger, or sadism may come up—and we want to practice saying yes to all of these. The overarching goal of all these practices is to develop awareness of present experience with acceptance.

• Recently, there has been a lot of interesting research on the effects of loving-kindness practices. It turns out that they build positive emotions and resources for people. They increase feelings of social connectedness. They actually change the brain in ways that correlate with developing more empathy and generosity. And it shifts us away from fault finding in ourselves and others. In one study, it even reduced back pain.

• For people who have experience in prayer traditions, loving-kindness practice can feel familiar because both prayer and loving-kindness practice generate similar feelings. The effects in the theistic rather than nontheistic context haven't yet been studied, but this is a very interesting area for future dialogue and research. In the mindfulness tradition, we're not necessarily asking for any external being or entity to do something; instead, we're simply trying to cultivate the feeling in our own heart.

Suggested Reading

Kramer, *Insight Dialogue.*

Lucas, *Rewire Your Brain for Love.*

Siegel, *The Mindfulness Solution*, chapter 8.

Surrey and Kramer, "Relational Mindfulness."

Questions to Consider

1. In what ways have you found that believing in your thoughts or perspectives can get in the way of connecting closely with others?

2. What is empathy, and what is the mechanism that enables us human beings to feel empathy for one another?

loving-kindness practice: A brief version of this foundational practice for cultivating acceptance, both toward the contents of our own minds and toward other people.

yes and no: A simple, brief exercise that can help us see more clearly our tendency to resist contents of the mind and shift to a more accepting attitude.

Attention and Empathy in Relationships
Lecture 6—Transcript

I'd like to share with you another story from early in my career as a clinical psychologist. This actually happened during my internship year. I was training at a facility that was then called Cambridge City Hospital. And it was a very good facility, but it was relatively poor. There were other Harvard teaching hospitals, like the Massachusetts General Hospital that had a lot of money from pharmaceutical contracts, and there was us treating the chronically mentally ill.

In the facility in which I worked was the old nurses' residence from the days when nurses lived on the hospital campus. And it had been built around 1900 and had high ceilings and very big open windows, but had fallen into disrepair. In fact, they were going to do a renovation, so I think maintenance had drifted to an even lower edge. And the scene was this room with high ceilings, peeling paint, a big black window because it was the evening time, and this is where I was working with a severely depressed young woman.

And she would come in and she would tell me, basically, that her life was hopeless. I had many tools that I had learned from graduate school and I was trying them all. I was thinking, well, this is anger turned against the self. She's had so many frustrations, hasn't been able to express herself—I'll try to help her express herself and that will help. No, this is actually learned helplessness. She's had so many experiences of frustration that what I need to do is help her to have some success in her life, and then she'll be able to come out of it.

Try as I would, nothing seemed to work. The harder I tried, the more she would convince me that her situation was hopeless. I remember leaving sessions and walking to my car and thinking, I was a good student. I could have gone into so many fields. This is clearly not my calling. But luckily, I had good supervision. And we started observing a pattern. Sometimes, after one of the particularly dismal sessions in which I left feeling quite despairing, she'd come back the next week and say, "Last week that was a little bit helpful."

I remember thinking, to you, maybe. I was ready to drive off a bridge, it was so depressing, frankly. And then, we started seeing a pattern that when we had these sessions that were particularly difficult, those were the next weeks in which she was feeling a little bit better. And what seemed to be happening was, if she could actually have me join her in her pain and actually feel the despair the she felt, that helped. That made her feel a little bit less alone, a little bit more understood, and a little bit hopeful.

Now even when relating to people who aren't particularly distressed, our capacity to be present and feel what they're feeling is very important for the relationship to go well. And the more intimate the relationship, the more this matters. Mindfulness practices can help us to be more fully present in precisely this way.

Mindfulness is a kind of training in being present. A friend of mine was talking to a hospice director and asking about people's reflections on their lives—and particularly if they have regrets. And the hospice director said that the number one regret that he hears isn't that people hadn't accomplished more or didn't have more exotic or stimulating experiences, but they regretted having not been more present for the everyday events of their lives.

Our normal state, especially in an era of smartphones, computers, and constant connectivity, is a kind of partial attention. We multitask. It distracts us from uncomfortable feelings. It makes us feel we can achieve more. But it leaves us more disconnected. Of course, we do have moments of full attention. Sometimes it could be simple things like threading a needle, or slicing a tomato, or walking on ice, or even watching a sunset, or perhaps empathizing with a grieving friend.

Sometimes danger can help. When we reach to get a tomato from a bin, we might do it with partial attention. When we slice it—more full attention. I mentioned earlier the Zen answer to sleepiness. Try meditating at the edge of a very deep well or a high cliff. Danger can highlight our level of attention. But often, just the intention to pay attention works, like listening to a symphony and having the intention to bring our full attention to it. Or deciding to turn our full attention to our friend or a loved one.

Concentration practices help to increase attention simply by repeatedly practicing paying attention to an object, and every time that the mind wanders, bring it back home to the object. Insignificant events can become vivid or rich. And we see this in our informal practice—brushing our teeth, showering, driving—if we bring full attention to these, they become very rich, very rewarding, and very full experiences in themselves, not obstacles or difficulties on the way to going to other things.

I had the opportunity to have the Dalai Lama join us at a conference at Harvard Medical School. And Jon Kabat-Zinn, who I mentioned before, who has done a lot to bring mindfulness practices into medicine, was talking with me about him. And Jon pointed out that when you're talking to the Dalai Lama, he feels fully present. It just doesn't feel like he's scanning the room, looking for the next networking opportunity.

And I had an opportunity to see him at another occasion when we were actually inviting him to come to this conference where we were seeing him as he was leaving a program at Emory University. And he travels with a security entourage. And first, he interacted with my colleague and I, discussing the meeting that was coming up at Harvard. And then, we went into another room where there was a group of undergraduate students, part of the club which was Students for a Free Tibet.

And these kids had been earnestly working to try to promote cultural autonomy in Tibet. And there was nobody there except my colleague and I, the security detail, and the Dalai Lama. And he took the time to go from student to student to student, giving them all his blessing, and talking to them about how important their work was because India placed on one side and China on the other side makes Tibet a natural bridge between these two great world powers. And it was just so moving to see him give full attention to these students. Now, the Dalai Lama says that it takes him about four hours a day of meditation practice to have this form of attention. But even if we do less than that, we can develop some of this ourselves.

Now, a very different famous person can also give us insight into how to be present. And this is Sigmund Freud. Even though many of his ideas came out of his cultural milieu and they don't stand up well to modern critiques—

and some of them people even find offensive—he did have a very useful suggestion for psychoanalysts that's relevant to our relationships generally. He suggested that a psychoanalyst should practice what he called "evenly hovering attention." And he defined that back in 1912 as "to listen and not to trouble to keep in mind anything in particular." Freud prescribed a kind of openness to whatever is happening in the other person, and that openness can go a long way toward enhancing relationships.

But Freud never explained how to develop this attitude. He didn't actually have a technology for it. Mindfulness practice helps us to cultivate this by practicing presence independent of content. Now, most of the time, we're interested in the content—Oh, what does that mean? Oh, what's that?—and labeling it and thinking about it. Mindfulness, instead, helps us to simply do open monitoring, to be present to whatever arises. And this develops what we can think of as a rare gift of wholehearted attention. Usually, in order to pay more attention, we turn up the volume in some way. We go for a much more interesting or more entertaining stimulus. With mindfulness practice, we can turn up our attention instead.

I remember during my first meditation retreat I was at the Insight Meditation Society up in Barre, Massachusetts. And it's a lovely facility. It's an old monastery. And there's a stone wall that must be 100 years old in front. And after several days of developing concentration and doing open monitoring and doing eating meditation and walking meditation and the like, I was sitting on the stone wall, feeling pretty focused, and an ant showed up. And I found the ant fascinating. It was going with its six legs and its antennae. And I just had this profound sense of the magic of it. That how, with this tiny little brain, it could coordinate all of these different activities at the same time. And it felt like fully fulfilling as the afternoon's entertainment. Now, if once we turn up our attention, an ant can be this fully engrossing, another human being that we're relating to can be quite interesting as well.

In addition to helping by helping us to simply be present, mindfulness practice also helps us to stay with discomfort. Remember the Zen master and sadistic general in the last lecture? Sitting with discomfort—being able to be run through with a sword without blinking an eye—strengthens this kind of mental muscle. And one way it gets strong is simply by being with the itch or the ache or whatever happens in our life and just feeling it and not moving.

The other way it helps is by seeing emotional events as impersonal uprisings or impersonal phenomena. And this helps us to develop affect tolerance, the ability to really be with feelings. Let me explain what I mean by this. Let's use a commonplace example. I have a friend and I think I've been generous to him. He does something that was pretty self-centered and I'm angry. In a normal state of mind, I would be going, I can't believe he did that to me after all I've done for him. What a jerk. It's not fair. He should apologize, et cetera, et cetera, et cetera.

And every time I had that thought, every time it goes through my mind, and it would probably pass through my mind repeatedly about how unfair his behavior was, I would have another wave of anger. If, on the other hand, I was doing mindfulness practice and being with this, I would simply notice—and I'm going to use words, but these are sensations, not narrated experiences—I would notice the tensing of these muscles, perhaps tightness in the chest, perhaps my respiration picking up, perhaps, if it was really bad, images of decapitating my former friend dancing through the mind.

But these would all be seen as impersonal events arising in the mind and body. And when they're experienced as impersonal events this way, they don't grab us in just the same way. We start to notice that the wave comes, the wave goes; the tension appears, the tension leaves. And it's not just anger—it could be fear, it could be joy, it could be sadness, it could even be lust. When we start to notice these as all simply neurobiological events rather than my precious feelings, they are transformed, and we're able to tolerate them at much higher levels.

When it's not personal, we have greater affect tolerance, the ability to feel this in greater intensity, greater pain tolerance. We even have the capacity to be with things like boredom, to be with aggression, to be with restlessness. And all of these things facilitate connecting with others. Because so often when relationships go poorly, what's happening is, where the other person is doing something, we find that uncomfortable and we feel a need to stop it.

Now, another thing that we see—and we see this very much in psychotherapy—is that other people can only really be close with us if we can tolerate both our feeling and their feeling simultaneously. Remember, the example that I said at the beginning of this lecture. It was only when I was able to be with her pain that we were able to connect. And she was able to get some relief from being together.

In the Buddhist tradition, one of the ways that we learn to tolerate these feelings is by noticing not only their impersonality, not just building up the muscle of tolerating discomfort, but also noticing that everything changes. We've talked about that before. But here, it becomes an asset, not just a problem. You ever wonder how long an emotion stays in the mind if not reinforced by a thought? Cognitive scientists say it lasts about 90 seconds.

Now, I don't know that you, but most of my emotions, particularly the difficult ones, last a lot longer than 90 seconds. And that's because they're constantly being reinforced by believing in the thought stream about them. There's a metaphor in the Zen tradition that I like a lot about this. They say, if you were to have a glass of water and to pour a teaspoon of salt in it and were to drink that water, it would be difficult. It would be unpalatably salty. But if you took that same teaspoon of salt and you dissolved it into a clear clean pond—no problem. You could drink of that easily. These practices help us to turn the mind into that kind of pond. And you see it in the Zen tradition. There are metaphors for that of being a still pond, of being a vast sky. They allow the mind to be able to accept all of the different elements and perturbations that arise and pass without getting caught in them and without getting stuck in a narrative about them.

So, evenly hovering attention is actually undefended, unconflicted, tolerant, and open attention. And we see in mindfulness practice that much of the time, we're actually defending against unpleasant experiences. We're trying to hold on to the good ones and push away the bad ones. Rather, what we're trying to develop here in our relationships is a kind of radical acceptance of all contents.

And being able to tolerate emotions in this way is necessary for developing empathy. Now, empathy is a particular kind of attention. You may recall,

I mentioned Carl Rogers at the beginning of the course. And he was a psychologist who did a great deal to help train other mental health professionals into how to establish a kind empathic resonance with our patients. And what he said about empathy is this: Empathy is "to sense the [other's] private world as if it where your own, but without losing the 'as if' quality."

Now, how does empathy work? Empathy works, as far as our neurobiologists now understand it, through the action of mirror neurons. Now, mirror neurons were first discovered in other primates. And what they would do is they would wire up the brains of primates and they would have those primates observe other members of their same species doing something. And they found that the very same brain areas that would have been activated if the primate him or herself we're doing this activity were activated by watching the other person do it.

And there are many examples of this that we can see as humans. For example, if you were to watch me drinking a glass of water or watch somebody else doing this and really attune to what's happening inside, you could probably sense a little bit of the experience of drinking happening yourself. An even more obvious example of this happens whenever we watch a scary or sexually explicit movie. In those circumstances, we're not involved in the action and yet our bodies react very much as though we were in the midst of it. So the way in which we sense what another might be experiencing is actually by sensing events in our own body. We sense in here what they might be feeling out there. And the greater our inner attunement and our tolerance of this, the greater our capacity to be empathic.

I mentioned earlier Sara Lazar's work on changes in brain structure that happened with meditation practice. Well, one of those is in the insula. There're parts of the insula that don't shrink with age. And the insula is very much involved in proprioception, which means feeling these inner sensations in the body. So when we can feel what's happening inside of us, we can understand others. It helps us to develop what modern psychologists now call *theory of mind*. And theory of mind is simply the awareness that other people don't live in my head, that they actually have different experiences.

But I can get a resonating feeling about their experience by tuning into some of my own. And this is critical for relationships, generally.

Acceptance is also critical for empathy. And how does mindfulness practice help cultivate acceptance? By simply seeing the judgments about ourselves and others like other thoughts, like itches or aches—simply coming and going. And this helps us to see ourselves and others more clearly. And when we can accept our own imperfections, our own difficulties, our own joys, our own sorrows, we become more accepting of others, and they feel our trust and acceptance.

One of my patients once put it like this to me. She said, " 'Love thy neighbor as thyself' is not just a commandment; it's actually a law of nature. That, if I can accept whatever is happening in myself, then I can love my neighbor. And I can't if I can't accept what's happening in myself because I'm going to reject the things that are brought up in me that I have difficulty with. And if I can fully accept the other, then I can fully accept myself."

Now, mindfulness practice also helps us to stay open-minded. And this is critical. There is a Greek myth about Procrustes. Now, Procrustes was a son of Poseidon, and he lived in a fortress that was along a major thoroughfare in ancient Greece. And every once in awhile when a passerby would come, he would invite them in to spend the night. And if it was evening, and they were tired, they often took him up on his offer. What the travelers didn't realize was that Procrustes had a bed, and the bed was of a fixed length. And in the middle of the night, if Procrustes felt that the traveler was too long for the bed, he'd make an adjustment. He'd come in and cut off the feet. If he felt he was too short, he'd come in and stretch them out. He also had a rack. And this became known, metaphorically, as the Procrustean bed.

Now, why did this myth propagate? And why do we still know it today? Well, it's because it has a certain resonance with a very basic psychological experience. This is what Jean Piaget, the pioneering cognitive scientist, called *assimilation* and *accommodation*. He pointed out that when young children are developing, they develop what he called *schemas* for the world. These are understandings of how it all works. It can be basic like that's a chair, and that's a bed, or this is what a good person is like, this is what a bad person is like.

And as we develop, we do one of two things: As we get new information or new data, we either assimilate it into our existing schemas, or we accommodate—we change those schemas to account for the new information. As we get older, we get better and better at assimilation and not so good with accommodation. We tend to see new things as, oh, yeah, that's just old wine in new bottles. I know all about that.

Now, that attitude doesn't actually work so well in relationships. Because in relationships, if we think we know what the other person's thinking, we know what they're feeling, we know where we're coming from—I'm sure you've had this experience—that can cause trouble. We do much better if we have a kind of radical uncertainty. And mindfulness helps us to have this uncertainty because we see all of our thoughts as simply coming and going. We don't trust them as much.

It's a little bit like jumping out of an airplane without a parachute. It's terrifying until you realize that there's no ground. All that's going to happen is the next experience, the next experience, and more uncertainty. This is famously expressed in a statement by Suzuki Roshi, the Zen master. He said, "In the beginner's mind, there are many possibilities. In the expert's mind, there are few." Now, of course, there are some beginners that don't really have beginner's mind, but we're trying to cultivate this kind of openness.

I often do an exercise with psychotherapists. And I ask them to reflect on what keeps them from being optimally present in relationships. And you might ask yourself this. What makes it hard for you to be open, present, to feel the other person's feeling, to have evenly hovering attention, to have beginner's mind? For each of us, it's different.

For one of us, it's, "Well, the person's talking about something that's upsetting to me and I don't like the upset feelings." For another one, it's, "It makes me anxious to feel so close." For yet somebody else, it might be, "Well, I disagree with them. And it's hard for me to have that disagreement." It's very useful to reflect on this, mindfully.

Now, early in the history of mindfulness practices, when they came to the West, and they were being taught in meditation centers, there was a lot of emphasis on concentration and open monitoring. Now, the third skill, the skill of acceptance, is gaining a lot more attention—and this is critical for relationships. Now one way to develop the skill of acceptance is to do acceptance practices. And one of those is called "loving-kindness practice." Let's try that together.

This is a loving-kindness practice, also called *mettā* meditation in the Pali. Because it involves visualization, it's usually easiest to do this with the eyes closed. Allow the eyes to close and just follow the breath through a breath or two to settle into the present moment. Then bring to mind somebody who is naturally loving and kind. This could be somebody you know in real life, like a friend or a loved one or a mentor. It could be more of a religious figure, like Mohammed, or Jesus, the Buddha, or Moses. It could be a spiritual teacher like the Dalai Lama, or Mother Teresa, or Martin Luther King—just somebody who naturally brings a sense of loving kindness to you when you think of them. It could even be an animal or a place in nature. Just envision this being and begin sending good wishes in your heart to this being.

There are traditional phrases that are often used for this. One set goes like this: May you be happy. May you be peaceful. May you be free from suffering. People often find that if they take their hands and take one hand and put it over their heart, and the other hand over that first hand, and apply a kind of gentle and loving pressure, it helps to evoke the feeling of loving kindness.

So try that for a moment. Envision this loving being and just to yourself say the words—May you be happy. May you be peaceful. May you be free from suffering. See if you can generate a little bit of the feeling by repeating the phrases. May you be happy. May you be peaceful. May you be free from suffering. May you be happy. May you be peaceful. May you be free from suffering.

Once you feel a little bit of that warm energy headed toward this loving being, imagine now that the being is with you and is wishing the same for you. Join them by turning the phrases toward yourself, again with the hands over the heart. May I be happy. May I be peaceful. May I be free from suffering. May I be happy. May I be peaceful. May I be free from suffering.

See if you can feel in your heart a little bit of that loving kindness toward yourself. May I be happy. May I be peaceful. May I be free from suffering.

Once you feel it toward yourself, pick somebody you care about, a friend, or a loved one, maybe somebody in need. Hold them in your heart and in your mind, conjure an image of them, and try sending the same loving kindness wishes to him or her. May you be happy. May you be peaceful. May you be free from suffering. May you be happy. May you be peaceful. May you be free from suffering.

Were we to practice this for a longer time, we could expand this out and send the same wishes to all sorts of other people and beings. To bring this to a close and bring our attention back to the present moment, I'm going to ring the bell. Listen to the bell from the beginning of the ring until it trails off into space and you can no longer hear it.

Now, I invite you to also take the time to do loving-kindness practice in a more focused and longer-term way. We've given an audio recording that you can follow, included in the course, and it expands out from what we've done in this brief exercise to be practicing loving kindness toward a broader community, toward the whole city, toward the country, toward the world, and ultimately all beings. And we'll also experiment in that longer recording with alternate phrases—May I be safe. May I be healthy. May I live with ease—or just using the beginnings of the words. And then, we'll practice using it even toward difficult people. And that becomes really interesting to try to generate a sense of loving kindness toward those who are difficult in our lives. It can be a very fruitful practice.

Now, in Buddhist traditions, these loving-kindness practices are designed to cultivate an open, quivering heart. And the image they often use is of a mother with a child. And whether the experience is joyous or painful, they say it's as a mother would feel toward her child leaving home to marry or pursue a profession, or as a mother would respond to her sick or injured child. This is the attitude of heart that we're trying to cultivate here. But of course, the mind can be a little ornery. And sometimes when we try to cultivate one thing, other things come up. In fact, ambivalence is pretty universal. I'm sure you've noticed this if you were ever in a pursue-ordistance relationship at some point in your life—where as soon as the other person who had been kind of disinterested was interested in you, suddenly they became less interesting. That kind of thing happens a lot. So what we want to do is realize that negative emotions may arise when we start to try to generate these loving-kindness feelings. Cynicism may come up. Anger may come up. Sadism may come up. And we want to practice saying yes to all of these. There's no need to become a saint here. The overarching goal of all these practices is to develop awareness of present experience with acceptance.

There's another little exercise that you can try—and it only lasts for a couple of minutes—that involves saying yes or no to experience and seeing how that affects the body.

For this exercise, begin by just settling into the body, taking a few breaths, and feeling whatever is happening in this moment. Feel all the sensations that are occurring here and now. Now try in your heart and your mind saying no to the sensations, as though you don't want these sensations to continue. See what that feels like, to try to stop the sensations. Just say no. Notice just what that feels like.

Then reverse it. Now say yes to the sensations, as though you're allowing everything to be just as it is. See how that feels in the body, to be welcoming and allowing to whatever you might be sensing or feeling. Notice the difference?

There's been a lot of interesting recent research on the effects of loving-kindness practices. It turns out that they build positive emotions and resources for people. They increase feelings of social connectedness—not a surprise there. They actually change the brain in ways that correlate with developing more empathy and generosity. And it shifts us away from fault-finding in ourselves and others. In one study, it even reduced back pain.

Now for people who have experience in prayer traditions, loving-kindness practice can feel familiar because both prayer and loving-kindness practice generate similar feelings. The effects in a theistic rather than a non-theistic context haven't yet been studied—and I actually think that that's a very interesting area for future dialogue and research, and I've been talking with theologians about this a bit.

In the mindfulness tradition, we're not necessarily asking for any external being or entity to do something. Instead, we're simply trying to cultivate the feeling in our own heart.

In the next lecture, we're going to look at a particular kind of empathy: empathy for suffering. And when it includes a wish to help, we call that *compassion*. And we'll see how mindfulness practices can help us to develop compassion both for others and for ourselves. Thanks.

The Science of Compassion and Self-Compassion
Lecture 7

E mpathy is very important for cultivating rich, meaningful relationships. But there's a particular type of empathy that researchers and clinicians are discovering is essential for any path to happiness: empathy for suffering—our own or the suffering of others—that includes a wish to help. We usually call this particular form of empathy compassion. Compassion, which leads to greater well-being, can be compassion toward ourselves when we're suffering or compassion toward others when they're suffering. Research shows that mindfulness practices generally, as well as focused compassion practices, can help us develop this ability.

The Evolution of Compassion
- To understand how compassion works, and what gets in its way, it's helpful to look at our neurobiology and its roots in our evolutionary heritage. We have three broad motivational systems that are all very useful for our survival and that interact with each other in different ways.

- The first system is our fight-or-flight system, which is focused on threats and is designed for protection and seeking safety. This system can be either activating or inhibiting depending on the circumstance. It can activate us to fight or flee, or it can inhibit us and make us freeze. The feelings that are activated by fight or flight involve feelings of anger, anxiety, and even sometimes disgust.

- The second system is our achievement/goal-seeking system, which involves our sense of drive, excitement, and even vitality. We see this activated when we're seeking pleasure—when we're achieving something. It's a very activating system, and the feelings that are associated with it are feelings of interest and excitement.

- The third system, which is particularly active in mammals, is the tend-and-befriend system. This is a system that has to do with feelings of contentment, safety, and connection. It's an affiliative system. It's a system that gives us feelings of soothing and creates feelings of well-being.

- All three systems are shared by all mammals, and each system helps with a certain aspect of survival. In addition, we're discovering that each system involves particular neurotransmitters and brain structures.

- The fight-or-flight system involves the activation and production of adrenaline, also called epinephrine, and noradrenaline, also called norepinephrine. This starts with activation in the amygdala, which is the almond-shaped part of the brain that's involved in figuring out whether a situation is dangerous or not.

- The second system, the drive system, involves dopamine. It also involves activation of the nucleus accumbens, which is the same brain area that is activated by crack cocaine, winning prizes, and achievement of all sorts.

- The tend-and-befriend system involves the neurotransmitter oxytocin. This is generated largely in the pituitary, which has fibers going into other parts of the brain. It's the tend-and-befriend system that allows for compassion. The problem is that the tend-and-befriend system is very easily overridden by the threat system and, to a lesser degree, by the drive system.

- When we're frightened for our own survival, we tend to tune out the needs of others. When we're drawn toward some goal or ambition, the same can happen. But when these other systems are quiet, then the tend-and-befriend system tends to flourish.

- Of course, sometimes the tend-and-befriend system prevails even when the other two systems are active. We're always very impressed when people put compassionate action above what seems to be their immediate needs. This can happen among soldiers in war, in strong love relationships, or even in parenting.

- Sometimes, of course, when people are acting heroically, it may be that they're being activated by their fear-based system. But sometimes it really is our compassion being able to overcome these other urges. Certain hormonal states can also make this happen.

Developing Compassion and Self-Compassion
- The word "compassion" comes from Latin and Greek to mean "to suffer with." Compassion means to suffer with another, and it includes a spontaneous wish to alleviate that suffering.

- In developing compassion, we can start with developing compassion for ourselves. This is one form of the broad scale of acceptance, and it is a very rapidly growing area of interest in research in psychology, neuroscience, and psychotherapy. Of particular interest is the analysis of how self-compassion affects our well-being.

- Self-compassion is quite different from self-esteem. Self-esteem is subject to narcissistic recalibration, which means that we normally compare ourselves to others who are sort of at our level and then think that we want to be at another level. But research shows profoundly positive benefits of self-compassion that aren't subject to these limitations.

- Kristin Neff and Christopher Germer are leading the charge in terms of teaching self-compassion and learning about its effects. They've identified that when things go wrong—when we suffer, fail, or feel inadequate—we experience a kind of unholy trinity of three things: self-criticism, which is often experienced as shame about failing in some way; self-isolation, which is often pulling back from others because we don't feel fit to be among others; and self-absorption, which often involves the production of narratives about how bad you are and that you can't believe you made that mistake.

- We can think of these three components as the activation of our threat response system. The self-criticism is our fight response and anger that we turn against ourselves. The self-isolation is our flight response—we want to pull back. And the self-absorption is our freeze response, just being stuck in a kind of paralysis.

- When we get into that unholy trinity, it adds insult to injury. Then, not only do we feel bad or have a painful feeling, but we also start to think that we are bad, and our sense of self starts to plummet. And there are many different negative narratives we develop about ourselves, including that we're alone or helpless.

- The antidote to this unholy trinity is developing self-compassion. When we feel self-criticism, we consciously cultivate self-kindness. When we feel self-isolation, we consciously cultivate common humanity, the awareness that we all have these experiences of loss and failure. And when we're self-absorbed, we can turn to mindfulness practice to bring our attention in to moment-to-moment experience and out of the persistent narrative about "me" and "mine."

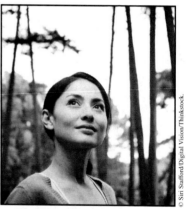
© Siri Stafford/Digital Vision/Thinkstock.

Self-compassion involves giving ourselves kindness and understanding.

- In laboratory research, psychologists have found that self-compassion is quite different from self-esteem and is completely unrelated to narcissism. In addition, research shows that self-compassion is positively associated with virtually every desirable outcome in terms of psychological well-being, including feeling good emotionally and having fewer physical ailments.

- Self-compassion is one of the acceptance skills, and we might also think of it as an equanimity skill. And it's interesting how it differs from other aspects of mindfulness skills. In open monitoring, if we're dealing with pain, we would take an attitude of feeling the pain with spacious awareness so that it can change. In self-compassion, the attitude is to be kind to yourself in the midst of the pain and that, too, will allow it to change.

- The central, albeit subtle, aspect of self-compassion practice is that we give ourselves kindness and understanding—not to feel better, nor to make the pain go away, but simply because we're in pain. This retains the overall framework of mindfulness of awareness of present experience with acceptance. We're not trying to get rid of the feeling, but we are trying to provide a sense of holding and comfort in the midst of it.

- Kristin Neff and Christopher Germer have developed a mindfulness self-compassion program that is eight weeks long and teaches various skills. By studying the effects of the program, they've identified five paths to self-compassion: physical, mental, emotional, relational, and spiritual.

Practices That Develop Compassion
- Mindfulness by itself tends to develop compassion. Compassion for ourselves tends to arise when we simply are open to our own suffering, and compassion toward others arises as we see that everybody else also suffers. Then, compassion arises naturally as we see our interconnectedness—as we step out of selfing and see the interconnectedness of all things.

- In Buddhist traditions, compassion and wisdom are seen as two wings of a bird or two wheels of a cart: One without the other doesn't work very well. If in trying to help a friend we have compassion without wisdom, we might lose the equanimity. We might be so identified with the sufferer, so desperate to try to fix the problem, that we can't provide a kind of holding. So, both are needed for compassionate action.

- Mindfulness practice can be used to develop wisdom, but other practices can be used specifically to develop compassion. Because it's difficult to open fully to the suffering of others, we usually use a stepwise approach. First, we develop concentration to steady the mind and allow it to be able to be with what happens. Then, we do loving-kindness practices and meta practices. These involve wishing ourselves and others well, but not necessarily with the attention to suffering or trying to do anything about the suffering. These can be a very good start to compassion practice.

- There are also some practices from Buddhist traditions that are designed specifically to develop compassion for others. One of these is called *tonglen*, which means "giving and taking," and it comes out of the Tibetan tradition. This practice is attributed to a Buddhist teacher named Atisa who lived in India in the 11th century. In the traditional practice, we inhale the pain and suffering of others and exhale kindness, warmth, and goodwill. This reverses our instinctual tendency to battle against emotional discomfort.

- In all of these practices, equanimity is important. This is the wisdom component, and it is about keeping perspective even as we're in the midst of "being with" someone else's suffering. To develop equanimity, you can simply try one of the following phrases: "Everyone is on his or her own life journey" or "I'm not the cause of others' suffering, nor is it entirely within my power to alleviate it."

Suggested Reading

Germer, *The Mindful Path to Self-Compassion.*

Gilbert, *The Compassionate Mind.*

Neff, *Self-Compassion.*

———, "The Science of Self-Compassion."

1. What are the three dominant human motivational systems, and how do they interact with one another? What are the implications of this for developing compassion?

2. What is self-compassion, and how does it differ from self-esteem?

equanimity phrases: Simple reminders that can help us to "be with" another person who is in pain, even if we can't make that pain go away.

giving and taking (*tonglen*): A compassion practice that can help us connect with a person or an animal that is suffering.

self-compassion letter: An effective exercise for generating self-compassion, particularly when we're feeling shame about something we've done or a perceived shortcoming.

soften, soothe, allow: A self-compassion exercise designed to help us find a loving relationship toward mental or physical pain that we find ourselves tending to resist.

The Science of Compassion and Self-Compassion
Lecture 7—Transcript

Empathy is vital for cultivating and maintaining rich and meaningful relationships. But there's a particular kind of empathy that researchers and clinicians are discovering is essential for any path to well-being. This is empathy for suffering—our own and the suffering of others—that includes a wish to help. We usually call this particular form of empathy *compassion*.

A lot of recent research is supporting the teachings of ancient wisdom traditions about compassion. It's confirming an idea that the Dalai Lama repeatedly emphasizes. He says, "If you want others to be happy, practice compassion. If you want to be happy, practice compassion."

This compassion, which leads to greater well-being, can be compassion toward ourselves when we're suffering or compassion toward others when they're suffering. As we'll see, research shows that mindfulness practices generally, as well as focused compassion practices, can help us to develop this ability.

To understand how compassion works and what gets in its way, it's helpful to look at our neurobiology and its roots in our evolutionary heritage. We basically have three broad motivational systems that were all very useful for our survival and that interact with each other in different ways.

The first system is our fight or flight system. And this is focused on threats and is designed for protection and seeking safety. This system can be either activating or inhibiting depending on the circumstance. It can activate us to fight or flee, or it can inhibit us and make us freeze. And the feelings we experience when we're in fight or flight, or activated by fight or flight, involve feelings of anger, anxiety, and even sometimes disgust.

The second system is our achievement and goal-seeking system. And this involves our sense of drive, excitement, even vitality. We see this activated when we're seeking pleasure, when we're achieving something. It's a very activating system. And the feelings that are associated with it are feelings of interest and excitement.

The third system, which is particularly active in mammals, is what's called our *tend-and-befriend system*. And this is a system that has to do with feelings of contentment, safety, and connection. It's an affiliative system. It's a system that gives us feelings of soothing and creates feelings of well-being.

Now all three systems are shared by all mammals, and each system helps with a certain aspect of survival. And we're discovering that each system involves particular neurotransmitters and particular brain structures.

The first, the threat system, the fight or flight system, involves the activation and the production of adrenaline, also called epinephrine, and noradrenaline, also called norepinephrine. And this starts with activation in the amygdala, which is, as we've mentioned before, that almond-shaped part of the brain that's involved in figuring out is a situation dangerous or is a situation not dangerous.

The second system, the drive system, involves dopamine. And it involves activation of the nucleus accumbens. Now in 1953, James Olds and Peter Milner implanted electrodes in the nucleus accumbens of rats. And they found that a rat would choose to press a lever which stimulated this. In fact, the rat preferred this even to stopping to eat or drink. It would press the lever until it died. Now this area is the same brain area that's activated by crack cocaine, winning prizes, achievement of all sorts.

The third system, the tend-and-befriend system, involves the neurotransmitter oxytocin. And this is generated largely in the pituitary, which has fibers going into other parts of the brain. And it's this last system, the tend-and-befriend system, that allows for compassion. The problem is the tend-and-befriend system is very easily overridden by the threat system, in particular, and to a lesser degree, by the drive system.

When we're frightened for our own survival, we tend to tune out the needs of others. We see this all the time in political advertisements. Which political ads are more effective? Those who say, "Beware of that awful candidate who's going to do terrible things to you and your loved ones"? Or the ones who say, "Vote for this person, they care about others"? Fear trumps compassion almost all the time.

When we're drawn toward some goal, some ambition, the same can happen. We all know of circumstances where our wish to accomplish something kind of got in the way of paying attention to the feelings of others. But when these other systems are quiet, then the tend-and-befriend system tends to flourish.

Though of course, sometimes the tend-and-befriend system prevails even when the other two systems are active. We're always very impressed when this happens, when people put compassionate action above what seems to be their immediate needs. Heroes putting their lives at risk for others do this. And this can happen among soldiers in war, in strong love relationships, or even in parenting.

Now sometimes, of course, when people are acting heroically, it may be that they're being activated by their fear-based system. For example, if I'm taking care of my kid who is in danger, it's simply I've drawn the line around who I am to be larger than me, but encompassing my child as well. So it's my fear that drives me into doing something. But sometimes it really is our compassion being able to overcome these other urges.

Certain hormonal states can also make this happen. There's a YouTube video that I recently saw. It's of a couple in Ireland who are on a farm. And they have some ducks and they also have a cat. And the duck, the mother duck, was sitting on the eggs waiting for them to hatch. And every day they'd go in to see whether they had gotten any ducklings yet. Well, one day they show up at the barn and they see the eggs but they're just the egg shells and no sign of ducklings. And the couple thinks—uh-oh, the cat. And they go, they start looking around to see what happened. And they're expecting to find a real tragedy. They go from barn to barn and then eventually, they come upon one barn and what they see is they see their cat and their cat is surrounded by kittens. The cat has just given birth. And mixed in with the kittens are the ducklings. And in fact, in the video you can see some of the ducklings are actually suckling at the cat.

So what happened in this circumstance was at the very moment that the cat encountered the ducklings she had a lot of oxytocin running through her body and that overcame her drive system which would probably have driven her to eat the ducklings. And instead, she took them in as her own. It's actually a very interesting story. She actually cared for them until—ducks apparently grow faster than kittens do—until the ducks became obviously too big for her to care for.

So what exactly is this compassion that the tend-and-befriend system allows us to experience? Well the word *compassion* comes from Latin and Greek. And in Latin, the first part of the word is *pati*, and that means "to suffer." And the second part—or the first part, I guess—is *com*, which is "with." So it's "to suffer with." And compassion means to suffer with another. And it includes a spontaneous wish to alleviate that suffering.

Now one of the ways that we can understand compassion with some nuance is to look at how compassion compares to some of its close relatives. We've already spoken about empathy. And empathy is feeling what another feels, but it's not necessarily feeling what another feels when they're suffering. We can feel empathy—joyous empathy—for somebody who's having a wonderful experience. And it doesn't necessarily include the wish to help, even if it's an empathic resonance to somebody else's suffering.

Sympathy is a little different. That's kind of curious. Sympathy is this kind of automatic reactive element to it, usually based on our own experiences of having been there before in some way. And it, too, may lack the wish to help.

Love is very close to compassion, but this word is very complicated for us because love brings up association to eroticism and sex, *eros* more broadly. And it may not include a sense of equanimity because when we feel love, there often is a sense of longing, or possession, or desperation that happens, which we don't usually associate with compassion.

Pity is interesting. Sometimes when we see the suffering of others, we feel pity. And pity involves a certain kind of distancing in a way. We're somehow superior. Pity is what happens when we think, oh well, those people had that medical problem because they smoked, or they didn't live well, or something like that—not like me.

And then finally, there's altruism. And altruism is really the behavioral part of compassion. And this is important: It's the way in which we have a wish to simply do something to alleviate the suffering of others.

Now in developing compassion, we can start close to home. We can start with developing compassion for ourselves. And this is one form of the broad scale of acceptance we've talked about. And this is a very rapidly growing area of interest in research in psychology, in neuroscience, and in psychotherapy. There are currently hundreds of peer-reviewed research articles, all that have come out in recent years, looking at self-compassion and how it affects our well-being.

Now self-compassion is quite different from self-esteem. We talked about the limitations of self-esteem before, that it's subject to narcissistic recalibration. Like the fellow who had established the $30 million business but then that wasn't enough, he needed more. And we see in our own narcissistic recalibrations that we normally compare ourselves to others who are sort of at our level and then think, I want to be at another level. For example, people in professional offices typically don't compare themselves to the maintenance people so much, but boy, can they get into comparative processes with people that are more or less at their same level. And there's the other problem of Lake Wobegone—we can't all be above average.

But as we'll see, research shows profoundly positive benefits of self-compassion that aren't subject to these limitations. I have a couple of good friends, Kristen Neff and Chris Germer who are leading the charge in terms of teaching self-compassion and learning about its effects. And what they've identified is that when things go wrong, when we suffer, or we fail, or we feel inadequate, we experience a kind of unholy trinity of three things. We experience self-criticism when things go wrong, and that's often experienced as shame about failing in some way. We experience self-isolation. We often pull back from others because we don't feel fit to be among others or it's too raw and too sensitive to be among others. And we experience self-absorption. We tend to get involved in narratives about how bad I am, I can't believe I made that mistake, and this kind of thing.

And we can think of these three components as self-criticism, self-isolation, and [self-]absorption as almost like the activation of our threat response system. The self-criticism is our fight response and anger that we turn against ourselves. The self-isolation is our flight response. We want to pull back. And the self-absorption is kind of our freeze response, just being stuck in a kind of paralysis.

What happens when we get into that unholy trinity is it adds insult to injury. Then, not only do we feel badly, not only do we have a painful feeling, but we start to think that we are bad, our sense of self, our sense of who we are starts to plummet.

And there are many different negative narratives we develop about ourselves. I'm defective or unlovable. I'm basically alone in the world. I'm helpless on my own. I'm fundamentally inadequate. I'll be abandoned. I'll be taken advantage of. I'll never get what I need. I'm a failure. The list is really endless.

So the antidote to this unholy trinity is developing self-compassion. When we feel self-criticism, we consciously cultivate self-kindness. When we feel self-isolation, we consciously cultivate common humanity, the awareness that we're all in this together and we all have these experiences of loss and failure. And when we're self-absorbed, we can turn to mindfulness practice to bring our attention into moment-to-moment experience and out of the persistent narrative about me and mine.

In laboratory research, psychologists have found that self-compassion is quite different from self-esteem and is completely unrelated to narcissism. In other words, it's not about feeling I'm better or worse than others, it's about figuring out how to take care of oneself during difficult times. And the research, it's almost getting boring because self-compassion is positively associated with virtually every desirable outcome in terms of psychological well-being. It's associated with feeling good emotionally, having low levels of anxiety and depression, having less shame and self-criticism, having fewer physical ailments. It's even associated with better immune system functioning; better heart rate variability—this is one measure of how quickly we can recover from stress whether our heart stays constantly jazzed up or whether it can adjust to the circumstances; more adaptive responses to academic value—this has been studied in schools a lot, and kids who are able to practice self-compassion don't get paralyzed by academic failure; lower rates of post-traumatic stress disorder in combat vets—combat vets who can be self-compassionate don't develop as much PTSD; and improved health behaviors including even eating more healthful foods.

Now as I mentioned, self-compassion is one of these third skills, it's one of these acceptance skills. And we might also think of it as an equanimity skill. It's interesting how it differs from other aspects of mindfulness skills. In open monitoring, if we're dealing with pain, we would take an attitude of "feel the pain with spacious awareness so it can change." What happens when we don't scratch the itch, don't make an adjustment for the ache, and simply stay with experience?

Self-compassion is a little different. It's "be kind to you yourself in the midst of the pain and that too will allow it to change." Open monitoring asks, what do you observe? What's happening in the moment? Self-compassion asks much more, what do you feel you need? What would allow for a sense of soothing and comfort at this moment?

So the central—and it's a little bit subtle—aspect of self-compassion practice is we give ourselves kindness and understanding not to feel better, not to make the pain go away, but simply because we're in pain—the way any good friend would, or like a parent does when they simply hold a child who is hurting. So this retains the overall framework of mindfulness of awareness of present experience with acceptance. We're not trying to get rid of the feeling, but we are trying to provide a sense of holding and comfort in the midst of it.

Kristen Neff and Chris Germer have developed a mindfulness self-compassion program and they've begun to study the effects. It's an eight-week program that teaches various skills. And they've identified five paths to self-compassion.

The first is physical: softening the body, not tensing up so much against pain. The second is mental: It's allowing thoughts to come and go—pretty much what we do in mindfulness practice. The third is emotional, which is a part of mindfulness practice but applied to emotions, which is simply befriending feelings, like, whatever comes up is going to be OK. The forth is relational, and this is instead of withdrawing into ourselves when we're hurting, finding a way to connect safely with others. And the fifth we could call "spiritual." It means commitment to something larger than ourselves. And we'll see, going forward, that this is important for well-being quite generally.

So let's try a little exercise that we can do together in which we can learn to soften, soothe, and allow.

This soften, soothe, and allow self-compassion practice was developed by my friend and colleague Chris Germer. Just find a posture in which you are alert and dignified, a kind of posture we've been using for other meditation practices. Start with a few breaths just to tune into whatever's going on inside. Notice all the different sensations in the body.

Now let your attention be drawn to any place in your body where difficult emotion can be felt, and see if you can sense where it can be felt most strongly—maybe some anger, some fear, or perhaps sadness. Soften into that location in your body. Let the muscles soften, like applying heat to sore muscles. You can try saying softly to yourself, "Soft. Soft. Soft." We're not trying to make the sensations go away, we're not trying to get rid of any feelings, we're just trying to be with them with a kind of loving awareness.

Now try to soothe yourself. Put your hand over your heart and feel your body breathe. Perhaps say some kind words to yourself, such as, "This is so painful. May I grow in ease, well-being, and acceptance." Just apply some loving touch to yourself. If you wish, you can also direct kindness to the part of your body that hurts most by placing your hand there, wherever that may be. Sometimes we feel emotions in one place or another. It may help to think of your body as if it were the body of a child you love, a child you're caring for. You can say kind words to yourself, just repeating, "Soothe. Soothe. Soothe."

Finally, we're going to allow the discomfort to be there. Abandon the wish for the feeling to disappear, for it to change, for pain to turn into pleasure—

just let the discomfort come and go as it pleases, like a guest in your home. To facilitate that you can repeat, "Allow. Allow. Allow."

So stringing this together, once we connect with the pain, we simply repeat to ourselves and send the feeling of "Soften. Soothe. Allow. Soften. Soothe. Allow." And you can use these three words like a mantra, reminding yourself to incline with tenderness toward your suffering. If you experience too much discomfort with an emotion, if it feels overwhelming, you can return your attention to the breath until you feel a little bit better able to attend to the difficult feeling. Then come back to "Soften. Soothe. Allow. Soften. Soothe. Allow."

You can end this practice with a few moments of breath awareness practice, just coming back into the body.

There's another exercise that we can try which involves writing a letter to ourselves from the perspective of somebody else.

This is a very simple yet powerful self-compassion practice that my friend and colleague Kristen Neff has developed. It's a self-compassion letter. Think of something that makes you feel badly about yourself, maybe an attribute or quality you don't like in yourself, or maybe it's something you did that perhaps you're ashamed of or feel guilty about. Now bring to mind a loving, accepting friend, someone who is a real pal—a real person (if you know them) who fits the bill, or an image of a loving other. Then write a letter to yourself from your friend's perspective. Right now, just imagine what the friend might say to you about the issue that concerns you. Can you do that for a moment? Chances are the friend will have a compassionate perspective. You can try writing an actual letter when you have the chance.

Mindfulness by itself tends to develop compassion. And it does this in a few ways. Compassion for ourselves tends to arise when we simply are open to our own suffering. And compassion toward others arises as we see that everybody else also suffers. And then compassion arises naturally as we see our interconnectedness. You know, as Lennon and McCartney put it, "I am he, as you are he, as you are me, and we are all together." We actually start to see this as we step out of selfing and see the interconnectedness of all things.

In Buddhist traditions, compassion and wisdom are seen as two wings of a bird or two wheels of a cart—one without the other doesn't really work very well. If we have wisdom without compassion, there's no heart in it. And if we're directing this toward another, our advice falls on deaf ears because it sounds hollow and it sounds intellectual. Of course, if in trying to help a friend we have compassion without wisdom, we might lose the equanimity. We might be so identified with the sufferer, so desperate to try to fix the problem, that we can't provide a kind of holding. So both are needed for compassionate action.

As we'll see a little bit later, mindfulness practice can be used to develop wisdom, but other practices can be used specifically to develop compassion. Because it's difficult to open fully to the suffering of others, we usually use a stepwise approach. First, we develop concentration to steady the mind and allow it to be able to be with what happens. Then we do the loving-kindness practices that we described before, the *mettā* practices. And these involve wishing ourselves and others well, but not necessarily with the attention to suffering or trying to do anything about the suffering. These can be a very good entrée to compassion practice.

We tried some loving-kindness practice before and I hope you have had the opportunity to follow the longer audio recording of this and really see what this is like. Those are the practices that use phrases like, "May I be happy. May I be peaceful. May I be free from suffering."

Now let's look at some practices from Buddhist traditions that are designed specifically to develop compassion for others. One of these is called *tonglen*. It comes out of the Tibetan tradition. And *tonglen* literally means "giving and taking." And this practice is attributed to a Buddhist teacher named Atisha who lived in India in the 11th century. And in the traditional practice what we do is inhale the pain and suffering of others and exhale kindness, warmth, and goodwill. And this reverses our instinctual tendency to battle against emotional discomfort.

As we've been incorporating it into Western psychotherapy, we've been making it a little bit easier by kind of inhaling compassion with the pain. So kind of taking the medicine with the toxin and then exhaling compassion because we find that oftentimes just trying to inhale the pain of others can feel a little bit overwhelming.

So let's do some *tonglen* practice together.

This is a variation on the Tibetan practice of *tonglen*, or "giving and taking." Begin by sitting comfortably with your eyes closed, and take some relaxing breaths. Just settle into the moment with allowing awareness. Scan the body for stress. Note any tension you feel anywhere. Note particularly any stressful emotions.

Once you've identified those in your own body, bring to mind a person, an animal, or even a place in nature for whom you'd like to develop more compassion. Now, aware of any stress you're carrying in your own body, inhale fully and deeply, drawing compassion inside your body and filling every cell with a sense of loving compassion. Then as you exhale, send compassion out to the person, animal, or the place in nature that you have in mind.

Simply continue doing this. Breathing compassion in, and breathing compassion toward the other out. Let your body gradually find a natural, relaxed breathing rhythm for this. Let's do it for a few more moments together. Compassion in toward ourselves and toward our own stress, compassion out toward the other who could use our care. Compassion in toward ourselves, compassion out toward the other who can use our care.

In all of these practices, equanimity is important. This is the wisdom component. This is about keeping perspective even as we're in the midst of being with someone else's suffering. There's a psychoanalyst by the name of Roy Schafer. And the language he uses is a bit vivid, but it captures what happens to us when we're trying to help others. He was talking about psychotherapists, but I think it applies to anybody. Most of us would rather think of ourselves as being a "breast of infinite capacity than a ravenously hungry parasite." We want to be somebody who helps. We want to be somebody who can put our own self-interest aside. And it can be hard for us to accept the limits of our capacity to help, both realizing that something may be too overwhelming for us and we have to pull back, and we might have to let go of our image of being the good friend or the good teacher, the good parent, son, daughter, even the good psychotherapist.

Now to develop this kind of equanimity there's a very simple practice we can try. And you can do this whenever you're with a person who's in pain and you notice yourself recoiling a little bit from the situation because it's hard to bear. You can simply try some phrases like this. "Everyone is on his or her own life journey." "I'm not the cause of others suffering, nor is it entirely within my power to alleviate it." "Though moments like this are difficult to bear, I may still try to help to the extent that I can." And this little exercise comes from my friend Chris Germer and I've used it with great help in moments when I'm in some way feeling an urgency that I have to fix the situation.

There's wonderful research that's come out recently on cultivating compassion for others. In one of them, they took 41 participants who logged onto a protected website and they were randomly assigned to a group that either received guided compassion meditation for 30 minutes a day, or to a group that received cognitive reappraisal training, which is just kind of CBT technique for thinking about your thoughts differently. And this went on for 14 days.

And the subjects in the compassion group were asked to contemplate and visualize the suffering of others and then wish for freedom from suffering for different categories of people. After the study, both groups were offered the opportunity to donate part of the money they had earned from the study to a charitable cause. The level of activity in brain circuits believed to be involved in generating positive emotion quite strongly predicted the amount of money that people donated, but only for participants in the compassion group.

So those who experience strong positive emotions in their training and directed that emotion toward alleviating the suffering of others actually acted most generously. Subjects who showed the biggest boast in activity in the insula, which we've talked about before, also donated the most money.

So I'd like to conclude this by sharing a little story. It's said in the ancient Jewish scriptures and texts, that what one should do with the Torah is to place the holy words on our heart. So a student asks a wise rabbi, "Why does the Torah say that we should place the holy words on our hearts?" And the rabbi answers that "because as we are most of the time, our hearts are a little closed. We place the words on our hearts so that one day when our heart breaks, the words will fall in."

In our next lecture, we're going to look at how to choose among these different practices we've been exploring. I'm hoping you've been practicing them along using the audio recordings on your own. And we're going to talk about how to modify these practices to fit your particular needs.

Tailoring Practices to Fit Changing Needs
Lecture 8

N ow that you have been exposed to a variety of different mindfulness and compassion practices, it will be helpful to step back and look at when each of the various techniques might be most useful to use. In this lecture, you are going to learn about how to choose among the different mindfulness practices that you have been exploring and how to modify the practices to fit your particular needs. You will learn how seven decisions can be helpful in modifying your practices to work with the situation at hand.

The Seven Decisions
- The question of which practice to use when and for whom is a cutting-edge area of investigation for mental health professionals who are using mindfulness practices in psychotherapy. Because different kinds of patients have such varied needs, clinicians want to be careful to introduce the most effective practices and, particularly, to avoid those that might be harmful for particular individuals at particular moments.

- While we don't yet have experimental research data to guide us, accumulating clinical experience is providing some direction. There are a number of choices that clinicians consider in their work. They can be useful for anyone doing mindfulness practice in deciding how to tailor our practice to our particular needs. There are seven decisions, as follows.
  - Which skills to emphasize

  - When to do formal or informal practice

  - Which objects of attention

  - Whether to take these in as religious or secular practices

     ○   Whether to work with life's difficulties in narrative or experiencing mode

     ○   Whether to stay at the level of relative or absolute truth

     ○   When to do practices that turn toward safety versus sharp points

Mindfulness Skills

- In regard to the first decision, there are three fundamental mindfulness skills. Some practices emphasize one more than the others. How might we choose among them? The three skills are concentration, which is used to refine the focus of the mind; open monitoring, which is used to see how the mind creates suffering; and acceptance practices, which are used to soothe and comfort us.

- Typically, most of us have to develop concentration first, because until we develop concentration, the mind is simply too scattered to be able to carefully observe what's happening in each moment. Once we have sufficient concentration, we can move on to open monitoring, or choiceless awareness. That's when we can broaden the field of awareness to pay attention to whatever arises in our consciousness.

- Then, if we notice a lot of resistance to the contents—if we notice that we are filled with self-critical thoughts, judgments, and resistance to certain aspects of what's coming up, that's when the loving-kindness or meta practices are so helpful, as well as the self-compassion practices and equanimity practices.

Formal versus Informal Practice

- There is a continuum of informal practices that we can do during the day, formal meditation practice, and intensive retreat practices. For most of us, it helps to pick a few informal practices—such as dog walking, showering, and mindful driving—and each time we are in those circumstances to practice them and to try to then pick regular times of the day for formal practices.

- For many people, it's helpful to engage in some kind of meditation class at a local meditation center once a week and to practice in the group as well as receive ongoing instruction.

- Retreat practice only makes sense if we're at a time in our life when we're feeling strong or not overwhelmed, because retreats tend to be rather intense and can be emotionally overwhelming. But they also have the potential to deepen our practice profoundly.

Objects of Attention

- When we do any practice, there are different objects of attention that we could use. Different objects tend to have different effects on the mind. A common object of attention is the breath. Others include the sensations of the feet touching the ground, sounds and sights, and the sensation of the air. We can think of these as a continuum, from the coarser to the subtler.

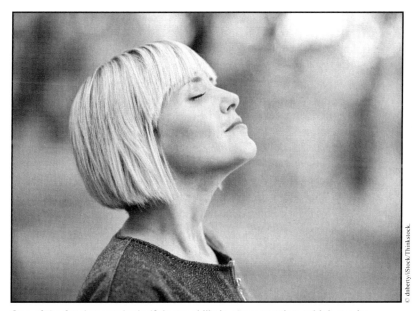

One of the fundamental mindfulness skills is concentration, which can be developed by paying attention to your breath.

- Many very intense experiences, such as heavy metal music, appeal to people, in part, because they create a sense of absorption. We are so brought out of our own thought stream by the intense sensations of the heavy metal concert, for example, that we're not worrying about our usual concerns. Intense sexual experiences can also function in this way.

- The problem is that when we're focusing on an object of awareness that's really, really intense, we tend not to see the subtle movements of the mind. So, we don't get a lot of insight into how the mind creates suffering for itself.

Religious versus Secular Practices
- Another choice point involves choosing a suitable style, which depends on our cultural background. Some of us are drawn toward spiritual or religious practices. These may be in a devotional tradition or theistic tradition. It can often be helpful to choose a practice that fits your own cultural orientation or belief system.

- For many people who aren't particularly religiously oriented, we can simply approach mindfulness practices from a very scientific standpoint. We can talk about neuroplasticity and discuss how these are exercises in intentional control training. There is no need to introduce a religious element into them. After all, the Buddhist psychology they come from is not a "religion" in the traditional Western sense of the word, based on doctrine, in that way.

- The only place where people get into a little bit of difficulty is if they come from traditions that try to prohibit certain thoughts and feelings from coming up in the mind. However, virtually all religious traditions have a loving and accepting element. It can be very helpful simply to find clergy who emphasize this aspect of the tradition, and then we can accept it even in a rather nonreligious way.

Narrative versus Experiential Mode
- The next choice involves the narrative versus experiential mode. This is relevant to psychotherapy, but it's also relevant to any of us

Lecture 8: Tailoring Practices to Fit Changing Needs

doing these practices. The narrative mode involves the stories we tell about ourselves. In the case of psychodynamic psychotherapy, they're stories about our earlier life history and what's happening in current relationships. In the case of behavioral traditions, how did we learn our particular beliefs? In the case of systemic or family approaches, how is it being maintained by the family, community, and culture?

- Instead of thinking about where your wave of anxiety, depression, or anger is coming from or what it is all about, experiencing mode is simply staying with the moment to moment. How is it felt in the body, and how is the mind responding to it? Is the mind trying to push it away, grasp it, or ignore it?

- There's an interesting balance. "Being with" experiencing mode, what we do in mindfulness practice is very, very useful for learning to be with difficult feelings. Yet stepping back and looking at things through narrative mode also can help us quite a bit.

Relative versus Absolute Truth

- A related decision has to do with whether to stay at the level of what we might call relative, or normal, human truth or to move to the level of absolute truth. The level of relative truth is simply the human story—our experiences of success and failure, pleasure and pain, longing for things that we don't have, hurt, anger, envy, joy, and even pride. These are the kinds of things that people come into psychotherapy talking about.

- Absolute truth refers to what are called in the Buddhist tradition the three marks of existence: *anicca*, which is the realization that all phenomena are in constant flux; *dukkha*, which is the unsatisfactoriness of experience; and *anatta*, which is the fact that we don't find any kind of enduring or separate self.

- We don't want to jump to the level of absolute truth when we haven't already processed things at the level of relative truth, but we do want to allow for the possibility that when we're caught in our human drama, we can also see it through the lens of the bigger picture.

Turning toward Safety versus Sharp Points

- The last decision—arguably the most important one—is about whether to turn toward safety or toward the sharp points. When people have been through difficult times or are overwhelmed, clinicians need to do a stage-based approach to treatment. They need to first establish a sense of safety, a sense of comfort, a sense of being held.

- Then, they can move on to starting to reintegrate things that have been split off, because the impulse to reintegrate is a good one. It's only when people allow all of their feelings to occur that they can become fully whole and fully present. But you can't rush it.

- Some mindfulness practices are quite helpful for turning toward safety, while others are helpful for reintegrating the difficulties, which in the Tibetan tradition is referred to as "turning toward the sharp points."

- Things that are helpful for turning toward safety are typically things with an outer, or distal, focus. When difficulty arises emotionally, it tends to be in the body. When we bring our attention outward, it works more readily for us. Examples of practices that can help us turn toward safety that have an outer focus include walking meditation, listening meditation, nature meditation, eating meditation, and open-eye practices.

- There are also other ways to turn toward safety that have an inner focus. These include mountain meditations, guided imagery, *metta* practice, and dialectical behavior therapy techniques.

- There's also a time when we want to turn toward the sharp points— when we want to try to reintegrate what we've pushed out of awareness. Then, we can use mindfulness practice as a kind of experiential form of treatment, where we start with something like the breath or another object of awareness and turn the attention toward anything that's unwanted or avoided, including a feeling or memory.

- Then, we simply notice how it is experienced in the body—whether it is experienced as pain, fear, sadness, or anger. We can see what arises in response to unwanted images or memories. We can even see what arises in response to urges toward compulsive behaviors, such as overeating or overdrinking. We can simply notice these events happening in the mind.

- Different people need different things, and any one of us needs different approaches at different moments in time. For example, we might go through a period where we've had a lot of difficulty in our lives and need loving-kindness practice or equanimity practice.

- Mindfulness of inner experience—simply spending a long period of time just staying with the breath or turning toward the sharp points—can be harmful when we're overwhelmed by traumatic memories, when we're afraid of disintegration or a loss of sense of self, and when people are suffering from psychosis. There are some practices that we could think of as life preservers, which are about using the practices that turn us toward safety and doing them in a very difficult moment. Usually, these involve some form of concentration practice that includes stepping out of the thought stream.

Suggested Reading

Germer, Siegel, and Fulton, *Mindfulness and Psychotherapy*.

Pollak, Pedulla, and Siegel, *Sitting Together*.

Siegel, *The Mindfulness Solution*, chapter 4.

1. What have you noticed in your meditation practice about the relationship among focused attention (concentration), open monitoring (mindfulness per se), and acceptance (loving-kindness, self-compassion, and equanimity) practices? When do you feel that one or another is more helpful?

2. Can you identify times in your life when mindfulness practices aimed at cultivating safety and stability would be more useful, verses times when turning toward the sharp points would be more helpful?

Tailoring Practices to Fit Changing Needs
Lecture 8—Transcript

Now that you've been exposed to a variety of different mindfulness and compassion practices, it may be helpful to step back and look at when each of the various techniques might be most useful to use. When we had the Dalai Lama at Harvard Medical School, my colleagues and I had thought it would be so wonderful—let's have him lead a group of 1,100 psychotherapists in some mindfulness meditation practice. So at the appointed time my colleague asked the Dalai Lama to please lead all of us. And he in his inimitable way started laughing. He thought, what will these silly people come up with next? Then he said, "I think some of you may want just one single meditation and a simple one that's 100 percent positive. That, I think, is impossible."

There are a whole lot of different outlooks toward oneself, toward suffering, toward the whole world. And because of that, in order to transform our destructive emotion, one goal, there are so many thousands of different meditations that are mentioned. He went on to say that, "Here, on the basis of my own experience, I can say that for one single type of meditation, it's effect is limited." After a little bit more discussion, he said this, he said, "Some other sort of companies, they always advertise some simple thing, something effective, something very cheap. My advertising is just the opposite. How difficult, and complicated!"

This question of which practice to use when and for whom is actually a cutting edge area of investigation for mental health professionals who are using mindfulness practices now in psychotherapy. Because different clients or patients have such varied needs, clinicians want to be careful to introduce the most effective practices and particularly to avoid those that might be harmful for particular individuals at particular moments. While we don't yet have experimental research data to guide us, accumulating clinical experience is providing some direction. Here are a number of choices that my colleagues and I consider in our clinical work. They can be useful for any of us doing mindfulness practice, in deciding how to tailor our practice to our particular needs.

There are seven decisions, and in the course of this lecture, I'll outline what all of them are about. The first one is which skills to emphasize between concentration, open monitoring, and acceptance practices. When to do formal or informal practice. Which objects of attention—when to pay attention to the breath, when to pay attention to other things. Whether to take these in as religious or secular practices.

Whether to work with life difficulties in what we could call a *narrative* or *experiencing mode*, and I'll explain that. Whether to stay at the level of relative truth, which is our every day look at the world, or absolute truth, truth as it's revealed through these practices. And finally, and most importantly, when to do practices that turn toward safety and give us a sense of safety and soothing, and when to do practices that help us to reintegrate bits of experience that are difficult, and we may have pushed out of awareness.

Let's start with the first choice. I mentioned earlier that there are three fundamental mindfulness skills. Some practices emphasize one more than the other. How might we choose among them? The three skills are focused attention or concentration. We use that to observe things clearly, to refine the focus of the mind. The second one is open monitoring, and that's to see how the mind creates suffering. The third is acceptance or loving-kindness practices, and this also might include compassion practices and equanimity practices. These are used to soothe and comfort us.

We can think of these as three legs of tripod. Typically, most of us have to develop concentration first. Because until we develop concentration, the mind is simply too scattered to be able to carefully observe what's happening in each moment. Once we have sufficient concentration, that's when we move onto open monitoring or choice-less awareness. That's when we can broaden the field of awareness to pay attention to whatever arises in our consciousness.

Then, if we notice a lot of resistance to the contents, if we notice that we are filled with self-critical thoughts, judgments, resistance to certain aspects of what's coming up, that's when the loving kindness or *mettā* practices are so helpful, as well as the self-compassion practices and equanimity practices, which we'll talk about in a little bit. We also talked about the continuum of practice—informal practices that we can do during the day, formal meditation practice, and intensive retreat practices.

For most of us, it helps to pick a few informal practices—like dog-walking, showering, and mindful driving, for example—and each time we are in those circumstances to practice them, and to try to then pick regular times of the day for formal practices—so to do them in the morning regularly or after work or in the evening. And for many people, it's helpful to engage in some kind of a class.

One great way to take up a regular formal practice pattern is to attend a meditation class at a local meditation center, and meet with people once a week, and practice in the group as well as receive ongoing instruction. A retreat practice only makes sense if we're at a time in our life when we're feeling like we're not overwhelmed, because retreats tend to be rather intense and can be emotionally overwhelming. But they also have the potential to deepen our practice profoundly.

Now when we do any practice, there are different objects of attention that we could use. So far, we've used mostly the breath for the longer practice. That's what you have in your recorded audio. But at the end of that audio, we also use other objects of awareness such as the sensations of the buttocks and the feet and the backs of legs touching the chair, sounds, sights, the sensation of the air, and different objects of awareness tend to have different effects on the mind. We can think of these as a rate on a kind of continuum from the more coarse to the more subtle.

At the coarse level, it's things like walking meditation. If we're doing walking meditation, my feet are touching the ground, and I'm stepping, lifting, stepping, that's a pretty vivid stimulus. Similarly, the sights and sounds of nature are pretty vivid or the taste of food as an eating meditation, or perhaps the sound of a bell. A little bit more subtle are things like the breath in the belly that arises and passes, or perhaps the use of a mantra (a repeated phrase), or a subtler still, the air at the tip of the nose as was offered as an alternative in the recorded audio of breath meditation.

Now I frequently ask groups of psychotherapists, who are mediators, I say, "Of you folks who meditate regularly, how many of you typically choose as your venue a heavy metal concert?" And naturally, none of the hands go up. But we might ask, why not? A heavy metal concert offers the opportunity for paying attention to a very vivid stimulus. There are burning guitars, there is loud music, there are flashing lights. And we could equivalently think of other things, like, do you usually go on roller coaster rides to meditate? Or go to an over-the-top expressive opera? And no, we don't usually go for things that are intense like this.

Actually many of those very intense experiences appeal to people in part, because they create a sense of absorption. We are so brought out of our own thought stream by the intense sensations of the heavy metal concert or of the roller coaster, that we're not worrying about our usual concerns. There are other things. Intense sexual experiences can function in this way. But the problem is that when we're focusing on an object of awareness that's really, really intense, we tend not to see the subtle movements of the mind, so we don't get a lot of insight into how the mind creates suffering for itself.

Now another choice point, the fourth, involves choosing a suitable style, and this depends on our cultural background. Some of us are drawn toward spiritual practices or religious practices. These may be in a devotional tradition or theistic tradition. It can often be helpful to choose a practice that fits your own cultural orientation or your own belief system.

I remember when I went to sit in my first silent meditation retreat, this is in mid-1970s, and I was kind of a countercultural person. As I described before, during the retreat you're not talking to the other participants. But there was this one group of guys who were dressed really oddly to me. They had on their brown robes tied with a belt—and there were a lot of hippies around in those days that had weird outfits, but this was obviously something different. I kept wondering, who are these folks and where are they from?

Well, at the end of the retreat, I got to ask them. It turned out that they were from a Trappist monastery that was down the block. They were following the tradition of Thomas Merton who had gone to the East to learn meditation practices to help in his monastic practices in the Catholic tradition. Among the folks who came and learned meditation was a fellow named Father Thomas Keating, and he developed something called "contemplative prayer." It's also sometimes called "centering prayer." This is in the tradition of what's called the *Lectio Divina*, which means "the holy reading of the scriptures." It's about opening the heart and mind, our whole being, to God or the ultimate mystery—but the world and experience beyond thoughts, words, and emotions.

So this is how they teach to do centering prayer—as you'll see it's a form of mindfulness practice. They choose a sacred word or symbol—in the case of centering prayer, it's usually from the Catholic liturgy—and they simply sit comfortably and introduce the sacred word, and begin to repeat the sacred word over and over, and have the word be the object of awareness. When the mind is distracted by a chain of narrative thought, the instruction is to ever so gently return the attention to the sacred word. They do this for however long a period of practice. Then they end with two minutes of silence, which is typically just being with the breath.

While this was originally designed as a Catholic practice, the words could really come from any tradition, and it could work quite well with any spiritual or religious tradition that resonates for you. There are also recently a lot of Jewish adaptations of this. Often, they'll use elements of the Kabbalah, which is this sort of mystical branch of Jewish tradition. These may overlook differences in worldview—and there have been some critiques about this, saying that basically some Jewish theologians thinking that they don't want too much of a wholesale adaptation of some of these Buddhist views, because they miss the relationship to a personal god. But these are catching on quite a bit.

It turns out that in the United States, Jews are 2.5 percent of the population—and only 1.5 percent of the Jewish population list it as a religion—but 25 percent of non-Asian Buddhists in America are of Jewish descent. Because there's such an interest in American Jewish populations in Buddhist practices, these are now practiced in a lot of different temples and synagogues.

In Islam, there are opportunities too. Some of these come from the Sufi tradition. These are the teachings of Rumi, who was a 13th century Persian mystical poet. You may know him for his followers who are the whirling dervishes, who do these dances where they spin around in white robes. They use the paying attention to the sensations of spinning as the object of awareness for a kind of mindfulness practice, and when the mind leaves the sensations of dancing, they come back to it over and over. And while Sufism has been rejected by certain people in Orthodox Islam, among somewhat more flexibly-oriented folks, there's a following of this.

And I also have a patient of mine who does more traditional Islamic practice, but he simply uses the prayers as you would use them in centering prayer as part of his practice. There are many opportunities for doing this that are compatible with people's religious beliefs and cultural orientation.

Now, of course, there are many people who aren't particularly religiously oriented, and then we can simply approach these from a very scientific standpoint. We can talk about neuroplasticity. These are exercises in intentional control training. As we've seen, there is no need to introduce a religious element into them at all. After all, the Buddhist psychology they come from is not really a religion in the traditional Western sense of the word based on doctrine in that way.

The only place where people get into a little bit of difficulty as I've seen it, is if people are coming from traditions that try to prohibit certain thoughts and feelings from coming up in the mind. Yet, virtually all religious traditions have a loving and accepting element. It can be very helpful simply to find clergy who emphasize this aspect of the tradition, and then we can accept it even in a rather non-religious way.

So the next choice involves narrative mode versus experiential mode. This is relevant to psychotherapy, but it's also quite relevant to any of us doing these practices. The narrative mode involves the stories we tell about ourselves—in the case of psychodynamic psychotherapy, about our earlier life history and what's happening in current relationships. In the case of behavioral traditions, how did we learn our particular beliefs? In the case of systemic or family approaches, how is it being maintained by the family, the community, and the culture?

Experiencing mode is different. Experiencing mode is, instead of thinking about, if I have a wave of anxiety, or a wave of depression, or a wave of anger, where is this coming from? What is this all about? It's simply staying with moment to moment how it's felt in the body. And how is the mind responding to it? Is the mind trying to push it away, grasp it, or ignore it?

I had a very interesting experience once, where in my teaching role, I had had a communication with somebody that unfortunately and unbeknownst to me in a phone conversation a student heard me say something, which I didn't say, and I wouldn't have said. But for whatever reason, there was this miscommunication. They were upset by it, and they were talking to other people in the program where I teach about it. I was upset that this miscommunication had happened. It was immediately after it happened that I went and was sitting a silent meditation retreat. But I was also teaching the retreat, so I had some opportunities for speaking.

But during the first day, I was mostly just participating as a participant. I was watching the waves come up. It would be a wave of shame that people are going to think that I'm a bad person. Who would say such a thing? Waves of anger—come on. Why didn't you come to me instead of talking to other people about it? Waves of fear that now I'm going to have to figure out a skillful way to process this, and I'm not sure what would be best.

At the end of the day, I had a few minutes to talk to my old friends, who were also co-leading the retreat. They said, "How have you been?" I said, "Well, I've been fine, except this incident happened." I found that in simply five minutes of talking to them in narrative mode of what the story was, the pain around it lifted. So it illustrated to me that there's this interesting balance. Being with experiencing mode, what we do in mindfulness practice is very, very useful for learning to be with difficult feelings. Yet stepping back and looking at things through narrative mode also can help us quite a bit.

A related decision has to do with whether to stay at the level of what we might call relative or normal human truth, or to move to the level of absolute truth. The level of relative truth is simply the human story, our experiences of success and failure, pleasure and pain, longing for things that we don't have, perhaps hurt, anger, envy, joy, even pride. These are the kinds of things people come into psychotherapy talking about.

Absolute truth refers to what are called in the Buddhist tradition the "three marks of existence." I've mentioned these before, but not in quite this language. They are *anicca*, which is the realization that all phenomena are in constant flux. In fact, it's not even that all things change, because to even think of things as things is a little bit too reified. There is *dukkha*, which is this unsatisfactoriness of experience. This is what has been poorly translated in the past as saying, "life is suffering." But a much better translation would be, "the mind often experiences dissatisfaction."

Actually, my favorite presentation of this comes from a great philosopher sage. She's actually a westerner. Sadly, she's passed away. You may know her work. She was called Roseanne Roseannadanna. Roseanne Roseannadanna used to say, "If it's not one thing, it's another," the sense that the mind is always unsettled about something. The third component of absolute truth is *anatta*, the fact that we don't find any kind of enduring or separate self. That's what we spoke about in an earlier lecture.

Now, of course, we don't want to force it. We don't want to jump to the level of absolute truth when we haven't already processed things at the level of relative truth. I'll give you an example. If a fellow were to come in to see me in psychotherapy, heartbroken, because he had been engaged to marry a beautiful, warm, erotically alive, intelligent, loving woman, who a few weeks before the marriage said, "I just can't go through with it"—if I were to say to him, "Well, don't you get it? It's *anicca*. All things change. What do you expect?" Or to say, "You know, the mind creates dissatisfaction no matter what our circumstances. Had you gone through with the marriage, you'd probably be dissatisfied about something else. Just ask a married person." Or to say that "the whole idea of and your fiancée as separate cells is illusory. We're all part of one big organism." That probably wouldn't be very sensitive, and it wouldn't be very helpful. We don't want to rush ourselves to this level of absolute truth, but we do want to allow for the possibility that when we're caught in our human drama, we can also see it through the lens of this bigger picture.

Now, the last decision is arguably the most important. This is the decision about whether to turn toward safety or turn toward the sharp points. Let me give you a little bit of history for this in the mental health field. All professions have made mistakes historically, and the mental health profession is no exception. Perhaps our biggest mistake came from clinicians extrapolating from their own experience and believing that it would be universal.

What happened—and this began I think in the 1950s and the 1960s—was the clinicians discovered in their own experience that part of what was healing, what they have discovered to be personally healing, was when there would be some kind of split-off affect—some feeling, some thought, even a memory, something that was painful and difficult to bear—and once they learned to be able to embrace it and to bear it, they felt a sense of transformation, a sense that, "Now I'm whole again. Now, I'm not fighting these things anymore. Now, I feel much better."

Unfortunately, what clinicians started doing was helping people who had been through serious forms of trauma, or didn't have a lot of safety, to start doing the very same thing. And what would happen is people would come into psychotherapy, and they would become overwhelmed. This is like what I was talking about before the idea that you have to clean out a wound first, and it gets worse before it gets better if we want to move toward healing— but it has to be under a condition where the person can recover. You wouldn't want to clean out the wound when somebody's working in a dirty field.

It took some time for clinicians to realize that when people have been through difficult times or they're overwhelmed, we need to do a stage-based approach to treatment. We need to first establish a sense of safety, a sense of comfort, a sense of being held. Once we have that, then we can move on to starting to reintegrate things that have been split off. Because, indeed, the impulse to reintegrate is a good one—it's only when we can take back in and allow all of our feelings to occur, as we've discussed earlier, that we can become fully whole and fully present—but you can't rush it.

It turns out that some mindfulness practices are actually quite helpful for turning towards safety, while others are helpful for reintegrating the difficulties, which in the Tibetan tradition is called "turning toward the sharp points." Things that are helpful for turning toward safety are typically things with an outer or distal focus. By distal, I mean distant from the mid-line of the body. Because when we feel feelings, we tend to feel them in here. When difficulty arises emotionally, it tends to be in the body. When we bring our attention outward, it works more readily for us.

One example is walking meditation. If I simply bring my attention to the sensations of the feet on the ground, it tends to ground me. In fact, in trauma treatment, these are called "grounding exercises." Listening meditation also works. To simply take time and listen to whatever sounds are arising, whatever sounds are passing. Nature meditation is a nice one. That's where we go out and take a walk or do some other activity, and simply pay attention to the clouds, to the sky, to the sensations of being out in the air. Or eating meditation, where we pay attention to the taste of food, or open-eyed practices generally are helpful this way.

There are also other ways to turn toward safety that have an inner focus. One of these is the mountain meditation. That one you have as an audio recording included with the course. The way that mountain meditation works is we imagine ourselves sitting as a mountain. We're in an environment, perhaps surrounded by other mountains, like a mountain range. What we do is we go through the seasonal changes, and it's a kind of guided imagery exercise.

We can experience all sorts of things. We can experience rain and snow coming. We can experience brilliant sky and sunshine. We can experience cold times—because we go through the whole year, it might be winter—and snow. We could have warmth and birds and bees, and all sorts of other activities. The idea that comes from this is it's really an equanimity practice. We start to identify with awareness itself. We start to, rather than be identifying with the contents of the mind, it's as though the mountain is there in awareness, while all these things come and go and change in and around us. I very much encourage you to try the practice. It can be very soothing, very comforting, particularly when we're going through hard times.

As we learn to identify with awareness itself, we then open much more to the full contents of the mind, even when they're difficult. Other practices that can be helpful are the loving-kindness practices we talked about before, or the *mettā* practices. "May I be safe. May I be healthy. May I live with ease." Or, "May I be happy. May I be peaceful. May I be free from suffering." This is an inner practice, but it provides a kind of soothing that gives us a sense of safety.

Finally, there are a number of practices that are derived from Dialectical Behavior Therapy, which is a form of treatment that's used for folks with borderline personality disorder, which means a lot disregulation of emotional states. These are very helpful for bringing us back into the present. They involve things like willing hands that we'll practice a little bit later, and developing a serene half smile, and things that make us feel safe even in the midst of difficulty.

Now, there's also a time when we want to turn toward the sharp points, when we want to try to reintegrate that which we've pushed out of awareness. Then, we can use mindfulness practice as a kind of experiential form of treatment. You will remember I talked about the narrative or the experiential. That's where we start with something like the breath or another object of awareness, depending on how frisky or focused the mind is. What we do is we simply turn the attention toward anything that's unwanted or avoided. This could be a feeling. It could be an image that comes to mind. It could be a memory. Then, we simply notice how is it experienced in the body—whether it be pain, or fear, or sadness, or anger, whatever it is—what's arising right now in the body? We can see what arises in response to unwanted images or memories. We can even see what arises in response toward urges, toward compulsive behaviors. So that if I have a feeling of I really want to get up and go the fridge, and get that piece of chocolate cake, or I really want to have a drink right now, we can simply notice these events happening in the mind as well.

Different people need different things, and any one of us needs different approaches at different moments in time. For example, when I'm choosing among the safety or the sharp points, it really depends on the day. Some days I might feel like I want to do some therapeutic work here with my mindfulness practice. Life's going OK. I'm stable enough. Let me turn toward anything that I seem to be resisting, anything that's giving me difficulty. Whereas on another day, I might think, gosh, I have a lot of things I have to tend to.

Life is chaotic. There's a lot of difficulty. Let me do more of these safety-oriented exercises.

And sometimes that's simply in the course of a day, or sometimes it's over a long period of time. We might go through a period where we've had a lot of difficulty in our lives where we think, you know, a lot of loving-kindness practice, a lot of equanimity practice. I just need to have some sense of stability here, and I'll do the integrative work later when I'm ready for it.

Now, I'd like to particularly emphasize when mindfulness of inner experience can be harmful—and by this, I mean when simply spending a long period of time just staying with the breath can be a problem: When we're overwhelmed by traumatic memories, as I've suggested. Also when we're afraid of disintegration or a loss of sense of self—and that may sound a little odd, but sometimes people go through periods in which they're noticing all the different parts that we've talked about before, but it's making them very anxious. And they're feeling, gosh, I don't know who I am anymore. And sometimes there's a sort of loss of sense of self that happens. I don't know if it's your feeling or my feeling that I'm experiencing. When people are having those kinds of difficulties, it's not a good time to do the turning toward the sharp points or the staying with the breath for a long period of time. And also, when people are suffering from psychosis, because it's just too easy to get caught in the narrative stream when this happens.

So there are some practices that we could think of as life preservers. And I want to give you an example from a clinical experience I had of how this could work. Basically, life preservers are about using the practices that turn us toward safety and doing them in a very difficult moment. And usually these involve some form of concentration practice that includes stepping out of the thought stream. I'll give you an example.

There was a woman who I'd been working with for some time. And she had had a really, really bad trauma history. When I first met her and started hearing about it, I started thinking initially, gosh, maybe she has trouble identifying what's real and what is it. Maybe she has a serious mental illness of some sort. Because the stories she was telling me about her childhood were so bad that I thought, this couldn't have happened, could it? Wouldn't a teacher have said something? Wouldn't a neighbor have done something? Wouldn't the police have been called? I'll spare you the details, but it was really horrible things.

Anyway, I came to know her over time. And I realized that there was a lot of internal consistency to her stories, that indeed probably what she remembered was the truth. Part of the way I discovered this or came to believe this is by hearing about other elements that fit together. For example, she had—I know this sounds terrible, but it's true—she had a brother who had committed suicide after he had done some terrible things. And there were other elements that all held together to make me believe that indeed this person did have a terrible, terrible childhood.

Anyway, because of this terrible past, she would be prone to all sorts of instability. And one day, she came into my office with a symptom that I've got to think is unique to the Boston metropolitan area. She came in and said that everywhere in her visual field that day she was seeing two- to three-foot-high Red Sox players, and they had the bats and the balls and the full regalia—a very unusual symptom.

Usually when somebody has a symptom like that, we think it has to do with an organic problem, drugs, or a metabolic issue. But in her case, I think it was just because of her bad trauma. And I started asking her what had happened. And indeed, she had had an experience earlier that day where somebody had spoken to her harshly. And because of the horrible violence she had been exposed to, this kind of thing would unnerve her. And I knew from past experience that it could produce all sorts of symptoms.

So after talking about that and coming to some understanding of it, I asked her if she'd like to try something different. And this is where the life preservers come in. I asked her to stand up at the window with me and look out. And outside the window, there was a tree—not a particularly bucolic tree, but nonetheless there was a tree. And I just asked her to look at the tree and bring her attention to it. And here's where the mindfulness instruction came in. I suggested that she look at the tree and not try to get rid of the Red Sox players—in mindfulness practice, we're not trying to get rid of anything—but rather to simply be with the tree and notice all of its textures, it's colors, and she could even describe them. And then we went on to look at the houses and other things. And ultimately, she started to feel somewhat calmer and importantly, somewhat safer.

She was still a little unsteady, so I asked her in between sessions—I was ending one session. I said, why don't you go walk around the neighborhood—it was a safe neighborhood and a nice day—and continue this practice of just bringing your attention out while allowing the Red Sox players to be there, but continuing to notice that there's the safe external reality. And she did this over time and came back after the next session. And she felt comfortable enough to drive home, felt pretty stable. She did that.

I called her up that evening and she was still having the experience of the Red Sox players, but she was feeling considerably calmer. I thought I better check in, and I called her the next morning, and the Red Sox players were gone. I don't know, maybe they had an away game, but they weren't bothering her anymore. And these kinds of things won't always work, but it's interesting to know that we can turn to these practices of the outer world in order to get a sense of safety.

So all of these decisions can be helpful in modifying our practices to work with the situation at hand. In our next lecture, we're going to look at some of the rapidly expanding research into how mindfulness practices affect the brain, how old notions that the brain matures around age 25 and just decays thereafter are being turned upside down by the results of research on mindfulness. Thanks for listening.

Modifying Our Brain Function and Structure
Lecture 9

W hat exactly do we mean by brain structure and function? And how do these relate to the idea of the mind? Different philosophical schools and approaches posit different relationships between the constructs of mind and brain. In this lecture, "mind" signifies the information being processed and our subjective experience in consciousness moment to moment. "Brain," on the other hand, involves what's going on in the underlying tissue structures. As you'll learn in this lecture, the mind changes the brain, and the brain changes the mind.

Studying the Brain: Neurobiology
- Neurobiological studies are often what draw people to mindfulness practice. They engage in mindfulness practice to improve aspects of their brain function, but they end up with a path to rather profound changes, even paths to psychological and emotional liberation.

- Also, by studying mindfulness and the effects of mindfulness on neurobiology, we get to see our mind as an impersonal process. We get to see that the thoughts and feelings that arise are actually just neurobiology unfolding.

- Increasingly, neurobiology also gives us the idea of possible new interventions—for example, neurofeedback. There are some studies in which they connect a computer to an imaging machine so that a subject can get real-time feedback on what their brain is doing in each moment, and as a result, they're better able to train their brain in certain ways.

- Scientists face many challenges in studying the neurobiology of mindfulness practices. What happens to our brain over time if we take up meditation practices? In psychological research, the momentary effects are called state effects, and the more long-lasting ones are called trait effects. State effects and trait effects reinforce one another. Both are challenging to measure.

- Some of the challenges in studying state effects include not knowing what the meditator is actually doing as we're observing them. Is he or she concentrating on the breath, enjoying a pleasant fantasy, or maybe even remembering to run an errand? Where exactly is the boundary between meditation and non-meditation?

- If you ask a question of a person while they're in an fMRI scanner, simply hearing and answering the question changes brain activity, so maybe we're simply measuring the person's response to the question.

- When we study trait effects, there are challenges there, too, because the way we study those is by looking at people who have been doing meditation over time and comparing them to people who haven't been doing meditation over time. But perhaps only certain people choose to meditate. Maybe the effects that we observe are because they're disproportionately vegetarian, or highly educated, for example. It's difficult to get random samples.

- A challenge that faces both state and trait studies is that we don't know if people can accurately report on their degree of mindfulness. A person needs some degree of mindfulness to be able to notice if he or she is being mindful. However, we're stuck with self-report. There are nine scales that are in use, and all of them ask people about their personal experiences and what they observe in their own minds.

- There are five factors in mindfulness practice, but these appear to be different depending on the experience levels. Some factors seem to develop more at lower levels of experience, and other factors seem to develop more at higher levels of experience.

- What might we use instead of self-report as a measure? Should we use the hours or years in meditation practice? It's a possibility. But we don't know exactly what the intensity of the meditation practice was or how well trained the person was.

- Also, until recently, we didn't have good active controls. In studies, we would assign people to a meditation practice or to a waiting list, but we couldn't tell if the effects that we were measuring were actually the effects of doing the meditation, or simply getting attention for being in the study, or participating in part of a group, or maybe being exposed to a new belief system. Sophisticated, high-tech equipment can't solve these kinds of problems.

- Despite these challenges, we are learning something about the neurobiological changes. There are several methods for being able to study what's going on in the brain. One set of methods measures electrical activity. Our chief instrument is the electroencephalogram (EEG), which is very sensitive to moment-to-moment changes. The problem is that the image we get is a bit blurry, so it's very difficult to tell exactly where in the brain activity is taking place.

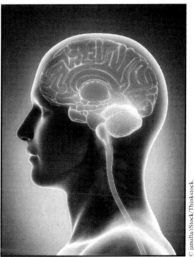

Research has shown that mindfulness practice leads to positive changes in brain function.

- The other way we can look at what's happening in the brain is through neuroimaging. There are three types: PET, MRI, and fMRI.

- Positron emission tomography (PET) detects radiation from emission of positrons. The reason it's not used very often anymore in meditation studies is that these positrons decay, and you can only actually record what they're doing during the period of time that they're decaying. So, you can only get very short videos of what's going on in the brain. Also, subjects aren't so keen about having radiation injected into them, so this has fallen a little bit into disuse.

- Much more frequently used is magnetic resonance imaging (MRI), which detects a radio frequency signal that's emitted by excited hydrogen atoms in the body. This method provides excellent imaging for soft tissue, including the brain. The resolution is quite clear. But an MRI only takes a snapshot, so we only see what's happening at a particular moment in time.

- Another instrument is functional magnetic resonance imaging (fMRI), which takes a series of MRI pictures one right after the other. The video is somewhat jerky because there are slow refresh rates for the frames, and the resolution isn't quite as good as an MRI, but you can see what's happening in the brain in real time. So, we can get a long video about what's happening in the course of meditation practice.

Changes in Brain Function

- Neurobiological research on mindfulness practice has taught us a lot about changes in brain function. The first area that we've noticed changes in is attention, which includes alerting, or becoming aware of a stimulus, such as a horn honking; and sustained attention, which is following a stimulus over time. Very closely related to sustained attention is the idea of conflict monitoring, which is about remaining focused despite distractions that are trying to pull our attention away.

- Research has shown that mindfulness practice improves both alerting and sustained attention. In fact, as little as eight weeks of training improved the detection of unexpected stimuli that were introduced in the laboratory, and it improved the ability to maintain attention on a stimulus over time.

- Mindfulness meditation practice also seems to stave off all sorts of normal cognitive declines that are associated with aging. Older meditators have been shown to outperform age-matched participants on an attentional blink task and on tasks assessing attention, short-term memory, perceptual speed, and executive functioning.

- Different types of meditation seem to yield different results in terms of electroencephalogram patterns, or brain wave patterns. Researchers are just beginning to investigate how different forms of meditation might affect the brain differently, but it's clear, at this point, that all of the different practices have measurable effects on our neurobiology.

- In addition, studies are showing that even within one type of meditation, different doses seem to have different effects.

- Mindfulness meditation activates parts of the brain that are essential for keeping our emotions in perspective and has the clinical effect of reducing excessive anxiety.

Changes in Brain Structure

- We used to believe that the brain reaches peak development at age 25 and deteriorates thereafter. However, the brain is much more like a muscle. If you use it, it bulks up; if you don't, it tends to wither.

- For example, professional musicians have more neuronal cell bodies, or gray matter, than amateurs in areas of the brain related to musical ability. And amateurs have more gray matter than people with no musical training. This is all evidence of brain plasticity. What we do with our attention really matters.

- Aging and pathology are usually associated with cortical thinning—with losing gray matter in the cortex. In 2005, Sara Lazar analyzed 20 long-term Western meditators and age-matched controls. They had, on average, nine years of meditation experience.

- Her team discovered that compared to age-matched controls, the meditators had thicker anterior insulae, sensory cortexes, and prefrontal cortexes. The differences in thickness were most pronounced in older subjects.

- The three regions affected by meditation practices were all thought to be involved in integrating emotional and cognitive processes. The opposite development—decreased volume in at least one of the affective structures, the anterior insula—has been strongly implicated in several pathologies, including post-traumatic stress disorder, social anxiety, specific phobias, and even schizophrenia.

- There are some limitations to this study. It had relatively small numbers, and people were only imaged once. And maybe people who have naturally thicker cortexes are more likely to practice meditation. Nonetheless, the findings fit expectations.

- The areas associated with paying attention to the breath and sensory stimuli, and areas associated with the integration of thoughts and feelings, had increased in thickness proportional to the amount of time people spent meditating in their lifetime.

- To get beyond these limitations, we need to do pre-post studies. We need to be able to randomly assign people to meditation or non-meditation groups. There has been one eight-week mindfulness course that was given to people with no meditation training, while a similar group was in a control group, and the researchers found increases in gray matter concentration within the left hippocampus and other areas.

- The hippocampus is involved not only in learning and memory, but also in emotion regulation. In fact, it gets smaller in depression and anxiety, and stress seems to shrink it. Altogether, researchers concluded that participating in eight weeks of mindfulness training was associated with changes in gray matter concentration in brain regions involved in learning and memory processes, emotion regulation, self-referential processing, and perspective taking—all valuable things to experience.

- Pre-post studies are showing that changes aren't just due to meditators being vegetarians or something else peculiar. Even when subjects are randomly assigned to mindfulness meditation or control groups, mindfulness training produces measurable changes in important brain regions.

Suggested Reading

Davidson, "The Neurobiology of Compassion."

Davidson, et al, "Alterations in Brain and Immune Function Produced by Mindfulness Meditation."

Hanson and Mendius, *Buddha's Brain*.

Lazar, "The Neurobiology of Mindfulness."

Lazar, et al, "Meditation Experience Is Associated with Increased Cortical Thickness."

Questions to Consider

1. How have scientists changed their understanding of neuroplasticity in recent years, and what does research on the effects of meditation tell us about how the brain develops over a lifetime?

2. What are some of the challenging questions scientists need to consider in studying the effects of meditation practice on the brain?

Modifying Our Brain Function and Structure
Lecture 9—Transcript

The last time I was in London, I asked my cab driver about his training and what kind of test he needed to pass in order to get licensed. It turned out he needed to know 25,000 streets and 20,000 landmarks. It took him three years to learn how to become a cab driver.

This stood in marked contrast to my own training as a New York City cab driver. I was asked to know 10 landmarks. I was told them all in advance. Two were the same—they were Madison Square Garden and Penn Station. For Yankee Stadium, I had to be able to say the Bronx, and for Shea Stadium, I had to be able to say Queens. And I only had to get 60 percent right, and I was able to take the test three times in one day.

The reason I was so curious about my cabbie's training wasn't just to compare it to my own experience, though. I was interested to hear firsthand because studies of London cabbie brains are often cited as evidence for experience-dependent neuroplasticity, the fact that different parts of our brains grow or shrink based on how we use them.

In the course of their training, compared with controls, London cabbies developed extra-large posterior hippocampi, parts of the brain that are associated with memory. And it's this sort of study that's prompted researchers to see how mindfulness practice might affect brain structure and function.

But let's back up a bit. What exactly do we mean by brain structure and function? And how do these relate to the idea of the mind, which we've been talking about throughout the course?

Different philosophical schools and approaches posit different relationships between the constructs of mind and brain. The way I'm using the terms, I mean mind to signify the information being processed and our subjective experience in consciousness moment to moment. Brain, on the other hand, involves what's going on in the underlying tissue structures. And what we're discovering is that the mind changes the brain, and the brain changes the mind.

Now, why do you think studying neurobiology or the brain might matter? Well, there's a number of reasons. Neurobiological studies are often what draw people to mindfulness practice these days. They think, oh, I'll be able to improve this or that aspect of my brain function or my brain structure. And they wind up, however, with a path to rather profound changes, even paths to psychological and emotional liberation.

There's a Zen kōan about this. Students are sent off to meditate on this and try to figure out what it means. "Intending to buy iron, they obtain gold." And one interpretation is people are drawn to these practices to try to fix something in their life, but what they wind up with is a rather profound personal and interpersonal transformation.

Also, by studying mindfulness and the effects of mindfulness on neurobiology, we get to see our mind as an impersonal process. We get to see that the thoughts and feelings that arise are actually just neurobiology unfolding.

Increasingly, neurobiology also gives us the idea of possible new interventions, for example, neurofeedback. There are some studies being done in which they connect a computer to an imaging machine so that a subject can get real-time feedback on what their brain is doing in each moment. And as a result, they're better able to train their brain in certain ways.

Now, scientists face many challenges in studying the neurobiology of mindfulness practices. And by reviewing them, we can understand that neurobiology better. The first question is, what do we want to look at? Are we interested in the momentary effects of mindfulness practice—in other words, what's happening in the brain while we're actually meditating—versus the enduring effects—what happens to our brain over time if we take up meditation practices? In psychological research, these are called *state effects* (the momentary ones) and *trait effects* (the more long-lasting ones).

Now, state effects and trait effects reinforce one another. Let's say we take up a behavior like mindfulness practice. Well, that's going to change the activity of the brain, and those changes in brain activity are actually going to change the structure of the brain. Then this changed structure of the brain is going to, in turn, change the activity of the brain, and this newly-revised activity of the brain is going to influence our behavior. So these things are reinforcing one another regularly.

So what are some of the challenges in studying the state effects? Well, there's a question of, what's the meditator actually doing as we're observing them? Is he or she concentrating on the breath, or perhaps enjoying a pleasant fantasy, or maybe even remembering to run an errand? Where exactly is the boundary between meditation and non-meditation?

If you ask a question of a person while they're in a scanner, simply hearing and answering the question changes brain activity. So maybe what we're measuring in terms of the moment-to-moment activity is simply the person's response to the question. These are difficult challenges.

When we study trait effects, the enduring changes, there are challenges there, too, because the way we study those is by looking at people who've been doing meditation over time and comparing them to people who haven't been doing meditation over time. But perhaps only certain people choose to meditate. Maybe the effects that we observe are because they're disproportionately vegetarian, or disproportionately highly educated. Or maybe it's because they've adopted a belief system.

And it's, of course, well nigh impossible to get random samples here. You can't very easily take a pair of identical twins, for example, and get one to meditate for 10 years and the other not to. Or for that matter, to randomly distribute people to 10 years of meditation practice or 10 years of a control group and study their brains afterwards. So these are tough challenges from a scientific standpoint.

There's a challenge that faces both state and trait studies, both the momentary studies and the "over a lifetime" effect studies: We don't know if people can accurately report on their degree of mindfulness. You may recall the Dunning-Kruger effect, where we discussed the way people who actually have less mindfulness practice experience tend to rate their level of mindfulness higher than people with more experience. And this is because a person needs some degree of mindfulness to be able to notice if he or she is being mindful, to notice what the mind is doing in each moment.

But if we didn't do self-report, what would the objective referent be? Currently, we're pretty much stuck with self-report. There are nine scales that are in use, and all of them ask people about their personal experiences and what they observe in their own minds. To complicate matters further, it turns out that they've found five factors, five elements in mindfulness practice, but these appear to be different depending on the experience levels. So some factors seem to develop more at lower levels of experience, and other factors seem to develop more at higher levels of experience.

If we weren't to use self-report scales, what might we use as a measure? Should we use the hours or years in meditation practice? It's a possibility. But we don't know exactly what the intensity of the meditation practice was or how well-trained the person was.

Also, until recently, we really didn't have good active controls. So what we would do is we would assign people to a meditation practice, or we might assign them to a waiting list. But we couldn't tell if the effects that we were measuring were actually the effects of doing the meditation, or simply getting attention for being in the study, or participating in part of a group, or maybe being exposed to a new belief system. And our sophisticated, high-tech equipment can't solve these kinds of problems.

Despite these challenges, we are learning something about the neurobiological changes. And we do this in part because we have several interesting methods for being able to study what's going on in the brain. One set of methods measures electrical activity. And our chief instrument here is the electroencephalogram or an EEG, and this is very sensitive to moment-to-moment changes.

The way we set up an EEG is we put hundreds—now, to do the high resolution kind—of electrodes all over the skull, and these electrodes can pick up very subtle movements in electrical activity. The problem with this is that the image we get is a bit blurry, because all of the electrical signals have to pass through the skull and pass through the skin.

So it's very hard to tell exactly where in the brain activity is taking place. On the other hand, the EEG is very sensitive to changes over time. We can see, in micro-detail, what's happening from moment to moment.

The other way we can look at what's happening in the brain is through neuroimaging, and there are essentially three types. First, there's PET scanning. That's Positron Emission Tomography. And it was used more in the early days. It detects radiation from emission of positrons. And the reason it's not used so often anymore in meditation studies is that these positrons decay, and you can only actually record what they're doing during the period of time that they're decaying. So you can only get very short videos of what's going on in the brain. Also, subjects aren't so keen about having radiation injected into them, so this has fallen a little bit into disuse.

Much more frequently used these days is Magnetic Resonance Imaging, or MRIs. What happens in an MRI is we're detecting a radio frequency signal that's emitted by excited hydrogen atoms in the body. And these are present in any tissue containing water molecules, including, of course, the brain. And using energy from an oscillating magnetic field that's applied at the appropriate resonant frequency, we're able to determine what's happening with those hydrogen atoms.

This provides excellent imaging for soft tissue, including the brain. The resolution is quite clear. But an MRI only takes a snapshot. So we only see what's happening at this particular moment in time.

The other instrument we have is called an fMRI, or a functional Magnetic Resonance Imaging machine, and this is like a video of an MRI. It takes a series of MRI pictures one right after the other. The video is somewhat jerky because there are slow refresh rates for the frames, and the resolution isn't quite as good as an MRI, but you can see what's happening in the brain in real time. And unlike PET scanning, which you could only do over brief period of time, you can do a functional MRI over 40 minutes or so. So we can get a long video about what's happening in the course of meditation practice.

So what have we learned? Well, we've learned a lot about changes in brain function. The first area that we've noticed changes in is attention. And this shouldn't be a surprise since, obviously, when we do meditation practice, the first thing we're doing is training the brain and training the mind to pay attention in a different way.

Now, attention has different components to it. It includes alerting, and that's becoming aware of a stimulus, like a horn honking or a baby screaming. And it also includes sustained attention, which is following a stimulus over time. Very closely related to sustained attention is the idea of conflict monitoring, which is about remaining focused despite distractions that are trying to pull our attention away.

We found that mindfulness practice improves both alerting and sustained attention. In fact, as little as eight weeks of training improve the detection of unexpected stimuli that were introduced in the laboratory. And it improved the ability to maintain attention on a stimulus over time.

A study of 3-month retreat participants—so these are folks who have spent the last three months doing sitting meditation, walking meditation, eating meditation, developing a lot of concentration—for those folks, they found reduced attentional blink. An attentional blink is the difficulty identifying a second stimulus when two are presented in rapid succession. If our minds aren't trained in mindfulness practice, we tend to miss the second one. But it turned out that the retreat participants tended to catch it.

A related study studied four Zen masters, people who had been at this for many, many years. And they showed that they had reduced habituation to stimuli. They hooked them up with an EEG, and they exposed them to clicking sounds. And people who aren't trained in meditation practice, after the first few clicks they start to zone out. They start not to notice the subsequent ones. For the Zen masters, each click was vibrant, had the same effect on the EEG over time. It's an interesting study in that it demonstrates that the Zen masters were developing what we're calling *beginner's mind*, this capacity to see each new event, each new experience, as though it's fresh and new rather than habituating to it.

Now, mindfulness meditation practice also seems to stave off all sorts of normal cognitive declines that are associated with aging. Older meditators have been shown to outperform age-matched participants, so other people of their same age but who haven't been meditating, on an attentional blink task, on tasks assessing attention, short-term memory, perceptual speed—how quickly they can recognize things—and executive functioning. Executive functioning has to do with decision making as to what's most relevant in a circumstance to pay attention to.

The investigators also reported that the typical negative correlation between age and sustained attention—as we get older, it's harder to follow a stimulus over time—wasn't present in Zen meditators.

A recent study addressed something a bit more sophisticated than this, a cognitive process that's more sophisticated called *fluid intelligence*. And fluid intelligence is our capacity to think logically and solve problems in novel situations independent of acquired knowledge. So it's our ability, really, to think on our feet rather than our ability to retain and recall facts.

And fluid intelligence involves analyzing the novel situation, identifying patterns and relationships that underpin the situation, and then extrapolating from these using our logical abilities. The study found that fluid intelligence declined more slowly in meditators than in age-matched controls.

And this is particularly crucial in today's world, where facts are easy to look up. You can Google anything. But interpreting them, figuring out what they mean, that's the challenge that we face. And it's nice to know that meditating can help to keep this faculty intact as we get older.

Now, different types of meditation seem to yield different results in terms of electroencephalogram patterns, brain wave patterns. In fact, Buddhist Lamas were asked to change from one type of meditation practice to another, and they wound up changing their brain wave patterns.

Let me tell you a little bit about brain wave patterns. They've been classified in bands based on frequency of brain waves. The fastest waves are called beta. And those occur when we're consciously alert, perhaps agitated, tense, and afraid—maybe too consciously alert in a sense. And those operate between 13 and 60 cycles per second, also called hertz.

A little bit slower are alpha waves. And those happen when we're entering states of physical and mental relaxation but are still quite awake and aware of our environment. And those are at 7 to 13 hertz. Slower still, we get into theta waves. And those are when we're beginning to really slow down, and we're beginning to move towards sleep and levels of reduced consciousness. And those happen between 4 and 7 hertz. And then there are the delta waves, and that's when we're headed into deep sleep. And those are at 0.1 to 4 hertz.

So deep relaxation, which occasionally happens during mindfulness practice, tends to be associated with high theta and delta waves, not surprisingly. What's interesting is that concentration and open monitoring, two of the three skills we've been talking about developing, they seem to be associated with high alpha and high beta waves. So that suggests that these states generally are highly-wakeful states.

And it's interesting because many people tend to think, oh, you know, meditation practice, that's all about calming down. Well, yes and no. It's about being calm, but it's also about being very alert. And among Tibetan monks, *mettā*, or loving-kindness practices, produce different patterns than other practices.

Now, to my mind, one of the most fascinating studies that's been done about brain wave activity and meditation, mindfulness meditation, was done by Richard Davidson at the Laboratory for Affective Neuroscience at the University of Wisconsin. I'd mentioned this study briefly earlier.

Over the years, he and his colleagues learned that when we're distressed, our brain activity tends to center on both the amygdala, that's the almond-shaped part of the brain that detects danger, and on the right prefrontal cortex, this region behind the forehead. And this region is particularly important for hypervigilance. An activity in one or the other areas tends to predict our daily moods.

So they did these high-resolution EEG studies, again, hundreds of electrodes around the skull, and they found that, in general, studying a broad population of people, there's a bell-shaped curve. And those folks who have more right prefrontal activation tended to be predisposed to clinical depression or anxiety. And those with more left prefrontal activation reported that their moods were rare or transient.

There's obviously a lot of survival value to right prefrontal activation because it's about hypervigilance. It's about being aware of the environment and scanning for danger. For psychological well-being, however, it's not so great. But historically, equanimity and feelings of peace didn't confer a big survival advantage.

So summarizing the differences between left prefrontal and right prefrontal cortical activity, when there's a lot of left prefrontal activity, people tend to report being happy, enthusiastic, and energized, kind of the opposite of depressed and anxious. And when there's right prefrontal activity, they're hypervigilant, depressed, or anxious. And this was studied initially in so-called normal individuals, also known as college sophomores, but it's since been replicated in older folks as well.

Now, what Richie Davidson found was after having tested 175 people in the lab and gotten that bell-shaped curve, he brought in a Tibetan Lama. And that Tibetan Lama had the most extreme value to the left in terms of left versus right prefrontal activation of anybody that had been measured to that point. Then they brought in other Tibetan monks over time, and they were all similarly very left-sided.

But Richie is a very good researcher, and he raised this question, he said, well, maybe it's people who have a lot of left prefrontal cortical activity are the ones who become monks in Tibet. Maybe we're simply measuring a pre-existing disposition.

So he got together with Jon Kabat-Zinn, and they took a group of stressed-out biotech workers and randomly assigned half of them to an eight-week mindfulness training course and half of them to just be on the wait list.

And before the course, everybody tipped right, because, indeed, they were stressed-out biotech workers.

After the course, the group that had gone through the course tipped left, but the others didn't. And the ones who had gone through the training had improved moods. They felt more engaged and more anxious. They also gave flu vaccines to both groups, and the immune response to the flu vaccine was much stronger in the folks who had been doing the meditation practice. So it appeared to help boost the functioning of our immune system.

If you were to look at the graphs that were published with this study, it's really quite striking. At time 1, before the mindfulness training course, the control group and the people who were going to go into the training looked very similar. At time 3, eight weeks after the mindfulness training course, you see dramatic differences between the leaning left on part of the folks who had been through the mindfulness training and leaning right for those who hadn't.

Now, another area of interest are regions of the prefrontal cortex, or the PFC, and this is associated with attention and executive decision making. And it's activated by a wide variety of practices. This is one of the few areas that have been examined in many different kinds of meditation. It turns out it's activated by Kundalini Yoga, by mindfulness meditation, but also by Tibetan Buddhist imagery practices, by Zen practices, and even Psalms recitation. So researchers are just beginning to investigate how these different forms of meditation might affect the brain differently. But it's clear, at this point, that all of these different practices have measurable effects on our neurobiology.

Now, other studies are showing that even within one type of meditation, different doses seem to have different effects. One study involved the anterior cingulate cortex or the ACC. And this revealed a particularly complicated, nonlinear response to meditation. Now, the ACC is involved in the integration of attention, motivation, and motor control. And this is what the researchers found. Non-meditators, complete beginners, show more activity in the ACC than Buddhist monks. OK. That suggests that meditation practice calms down the ACC. But they found that more regular, non-monastic meditators, laypeople who have been at this, show even more activity in the ACC than the non-meditators. So why does a lot of meditation on the part of monks yield very low ACC activity, trying meditation for the first time yields a bit more, but moderate experience shows the most ACC activity?

Well, one hypothesis is that for the monks, attention and motor control has become effortless. They become so good at it that they don't need a lot of activation of this part of the brain. While regular meditators know how to activate these circuits, but they have to still exert a lot of efforts to do it. And perhaps the novices show less activity because they don't really know at all how to activate these attention and control circuits. Clearly, we're just at the beginning of understanding how these things might work.

Now, the insula is a part of the brain that's associated with interoception or proprioceptive awareness, visceral or gut feelings, and it processes transient body sensations. We found that it's activated during mindfulness meditation. I mentioned earlier that it's important for empathy. It deals, in particular, with our visceral responses to the feelings of others and simulating inside what we're imagining is happening in another person, probably through the action of mirror neurons. And the fact that it's activated in mindfulness meditation suggests that mindfulness meditation should indeed help us to respond more empathically to others.

Now, there's been a recent study of patients with generalized anxiety disorder. And this study stands out because it used a really good control group, and it looks at the interface between neurobiology and a clinical disorder. Now, generalized anxiety disorder means pretty much being afraid of everything. It's not like a specific phobia, where you're afraid of snakes or dogs, perhaps, nor the kind of thing like difficulty with public speaking or going on airplanes. It's when we tend to feel fearful across the board.

Now, I've mentioned the amygdala. That's the almond-shaped part of the brain that's responsible for determining if stimuli are dangerous or not. Is it a lion, or is it a beige rock? Well, folks without anxiety problems and anxiety patients were both shown pictures of angry, neutral, and happy faces while in a functional MRI machine. And the anxiety patients showed higher amygdala activation than the people without anxiety in response to neutral but not angry faces. And that suggests that ambiguous stimuli—a neutral face where you can't quite tell what they're feeling—elicits a stronger fear reaction in these generalized anxiety disorder folks than it does in normal people.

And the anxiety patients were then randomized to either an eight-week mindfulness training or a stress reduction program. And the nice thing about this study was the stress reduction program was identical in structure—same amount of time, same amount of time in various activities—it was just instead of doing mindfulness training, they were training in other things. The amygdala reaction to neutral faces decreased more in the mindfulness meditation group than in the stress reduction group.

Now, the prefrontal cortex is part of the brain that evaluates emotional responses and regulates emotions. It thinks, yes, it does look like a lion, but lions aren't generally found around here, so it's probably a beige rock. And the researchers found that the activation of the prefrontal cortex, as well as the connectivity between the amygdala and the prefrontal cortex—suggesting the prefrontal cortex is regulating the effects of the amygdala—increased significantly more from before the intervention to afterwards in the mindfulness group, but not in the stress management group. Also, scores on measure of anxiety were lower in the mindfulness group.

So here, we see that mindfulness meditation activates parts of the brain that are essential for keeping our emotions in perspective and has the clinical effect of reducing excessive anxiety.

So now let's talk about brain structure. This is where the experience of my London cabbie comes in, because this is about experience-dependent neuroplasticity. I mentioned before that when I was in training many years ago, we used to believe that the brain reaches peak development at age 25 and deteriorates thereafter. Actually, the brain is much more like a muscle. If you use it, it bulks up. If you don't, it tends to wither.

And a lot of data beyond London taxi drivers' experiences has been accumulating. For example, people who learn to juggle and are scanned in an MRI, and three months later are scanned again, show changes in areas that detect visual motion.

Also, we see this in musicians. Professional musicians have more neuronal cell bodies or gray matter than amateurs in areas of the brain related to musical ability. And amateurs have more gray matter than people with no musical training. This is all evidence of brain plasticity. What we do with our attention really matters.

So remember why hair thinning isn't such a big deal? It's because aging and pathology are usually associated with cortical thinning, with losing gray matter in the cortex. And there was this landmark study in 2005 by my friend and colleague Sara Lazar at Mass General Hospital. She took 20 long-term Western meditators and age-matched controls. They had, on average, nine years of meditation experience. I was actually a subject in this. I wanted to give you an idea of what it felt like to participate.

I was slid headfirst, lying down, into a big MRI machine. And then a mirror was suspended above my eyes so I could see out through the opening where my feet extended into the outside world. And I could see written instructions. Then they turned on the machine, and it started this very loud, rhythmic clunking, and I was asked to do breath awareness practice. It was a bit challenging at first to meditate given the loud, rhythmic clanking. But after a while, it became just another stimulus, and I was able to develop some concentration. But one of the challenges they have in doing this kind of research is how to get experienced meditators not to practice meditation. Because when you've doing this for years, if you lie down somewhere, the natural tendency is to start following the breath.

So they had us try doing two different non-meditative activities. They had us lying there "doing nothing," and then they had us generating random numbers. And generating random numbers genuinely felt like a different state of consciousness than following my breath or trying to do nothing. Trying to do nothing was actually the hardest.

So what did Sara and her team discover? Well, they discovered that compared to age-matched controls, the meditators had thicker anterior insula, sensory cortex, and prefrontal cortex. And the differences in thickness where most pronounced in the older subjects. If you saw graphs of these, you'd see, in the meditators, going from age 20 up to age 50, things were pretty even. But in the non-meditators, you saw them decline. You saw thinning happening in these various areas.

Now, the three regions affected by meditation practices were all thought to be involved in integrating emotional and cognitive processes. The opposite development, decreased volume in at least one of the affective structures, the anterior insula, has been strongly implicated in several pathologies, including Post-Traumatic Stress Disorder or PTSD, social anxiety, specific phobias, and schizophrenia even. So we start to see that what's being maintained here when it shrinks is often associated with real difficulties.

Now, there are some limitations to this study: It had relatively small numbers, people were only imaged once, and maybe people who have naturally thicker cortexes are more likely to practice meditation. Nonetheless, the findings did fit expectations. The areas associated with paying attention to the breath and sensory stimuli and areas associated with the integration of thoughts and feelings had increased in thickness proportional to the amount of time people spent meditating in their lifetime.

To get beyond these limitations, we need to do pre-post studies. We need to be able to randomly assign people to meditation or non. And there has been one eight-week mindfulness course that was given to people with no meditation training, while a similar group was in a control group, and the researchers found increases in gray matter concentration within the left hippocampus and other areas.

Now, the hippocampus is involved not only in learning and memory, but also in emotion regulation. And in fact, it gets smaller in depression and anxiety, and stress seems to shrink it. So altogether, researchers concluded that participating in eight weeks of mindfulness training was associated with changes in gray matter concentration in brain regions involved in learning and memory processes, emotion regulation, self-referential processing, and perspective taking, all valuable things to experience.

So we're seeing that pre-post studies are showing that changes aren't just due to meditators being vegetarians or something else peculiar. Even when subjects are randomly assigned to mindfulness meditation or control groups, mindfulness training produces measurable changes in important brain regions.

In our next lecture, we're going to look at how mindfulness practices can help with a common problem in modern life—feeling lonely, isolated, or alienated from others. Thanks for listening.

Solitude—An Antidote to Loneliness
Lecture 10

Much of our psychological distress—and, in fact, many clinical disorders—are either caused or exacerbated by our sense that we're alone with it or that the problem itself marks us as defective, perhaps even unfit to participate in the human family. This can happen because of many factors, from being the victim of sexual or physical abuse to struggling with anxiety or depression. One reason why therapy groups can be so effective in helping people deal with their difficulties is that it helps us not feel so alone. Luckily, mindfulness practices can also help ease our sense of isolation.

Suffering in Isolation
- There's a problem in consumer economies, because the way in which we sell things to one another is by promising, in essence, happiness to the person that uses our product or service. One of the results of this is that we think if we're not happy, then it's our fault. This extends to things far beyond buying consumer products, including our choices about our spouse, career, and place of residence.

- Our psychiatric diagnostic system, unfortunately, just exacerbates the problem. We tend to think that if people are suffering, it must be because they're sick. This emphasis on individuality, as well as this emphasis on trying to acquire happiness, tends to create loneliness and alienation. We feel a chronic disconnection, and it results in a loss of energy and meaning for a lot of people—all sorts of negative self-images.

- Historically, religious belief and participation in religious groups helped us feel more connected. But that seems to be declining in modern cultures. People no longer have these natural senses of connection to community that we want to have.

- Mindfulness can help generate empathy and compassion, and both of these help us support intimate relationships. There's a school of psychology called relational-cultural theory that grew out of a feminist critique of conventional psychology. It was the work of Jean Baker Miller and Irene Stiver. They focused on the benefits of mutual connection rather than focusing on individual autonomy and individuation.

- They identified several different benefits of mutual connection. When people are connected to one another, they have more energy and vitality, a greater capacity to act, increased clarity, and enhanced self-worth (or self-efficacy). There's a natural desire and capacity for more connection. And we can use mindfulness practice to develop just this sense of connection.

- In our mindfulness practice, when we're with another human being, we try being aware of three objects of awareness. First, we are mindful of the sensations, thoughts, and feelings that are happening in "me." Second, we can be mindful of the words, body language, and mood of the other. Third, we can be mindful of the flow of relationship.

- When we do mindfulness practice, and we become aware of what's happening in "me" and in "you" and feel the sense of connection or disconnection, we tend to be able to adjust the relationship. When there's more of a sense of disconnection, we tend to find a way to come back together.

- Interpersonal connection fosters awareness of what Zen master Thich Nhat Hanh called "interbeing"—a connection to something larger than ourselves. We experience interbeing on many levels. It could be being part of a family, part of a neighborhood, or part of the natural and human world. It's a natural consequence of seeing our "self" clearly and noticing that this is simply an impermanent, ever-changing process that's wholly interconnected with the environment.

- This sense of interbeing has been noticed by human beings from time immemorial. In theistic terms, it's very often described as everything being part of God or "the divine." In nontheistic terms, it's seen much more in terms of everything being part of a universe of matter and energy or an ecological system.

- Religious mystics throughout the ages have noticed that our narrative, word-based thought tends to obscure this reality, the fact that we're living in the thought stream. What we're noticing through mindfulness practice is that, most of the time, we're simply living in this narrative about "me" and about what "I" want. Developing language for the separate objects in our experience is what obscures the reality of interbeing, or interconnectedness.

Suffering Together
- Through mindfulness practice, as the thought stream starts to become less and less relevant, we actually feel, in a moment-to-moment way, the interconnectedness of all things. This sense of interconnection, which mystics from various traditions have identified with their own cultural language, is what becomes available to us with mindfulness practice, and it gives us a profound sense of connecting to the larger world and to one another.

- Connecting to others and suffering together is central to all relational healing—to medicine, to the ministry, to parenting, and even to marriage and friendship. Appreciating the impersonal and universal quality of pain is part of how we do this, because we need to learn how to open to the other's pain as we open to our own. That's the power of therapy groups.

- There are many studies of the effects of mindfulness on relationships. Qualities of marriage were reportedly improved with mindfulness training adapted to couples. In addition, mindfulness practice improved stress-coping skills so that couples were able to handle difficulties in a way that didn't devolve into a fight. In addition, mindfulness improved day-to-day ratings of marital closeness and satisfaction.

- Other formal studies show that mindfulness skills enhance relationships, in part by helping us differentiate the experience of emotion from the enactment of emotion. This involves having a moment to take a breath before reacting. We're only able to do this if we have the capacity for increased affect tolerance. Being able to bear the other's upset feeling as well as our own is critical for this.

- The other thing that we get from mindfulness practice is we simply become aware of this full range of emotional experience, which is so important for empathy. Insula activation enables us to feel the mirror neuron activation and the awareness of the effects of the emotional exchange on the relationship.

Solitude

- One of the things that mindfulness practice allows us to do is be alone. And we don't often think about this in the modern world, but solitude can be a very, very powerful tool for not only developing our own awareness and appreciation of interbeing, but also for connecting us to others. The tendency for "I, me, me, mine" is dissolved somewhat in experiences of solitude.

- Isolation being a negative thing may be hardwired among us. After all, we're social primates. We evolved in groups, tribes, and bands. And when we're part of a group, to be separated from that group can be quite threatening. This is in part because we needed one another to survive in a hostile environment.

- Many of us live in urban environments, where we have few moments without interpersonal stimulation. So, being alone can bring up all sorts of difficult feelings for us. It can be quite disorienting.

- Sometimes being alone means feeling like a loser—feeling that lovable people aren't alone and that only losers are alone. When we're alone, the self can feel very threatened, in part because we think of ourselves as having been ostracized from the human family.

- It's also difficult because we know from child development that it's contact with others that provides our sense of emotional regulation. We use others to modulate our moods when we're having a hard time. It helps us create our sense of identity. And while Buddhist psychology is interested in dismantling that, most of us are kind of attached to our identity, which means that the other provides the protection of the primate troop or human group.

- In the modern day, many people are never alone, because they never have any time without their television, radio, or cell phone. This robs us of an opportunity to develop quite a lot of important skills.

- Most religions have recognized that solitude has enormous potential for spiritual development. And one common thread in spiritual development across many different religious traditions is the appreciation of interbeing. Almost all traditions have hermits, monks, nuns, or wandering ascetics, all of whom remove themselves from the hubbub of daily life in order to, in essence, experience interbeing.

- In doing this, they go through phases in which they face loneliness. Most serious inner explorers have had deep loneliness. They come face to face with feelings of being unloved, being alone, realizing that this life cycle is impermanent and that death is coming, and realizing that meaning is socially constructed. We see this in the stories of Jesus, Laozi, and the Buddha—all of whom went off alone to find paths to well-being.

- We can even have this experience in the course of our ordinary meditation practice. There's this tradition of noble silence, which involves not talking to others, not making eye contact, not doing all of the various things we do to interact. Even in the presence of a community, having this solitude gives a profound sense of interconnection as well as connection to one's own experience.

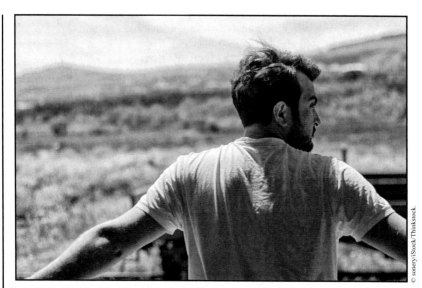
Mindfulness practice allows us to be alone, and solitude is important in relationships. We have to be comfortable with ourselves before we can be comfortable with other people.

- Loneliness is quite different from solitude. When we're lonely, we're longing for contact, and we see our aloneness as a mark of failure. We think that we're the only one. We feel vulnerable and unloved. And loneliness is usually imposed, not chosen.

- Solitude, on the other hand, is about valuing "being with" oneself, choosing it, and recognizing that it's part of our common humanity. Mindfulness—by reducing the self-focus and increasing our interest, curiosity, and awareness of interbeing—supports solitude over loneliness. It makes it so that when we're alone, we're much more likely to experience it as solitude than as loneliness.

- Our capacity for solitude is very important for intimacy, because if you can't be with yourself, alone, then you're not going to be able to be with another person.

- Solitude, at its most gratifying, connects us to the world outside of ourselves. And by removing the moorings of identity that we usually get in our social life, we have the option of seeing our part in the larger world, and this connects us to the big picture.

Suggested Reading

Brach, *Radical Acceptance.*

Kornfield, *A Path with Heart.*

Surrey and Jordan, "The Wisdom of Connection."

Tillich, *The Eternal Now.*

Questions to Consider

1. When in your life have you felt most lonely or alienated from others? What were the personal or cultural beliefs that contributed to your sense of isolation?

2. Try the breathing together exercise, either with another person physically present or with another person held as an image in the mind. Reflect on what happens. Did you feel more connected to the other person? What might keep you from feeling this connection more fully at other times?

Solitude—An Antidote to Loneliness
Lecture 10—Transcript

I'd like to share with you a well-known Buddhist teaching story. It's a painful tale, but it illustrates the importance and the universal truth about the value of connecting with others.

It's said that in the time of the Buddha, there was a woman who was nearly psychotic with grief because she had lost her only living son. And she was carrying his lifeless body, wailing, wandering around the village asking for help. And her friends and neighbors, they felt at a total loss. They felt her pain, but didn't know what to do until one gentleman suggested that she go over to the next valley, where a great teacher was camped out with his followers. So she did. She went over there and in the next valley, she found the Buddha surrounded by his monks.

She spoke to some of the monks and explained her situation and said, "Might I have a meeting with the great teacher?" And they arranged it, and she came and met with him. And she said, "I can't bear this. I just can't bear to be without my son. Can you possibly help me? Can you bring him back to life?" And the Buddhist said, "Well, I think I can help." And she said, "Tell me, tell me, what do I need to do?"

And he said, "Here's what you need to do. I need you to go back to the village and go to a neighbor's house and get from them a mustard seed, and then bring that mustard seed back to me." And mustard seeds, in the days of the Buddha, were extremely common. They were like salt and pepper or flour might be in a modern Western home. And she said, "Certainly, certainly, I'll go right away."

And as she turned to leave, he said, "Just one more thing. Just make sure when you get the mustard seed that you get it from a house where people are not suffering from some kind of a loss." She says, "OK, OK, I'll go." And she heads off to do that.

She comes back to the village and goes to the first neighbor's house, knocks on the door. The neighbor opens the door. She tells her story. And they're, of course, moved and willing to get the mustard seed right away. They come back with the mustard seed.

And she says, "Oh, oh, just one thing. I have to ask you, are you suffering here because of some sort of loss?" And the gentleman says, "Well, sort of. Our nephew, you see, he went off to town several days ago, and he was supposed to just transact some business and come right home. But he hasn't come home yet. And this isn't like him. He's a responsible young man. So we're worried that perhaps he was beset by bandits."

She thanked him and went on to the next house. At the next house, knocks again, tells her tale again. They come. They bring a mustard seed. She asks her question. They say, "Oh, well, you see, it's my aunt. She's actually here in the back room right now. And the doctor came yesterday, and he's not sure what's wrong, but he doesn't think she's going to last very long. We're really quite distressed about this."

And this is how the story unfolds. She goes from household to household. In each household, she receives a mustard seed, and in each household, she receives a story. And it's said that at the end of her rounds, after she had visited all of the houses in the village, she went back to the Buddha and said, "Thank you. I think I'm beginning to understand." And as the tale goes, she went on to become a great teacher in her own right.

Now, muster a psychological distress. And actually, many clinical disorders are either caused or exacerbated by our sense that we're alone with it, or that the problem itself marks us as defective, perhaps even unfit to participate in the human family. And this can happen from anything, from like being the victim of sexual or physical abuse, to even struggling with anxiety or depression. It's one reason why therapy groups can be so effective in helping people to deal with their difficulties. It helps us to not feel so alone. Luckily, mindfulness practices can also help to ease our sense of isolation.

Now, there's a problem in consumer economies generally, because the way in which we sell things to one another is by promising, in essence, if you buy my product or use my service, you're going to be happier. Now, other kinds of economies have their own difficulties, but this is a difficulty we certainly experience in ours.

And one of the results of this is we think if we're not happy, it's our fault. After all, when I'm marketing my own presentations that I do for mental health professionals, or even when the folks were marketing this course, the idea is if you have this experience, you're going to feel better. That's naturally how we sell things to one another.

But then if we find we're not happy, that becomes a real problem. And we start to think, I must have done something wrong. For example, if I'm watching, say, a Pepsi commercial, and everybody is smiling and laughing and playing volleyball on the beach, and that's not my experience, I, in essence, feel, what's wrong? I should have bought Pepsi instead of Coke, right? Or worse, if we did make the so-called right choice, then we think it's some kind of inherent weakness.

And this extends to things far beyond buying consumer products. We start to think, if only I had chosen a different spouse, if only I had chosen a different career, if only I was living in a different part of the world, then I'd be happy. It must be my fault that I've made a mistake like this.

And our psychiatric diagnostic system, unfortunately, just exacerbates the problem. We tend to think that if people are suffering, it must be because they're sick. And if you looked at the *Diagnostic and Statistical Manual* that we use for diagnoses, it covers absolutely everything a human being might experience.

So this emphasis on individuality, as well as this emphasis on trying to acquire happiness, tends to create loneliness and alienation. We feel a kind of chronic disconnection, and it results in a kind of loss of energy and meaning for a lot of people, all sorts of negative self-images. Think about what it was like as a kid. For so many of us, if we were alone on a Saturday night, and we assumed everybody else was out at the party, the thought processes goes to, what's wrong with me? Am I unlikeable? Am I unlovable?

Now, historically, religious belief and participation in religious groups helped us to feel more connected. But that seems to be declining in modern cultures. In the United States, for example, in 1950, only 2 percent of the population self-reported that they were religiously unaffiliated. By 2010, it was up to 16 percent of the population. And by 2012, if we look at younger people between the age of 18 and 39, 32 percent of the population says that they're unaffiliated. People no longer have these natural senses of connection to community that we once had.

So how might mindfulness help us with this? Well, we've discussed already how it can help to generate empathy and compassion, and those both help us to support intimate relationships. In this lecture, we're going to explore further how to use mindfulness and compassion practices to facilitate communication and connection, as well as to facilitate the capacity to be alone, which, as we'll see, is really necessary for being able to feel connected to others and connected to the wider world.

Now, there's a school of psychology called "relational-cultural theory" that grew out of dissatisfaction with the prevailing models that we had. And it came from a feminist critique, and it was started at Wellesley College. There's a center for psychology of women there. And it was the work of Jean Baker Miller, Irene Stiver. Many of you may know Carol Gilligan's work. She wrote a very well-known book called *In a Different Voice*, about how girls really are different in the world than boys.

And what they focused on here were the benefits of mutual connection rather than focusing on individual autonomy and individuation. And at the Stone Center, they identified several different benefits of mutual connection: that when people are connected to one another, they experience more energy and vitality; they have a greater capacity to act; they have increased clarity; the words they use as they say, "enhance self-worth," but I would say "enhance self-efficacy"—the feeling that I can handle life's challenges; and there's a natural desire and capacity for more connection that comes out of this.

Now, one of my friends and colleagues, Jan Surrey, has suggested a way that we can use mindfulness practice to develop just this sense of connection. And she suggests that in our mindfulness practice, when we're with another human being, we try being aware of three objects of awareness. First, I could be mindful of the sensations, thoughts, and feelings that are happening in me, as we normally do as we've been doing meditation practices. Then I can be mindful of the words, body language, and the mood of the other, of whoever I'm with at the moment. And then I could be mindful of the flow of relationship.

Now, let me explain this last part because it's a little bit tricky. We don't usually think about this so much. The best way I can illustrate this is from what happens very often in couples therapy. Many, many psychotherapists have had this example. And if I can use a kind of conventional heterosexual couple, typically what happens is it was the woman's idea to come into treatment. And she's sitting there with her husband, and she's really at her wit's end. And she's saying to her husband, "Honey, I just hate it. Every time I have some kind of difficult emotional experience and want to communicate with you, you disappear."

And the husband, really feeling quite confused, turns to his wife and says, "But sweetheart, I'm sitting right next to you." And the woman can't believe it. She rolls her eyes and she just says, "I don't mean you disappear geographically, you ninny. I mean you disappear emotionally." And the husband says, "But I'm here with you, honey. I'm listening." And they have this disconnect, because he really doesn't know what she is talking about. She's talking about this felt sense of connection or disconnection, and he doesn't really have a good, nuanced sense of what that's even about in a relationship.

When we do mindfulness practice, and we become aware of what's happening in me, what's happening in you, and this felt sense of connection or disconnection, we tend to be able to adjust the relationship—that when there's more of a sense of disconnection, to finding a way to come back together.

Now, there's a very powerful mindfulness exercise that's being used in recent years. It's not one that comes out of the Buddhist traditions. It's really a Western innovation called "breathing together." And the full practice is available for you as an audio recording included with the course, and I very much encourage you to try it.

What you do in this practice is, ideally, you do it with another person. And it can be somebody who you know well, or somebody you don't know so well. Perhaps it's somebody who's watching the course with you and has had some meditation experience at this point. Now, if you don't have the opportunity to do it with a physically present partner, it can still be done with a mental image of the other. You can simply call to mind another person who matters to you that you'd like to do this with.

This is the way the practice works. You're going to begin by practicing meditation, a breath-focused practice, facing one another with the eyes closed and simply notice the feelings that arise and pass. And the instructions for this are on the audio recording. What most of us notice is that it feels differently to us to be with our breath simply knowing that there's another human being across from us being with his or her breath.

And then what we do is we open the eyes a little bit, and we look at the other person's midsection or belly, just so that we can see the other person's breathing. And we try being with our own breathing as we notice the other breathing. That can be quite powerful simply to feel that we're in this together.

Then finally—and you'll be guided for this step by step in the audio recording—we start to go through the lifespan together, to consider our own experience and the experience of the other person beginning as a baby, wholly dependent on others, and having good fortunes and bad fortunes. Because, of course, we all have had good fortunes and bad fortunes at every stage in our development. And we go all the way through the life cycle, going to school, graduating, entering into family life, and all the way to the end of life. And as we do this together, we start to notice that, gosh, every one of us has in common joys and sorrows, victories and defeats, at every stage and at every transition.

I invite you to try this exercise because it can be very powerful. It's being used a lot in couples therapy these days, although you don't have to do it with somebody you're intimately involved with—it can be done with a friend or even an acquaintance. I often do it with groups. And it can be done with a stranger and be quite moving.

Usually what comes up is a kind of sadness about mortality, because we go through the whole life cycle and realize we're all in this together, but then an appreciation for the fact that we're all in this together. We all very much have in common this experience of birth, of going through so many joys and sorrows at every single developmental stage. And we start to notice how the way in which we understand other people is by connecting with what happened to us at those stages. In the Buddhist tradition, they talk about the 10,000 joys and sorrows as being the experience of living a life.

Now, this sort of interpersonal connection fosters awareness of what we might call *interbeing*. That's Thích Nhất Hạnh, the Zen master's word for this connection to something larger than ourselves. And we experience interbeing on many levels. It could be being part of a family, part of a neighborhood, part of the natural and human world. And it's a natural consequence of seeing ourselves clearly, as we've spoken about before, noticing that this is simply an impermanent, ever-changing process that's wholly interconnected with the environment, part of the superorganism of other human beings, and even the larger ecological system.

Now, Aldous Huxley used to talk about the perennial philosophy, because this sense of interbeing has been noticed by human beings from time immemorial. In theistic terms, it's very often described as everything being part of God or everything being part of the divine. In non-theistic terms, it's seen much more in terms of everything being part of a universe of matter and energy, atoms and molecules, or an ecological system, or the natural world.

Now, what many people have noticed—Huxley among them, and religious mystics throughout the ages—is that our narrative word-based thought tends to obscure this reality, the fact that we're living in the thought stream. What we're noticing through mindfulness practice is that, most of the time we're simply living in this narrative about me and narrative about what I want—that actually, the words are what obscure the reality of interbeing or interconnectedness.

Now, some people have even interpreted the Genesis story, the story of the Garden of Eden, as being about this, because in that story, Adam and Eve wind up eating of the Tree of Knowledge, right? And what is the Tree of

Knowledge? The Tree of Knowledge is about learning to distinguish good from evil and, in essence, separating this from that, to be able to say, this is me, that's you, that's a tree, that's a frog. And in developing language for the separate objects in our experience, we lose awareness of interbeing.

One of the things that happens through mindfulness practice, and you may not notice this initially, you need some depth of practice to get this, is as the thought stream starts to become less and less relevant, we actually feel, in a moment-to-moment way, the interconnectedness of all things.

When this first happened to me, I remember it was probably when I was in college, and I remember walking across campus. And I know this may sound peculiar, but it was as though there was no separation from what I thought of as my mind and the experience of the interconnected larger universe. It was as though walking through the trees, walking through the pathways, was like walking through my own mind.

And this sense of interconnection, which mystics from various traditions have identified with their own cultural language, is what becomes available to us with mindfulness practice, and it gives us a profound sense of connecting to the larger world and to one another.

Now, connecting to others and suffering together is central to all relational healing, to medicine, to the ministry, to parenting, even to marriage and friendship. And appreciating the impersonal and universal quality of pain is part of how we do this. Because what we need to learn how to do is to open to the other's pain as we open to our own in suffering together. That's what happened in the story of the mustard seed. That's the power of therapy groups. There's even a form of interpersonal mindfulness practice called "insight dialogue" that was developed by a fellow named Gregory Kramer who had many years of meditation practice, which is entirely about different exercises that are like the breathing together exercise in which we simply see all of our practice as an interpersonal practice.

There are many studies of the effects of mindfulness on relationships. And no surprise, they help. Qualities of marriage were reportedly improved with mindfulness training. It was adapted to couples therapy. People had improved stress-coping skills. They were able to handle difficulties in a way where it didn't devolve into a fight so easily. And mindfulness also improved day-to-day ratings of marital closeness and satisfaction.

It even works well for divorce. I have three friends that I've taught with on a number of occasions. And they're named Bill Morgan, Stephanie Morgan, and Susan Morgan. And when they're introduced, or when they show up on the brochure advertising the program, people are often curious, how did we wind up with three Morgans?

Well, here's the story. Bill used to be married to Stephanie. And they were married for many years, and they ran into difficulties as often happens, and they decided to separate, and then eventually to divorce. And it was a difficult period. They were both part of this group of people that I mentioned a while ago that for 30 years have been investigating mindfulness in psychotherapy in the Boston area. And for a little while, they weren't able to both participate in the group at the same time. They would alternate.

But they were both very serious about this mindfulness practice. And they were actually able to work with the difficult feelings about the divorce in such a way that they saw it as their own issues rather than all about being the other person's fault. Eventually, Stephanie remarried. Bill remarried somebody, who is now Susan Morgan. And the three of them are actually good friends and are able to interact with one another.

Now, that can happen outside of mindfulness practice. But I think it's an illustration of the power of these practices to help people to step out of their immediate desires, out of their narratives about selfing, and just see the whole picture and tolerate difficult feelings as they arise that allow them to have this kind of relationship together.

Other formal studies show that mindfulness skills enhance relationships, in part by helping us to differentiate the experience of emotion from the enactment of emotion. This involves having a moment to take a breath before reacting. You may have noticed in your own relationships that almost all the times when things go wrong it's because a feeling arises, and we immediately act on it and express something. And oftentimes, it just throws gasoline on the flames and things get worse.

And we're only able to do this, to not immediately express it, if we have the capacity for increased affect tolerance, the ability to be run through with a sword without blinking an eye. And being able to bear one another's upset feeling as well as our own is critical for this.

Now, the other thing that we get from mindfulness practice is we simply become aware of this full range of emotional experience, which is so important for empathy. We talked about the insula activation that's involved in this earlier. And it enables us to feel the mirror neuron activation and the awareness of the effects of the emotional exchange on the relationship.

Now, I mentioned earlier that one of the things that mindfulness practice allows us to do is actually allows us to be alone. And we don't often think about this in the modern world, but solitude can be a very, very powerful tool not only for developing our own awareness and appreciation of interbeing, but for connecting us to others. The tendency for I, me, me, mine, is actually dissolved somewhat in experiences of solitude.

I remember visiting Athens a number of years ago, and in the agora, in the marketplace, they had an exhibit of ostracon. Now, ostracon were these pottery shards on which a person's name was written down in ancient Greece if they had to leave the community, if they were going to be ostracized. And it was used in ancient Greece to try to regulate society and regulate people's social behavior. Basically, if you violated the rules, you were out.

Now, paleontologists suspect that this custom goes way, way back, because they find isolated campsites outside of the main settlement in prehistoric times. And the assumption is, these were folks who themselves were ostracized early on.

And this may well be hardwired among us. After all, we're social primates. We evolved in groups and tribes and bands. And when we're part of a group or a band or a tribe, to be separated from that group can be quite threatening. This is in part because we needed one another to survive in a hostile environment.

Now, many of us also live in urban environments, where we have few moments without interpersonal stimulation. So being alone can bring up all sorts of difficult feelings for us. It can be quite disorienting.

I mentioned the problem of being alone on Saturday night as a teenager. Sometimes being alone means feeling like a loser, feeling that, well, lovable people, they're not alone. Only losers, only rejects are alone. And when we're alone, self can feel very, very threatened in part because we think of ourselves as having been ostracized from the human family.

It's also difficult because we know from child development that it's actually contact with others that provides our sense of emotional regulation. We use others to modulate our moods when we're having a hard time. It helps us to create our sense of identity. And while Buddhist psychology is interested in dismantling that, most of us are kind of attached to our identity, thinking oh, I'm Ron. I'm a psychologist. I'm a dad, those kinds of things. You know, I tend to cling to them. And it means the other provides the protection of the primate troop or the human group.

Now, in the modern day, many people are never alone, because they never take any time without the television, the cell phone, my iPod. I'm busily texting, emailing, or perhaps playing video games and interacting with other imaginary figures in that way. And this actually robs us from an opportunity to develop quite a lot of important skills.

Now, most religions have recognized that solitude has enormous potential for spiritual development. And here, I'm going to look across many different religious traditions and say that one common thread in spiritual development is this appreciation of interbeing. And we see almost all traditions have hermits, and monks, and nuns, or wandering ascetics, all of whom remove themselves from the hubbub of daily life in order to, in essence, experience interbeing.

And in doing this, they go through phases in which they face loneliness. Most serious inner explorers have had deep loneliness. They come face to face with feelings of being unloved, of being alone, realizing that this life cycle is impermanent, that death is coming, and realizing that, in a certain way, it's meaningless—that meaning is socially constructed. And we see this in the stories of Jesus, of Lao Tzu, of the Buddha—they all went off alone to find paths to well-being.

Here's what's written about some of them. This is about Jesus from Matthew. "And when he had sent the multitudes away, he went up into a mountain apart to pray: and when the evening was come, he was … alone." And it's said that he spent 40 days and 40 nights alone. And what it says in Mark is, "And he was in the wilderness for 40 days, tempted [by] Satan; and [he] was with the wild beasts; and the angels ministered [to] him."

We'll see that the same theme occurs with other great spiritual leaders. Lao Tzu said, "Ordinary men hate solitude. But the master makes use of it, embracing his aloneness, realizing he is one with the whole universe."

And the Buddha is said to also have gone into solitary meditation under the Bodhi Tree for some 49 days and nights. Apparently, 40 meant a very long time in the Axial Age, when both the Buddha and Jesus lived. And it's said that that's where he attained enlightenment. And what he said was, "I will not leave this spot until I find an end to suffering." And under the Bodhi Tree, what's reported is he said this, "Having tasted the sweetness of inner solitude and calmness, he who lives by the Dharma [the natural law] is free from fear and suffering."

Now, we see this in radical forms in the Tibetan tradition. There's this tradition of going off into a hut and living completely isolated for many years. And here's what a woman, Alexandra David-Neel, who in 1924 went from England to study with the Tibetan Lamas, here's what she said. She said,

Words cannot convey almost the almost voluptuous sweetness of feelings experienced when one closes the door of one's *tsams khang* [that's the hermitage hut] … or when one looks down from the heights at the first wintry snow heaping up in the lower valleys, creating for months around the hermitage an impassable white and cold rampart.

Now, we can even have this experience in the course of our ordinary meditation practice. There's this tradition of noble silence, which is not talking to others, not making eye contact, not doing all of the various things we do to interact. And I can tell you from my own experience in retreat that even though we're among other people, having this solitude gives a profound sense of interconnection as well as connection to one's own experience—and these experiences open up—of really feeling part of interbeing.

Now, loneliness is quite different from solitude. When we're lonely, we're longing for contact, and we see our aloneness as a mark of failure. We think we're the only one. We feel vulnerable and unloved. And loneliness is usually imposed, not chosen.

Solitude, on the other hand, is about valuing being with oneself, choosing it, recognizing that it's part of our common humanity. Mindfulness, by reducing the self-focus and increasing our interest and curiosity and awareness of interbeing, supports solitude over loneliness. It makes it so that when we're alone, we're much more likely to experience it as solitude than as loneliness.

Now, our capacity for solitude is very important for intimacy, because if I can't be with me, alone, I'm not going to be able to be with you. And we've all seen this in relationships. You see it somewhat more in younger people, but it can happen when we're older as well.

If I feel like I desperately need to be with you to feel OK, then as soon as we have some kind of disharmony, as soon as you're not quite with me, or you're angry with me, I collapse, and I have a desperate need to make you be different. And I don't have the flexibility to really listen to what's going on. In fact, this kind of desperation can sometimes lead to power imbalances, where one person will basically give away more and more of his or her rights in the relationship just because they're so desperate not to be left.

Solitude, at its most gratifying, connects us to the world outside of ourselves. And by removing the moorings of identity that we usually get in our social life, we actually have the option of seeing our part in the larger world, and this connects us to the big picture.

So I ask you to take a moment to reflect on what connects you to the big picture. What helps you to identify with something larger than yourself? Is it nature? Is it friends and family and community? Perhaps it's a time with a spiritual teacher, somebody who's so interconnected him or herself that just being in their presence brings up this feeling for you? Or is it a connection to a religious figure or tradition, Jesus, the Buddha, Mohammed, Moses, Lao Tzu?

And what activities help you feel connected to something larger than yourself? Is it prayer? Have you found this yet through meditation or mindfulness practice, or perhaps spending time in nature talking with a friend, hugging an animal, reading scripture, or producing art? We want to inquire and notice what helps us so that when we're in solitude, we have this experience of interbeing.

And when we can be with ourselves, then we can really be with others, because if I can tolerate my own experience, then whatever happens in you, I can both be there with and for you. As Paul Tillich put it, "One hour of solitude may bring us closer to those we love than many hours of communication."

So in our next lecture, we're going to talk about connecting with a particular type of person: children and adolescents. Thanks for being here.

Connecting with Children and Adolescents
Lecture 11

C hildren live in different cultures from adults, even if they are raised by their biological parents. They have different understandings of how the world works and different ways of coping with difficult situations. Therefore, mindfulness practices, which are typically geared toward adults, need to be modified to mesh with the culture of the child. In this lecture, you will learn how mindfulness practices can help adults enter the child's world and how various practices can be tailored to fit the child's world.

Differences between Children and Adults

- Compared to adults, children live in a culture with a different sense of time. The younger the child, the more he or she tends to live in the present. Children are able to remember the past in a way that they can't when they're younger, and this continues until they reach adulthood, when they are virtually never in the present. They're always thinking about the past and the future.

- Children often also have a different sense of reality. The younger the child, the more he or she lives in fantasy. Selma Fraiberg, who is one of the leading clinicians studying younger children, called these the magic years, in which fantasy and reality are fluidly intermixed in younger children.

- They also have a different use of language. The younger the child, the less his or her world is created by words and concepts. They're involved in moment-to-moment sensory experience. As they get older, they become more attached to language.

- In a certain way, children have more of a beginner's mind. They're more fresh and open to experience. By cultivating a beginner's mind, mindfulness practices help us to enter their world. They help bring us into the present. They help us see reality as fluid, because we're not so attached to our particular thought forms. And they help us to be less attached to words.

- What is the difference between work and play? Work is more goal oriented than play. Work, of course, we do based on others' demands, rather than whatever is arising internally, like we do with play. And work definitely favors results over process, while play favors process over results.

- We can think of play as being the work of children, but many of us forget how to play as adults. We become so focused on goal orientation that it's difficult for us to fully participate with children.

- Mindfulness practices can help us with this, because they develop a kind of playfulness. They can help open us up to nonverbal communication, and they can facilitate "being with" silence, because often children just want to be silent and have us be with them. They can also help us tolerate repetition, which is sometimes involved when children are playing. For example, a child might repeatedly request that you read *Goodnight Moon* to him or her.

How Mindfulness Helps Caregivers

- There is a tremendous amount of research that shows that it is, in essence, adult presence that regulates children's arousal and helps children learn their own emotional regulation skills. In other words, adults provide emotional regulation for children. If we are with an upset child and we get upset about their being upset, it tends to go poorly. But if we can accept distress, the children we are with can accept distress. This inner stability is particularly essential when words aren't as powerful.

- In the Buddhist tradition, it is said that if you practice mindfulness diligently enough, you'll become aware of what are called mind moments, which are the shortest periods of time that the mind can be conscious of. We can't think about being responsive to children; we have to develop this kind of inner attunement and stability.

- Mindfulness can help caregivers provide the kind of environment that children need to flourish. Caregivers have to support firm, consistent, and appropriate limits and to be able to be empathic, connected, and loving. However, this is much easier said than done.

- Mindfulness practices can help us to respond more appropriately to misbehavior—to not make so many of the automatic errors that get us into trouble. It's very difficult not to get angry and act out of anger when children misbehave. Action so quickly follows affect that we don't even have vocabulary for the difference between feeling anger and enacting anger. Mindfulness practices allow us a moment to take a breath, which can be essential for responding effectively to children.

- Children enroll adults in very sophisticated behavior-modification programs. They basically train us to yell and to give in. In fact, we get positively reinforced every time that we give in. Children enroll us in these projects quite regularly. And they have pretty big brains. They can devote about 100 percent of their resources toward training their parents. This is why their behavior-modification programs typically work out so much better than ours do.

- Most of our parenting mistakes occur when we take our children's behavior personally. Our errors are compounded by self-hatred over what Trudy Goodman calls parenting crimes, which are all the things that we do in raising children that we absolutely can't believe that we did.

- Convicting ourselves of parenting crimes is rarely helpful. Mindfulness—particularly acceptance—can help us begin to let go of these judgments. Mindfulness can help us just notice the feelings and thoughts arising, and it can help us relate to our child as we might relate to another person's child, where we might not take it so personally.

Mindfulness Exercises for Children

- Mindfulness practices for parents and other caregivers can help them take care of children. There are also practices that we can teach to children directly. There is a wealth of these that has been developed, but you can also invent your own.

- The basic principle is to think about how children are different from adults and how you have to adjust the practices to meet their needs. One way that children differ from adults is that they tend to have a shorter attention span. So, in general, the mindfulness practices we're going to design for children are going to be shorter than the ones we would do for adults.

- Another way that children are different is that they tend to like more vivid stimuli. Children are going to gravitate more readily toward coarse stimuli, like the sensations of walking meditation or eating meditation, versus more subtle ones, like the sensations of the breath in the body or the tip of the nose.

- When we design environments for young children, they often have bright, primary colors and very clear shapes. These stimuli generally resonate well with children, especially compared to the subtle shapes and pastels that attract adults.

- One of the mindfulness exercises we can do with children is called three breaths. This is analogous to something called the three-minute breathing space, which is part of the system known as mindfulness-based cognitive therapy. When we're with a child, you can say, "Stop whatever you're doing just for a moment and take three breaths." Then, you simply ask the child, "What did you notice happening in your mind and body during that time?"

- This simple exercise helps to tune children in to their current sensations—to what's happening on a body level and what thoughts are arising and passing. Most of the time, children never take a moment to look inside. This is a very simple exercise that can be done with virtually any children.

- Another exercise is called apple meditation, which is very similar to eating meditation and uses an apple. We can take this as an opportunity for inquiry into inter-being and ask the child, "Where did the apple come from? How did it get to the store? Where did the tree come from? What nourished the tree? How many people have helped the apple to arrive in your hand?" Following that inquiry, we simply eat the apple as an eating meditation, paying attention to each bite and the sensations.

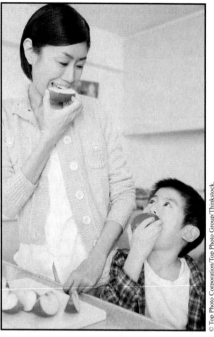

© Top Photo Corporation/Top Photo Group/Thinkstock.

Apple meditation, the practice of eating an apple mindfully, can be very rewarding.

- We can also modify loving-kindness practice to work with children. You tell the child, "Remember something you did that makes you feel glad inside. Send a smile into your whole body, and let the feeling of happiness, peace, kindness, and love spread from your heart through your whole body."

- Then, much as we do with other loving-kindness practices for grown-ups, we send these feelings to other people in the family. Sending them to a pet works well with children, or they can send them to a friend. Then, they can send them to their whole class, to their neighborhood, to the country, or even to the whole world.

- Another practice that is great to use with children is called the bell-in-space meditation, which basically uses a bell as a vivid object of awareness. In addition to these practices, you can invent your own practices. And the younger the child, the shorter the time and the more intense the stimulation should be. The older the child, the more you can use practices that are like those we use for adults.

Suggested Reading

Goodman, "Working with Children."

Goodman, Greenland, and Siegel, "Mindful Parenting as a Path to Wisdom and Compassion."

Kabat-Zinn and Kabat-Zinn, *Everyday Blessings*.

Siegel, *The Mindfulness Solution*, chapter 12.

Questions to Consider

1. In what ways is the culture or world of children different from that of adults? How might mindfulness practices help us enter their world?

2. In your experience caring for children, in what circumstances have you found yourself becoming most unproductively reactive? How might mindfulness practices help you have a more skillful response?

Mindfulness Practice

apple meditation: A version of eating meditation suitable for children that uses a vivid object of awareness and encourages reflection on the interrelated nature of all things.

bell in space: An easily accessed mindfulness practice for children. They can be given the instruction to count the bells (which may help younger children to remain attentive) or simply to listen to them.

loving-kindness practice for children: An adaptation of this foundational practice for cultivating acceptance using language and imagery suitable for children.

three breaths: A very brief exercise suitable for children to help them notice their experience in the present moment.

wake up your senses: A brief practice for children designed to help them step out of the thought stream and become conscious of bodily sensations.

Connecting with Children and Adolescents
Lecture 11—Transcript

For about 25 years, I worked in child community mental health, most of that time, as the Chief Psychologist of a mental health center that treated people from diverse cultures, as well as diverse economic backgrounds. And in that kind of environment, we pay a lot of attention to culture. And one of the things that occurred to me is that kids actually live in different cultures from adults, even if the child is raised in a family that's his or her biological parents, and in a consistent ethnicity.

Kids, for example, live in a culture with a different sense of time. And the younger the child, the more they tend to live in the present. I remember when my own twin daughters were around age two, and were starting to get into that phase that's often affectionately called the terrible twos, I asked a friend of mine that I was teaching a course with, who is a developmental psychologist, "What's up with this? What's going on?" And she said, "The way I understand it, is it's simply cognitive maturation that results in the terrible twos."

I said, "How does that work?" And this is what she explained. If I have a child who is about one year of age, and the child is beginning to be upset, or cranky, or crying, or difficult, we might say, "Oh, look at Teddy." And the child turns his or her attention to Teddy. "Teddy's dancing!" And after a few moments, the problem is solved. But once a child reaches the level of cognitive development that you get around age two, and the child starts to fuss, and they might have language by now and they start to complain, and you say, "Hey, look at Teddy. Teddy's dancing!" And the child looks at Teddy, and they say, "Now give it to me." What happens is kids are able to remember the past in a way that they can't when they're younger. And this continues throughout the developmental lines, and the developmental life cycle, until they reach adulthood. And by the time kids reach adulthood, they are virtually never in the present. They're always thinking about the past and the future, like the rest of us.

Kids often also have a different sense of reality. The younger the child, the more they live in what we might call fantasy. Selma Fraiberg, who is one of the leading clinicians studying younger children, called these the "magic years" in which what we think of as fantasy and reality are fluidly intermixed in younger children.

And they also have a different use of language. The younger the child, the less their world is created by words and concepts. And we know this. They're involved in moment-to-moment sensory experience. When we play with a very young child, they're often just playing with the dolls or the dinosaurs or the cars, or whatever it might be, and they don't need to talk a great deal. As they get older, they become more attached to language.

Now you may recall Suzuki Roshi's famous line that "in the beginner's mind, there are many possibilities; in the expert's mind, there are few." In a certain way, kids have more of a beginner's mind. They're more fresh. They're more open to experience. Mindfulness practices, by cultivating beginner's mind, actually helps us to enter their world. It helps to bring us into the present, which is where the kids are living. It helps us to see reality as fluid, because we're not so attached to our particular thought forms. We see thoughts as coming and going, coming and going. So the difference between the narrative that we associate as reality, and the narrative that we associate as fantasy, becomes less important. And they help us to be less attached to words. And this makes it much easier to be really intimate with kids.

Now, I often ask groups of psychotherapists, what's the difference between work and play? And they come up with different ideas. I ask you to think about that for a moment. Can you think about, what are some of the qualities of work that are different from qualities of play? Most people come to the conclusion that, well, work is definitely more goal-oriented. After all, there's a product at the end of it. It's about doing something. It's not about just being there. The idea is to be producing something. Work, of course, we do based on others' demands, rather than whatever is arising internally. And work definitely favors results over process, while play really favors process over results.

Of course, we can think of play as being the work of kids—and indeed, it is what they do with much of their time—but many of us forget how to play as adults. We become so focused on goal orientation, that it's hard for us to be with kids, and to fully participate with them, and follow them in whatever enjoyable, fantastic activity they're involved in.

Mindfulness practices actually can help us with this. Because mindfulness practices, by helping us to step out of the thought stream, and be in the present moment, develops a kind of playfulness. The Dalai Lama, for example, if you spend any time with him, he's always laughing. He sees humor and folly in all sorts of matters, including very serious ones. So because of this, mindfulness practices can help us to connect with kids. They can help to open us to non-verbal communication. They also help us to be with silence, because oftentimes kids want to just be silent, and have us be with them.

I don't know if you were ever involved with bedtime rituals, or you have been involved, with the child. For example, they wash up and it's time for reading them a story of some sort. And the child is really, really excited, because they really, really want to have the 239th reading of Goodnight Moon. And as an adult, we may be thinking, well, sweetheart I kind of know how that one turns out. How about this book you haven't heard? They say, no, no, no, I really want Goodnight Moon. Because, for them, it's fresh each time. They're able to approach it with beginner's mind. Even though, cognitively, they now how the story turns out.

If, in the course of our meditation practice, we can develop interest and curiosity in the one-thousandth breath that's arising in the body during this course of meditation, then we can certainly get interested in the 239th reading of Goodnight Moon. It helps us to be present. And we know this intuitively. People who are really good with kids are able to be with kids in these ways.

Now I learned something else in my years in community mental health, working with kids. It seemed to me that if I were an excellent therapist, and was having a really good day and I could resolve, let's call it one unit of distress or past trauma in a 50 minute session with a child that I had a great working relationship with. But if that child went home and accumulates, let's call it one-and-a-half units of distress in between sessions, what's the trajectory going to look like over time? Not so good.

The alternative is to, in essence for children, supply sufficient light, sufficient water, fertilizer. Don't pluck them up by the roots, and most kids will thrive. Now of course, there were children, and we ran across these, who had had traumatic experiences, or periods of deprivation that were so serious, that even putting them in a nurturing and enriching environment, they needed other kinds of work to help to process what had happened in the past. But an awful lot of kids, if we simply construct a salutary environment around them, they start to do quite well.

So one of the things that we started doing in child community mental health was to shift from thinking that what we're trying to do is treat children, to trying to provide environments around children that were going to foster their wellbeing. And the idea was to basically help parents, and teachers, and other caregivers, to be present for kids in a way that was going to be helpful for them. And there's a tremendous amount of research that's come out that shows that it's, in essence, adult presence that regulates children's arousal, and helps children learn their own emotional regulation skills. Let me give you an example from a very different arena of how this works.

Thích Nhất Hạnh tells a story about people fleeing Vietnam at the end of the Vietnamese War. And it was a terrible scene. They were being hurried onto these refugee boats. Often, they had no idea where their family or friends were. Very often, they had experienced some kind of horrible, horrible trauma, seen terrible things in combat, seen people do abusive things to one another. They really didn't know much about their destiny.

They had heard rumors that the boats were often subject to pirates, and they were headed off to uncertain shores. There weren't even clear agreements about which countries were going to let them in. This was a very rough circumstance. And these boats were overcrowded, to boot.

Now, what Thích Nhất Hạnh reported—and he heard this from refugees who had had this experience—was that people's sense of well-being was determined in large part, by who they were near on the boat. Let's say there was a person on one of these refugee boats who had a sense of center to them. Perhaps they were a monk or a nun, who had done a great deal of mindfulness practice. Perhaps they were simply somebody who had come across and developed a sense of equanimity from other pathways.

And what you could see is, on the boats, if there was somebody who had this kind of equanimity, there would be kind of concentric circles of other people around this person, who were more or less centered, who were more or less feeling a sense of being OK. Conversely, if there was somebody who was flailing about, in anxiety or anger, or some other form distress, you could see concentric circles around that person, of people looking more distressed.

Now in the same way that it functioned on the refugee boats, adults provide this kind of emotional regulation for kids. We know this. If we are with an upset child, and we get upset about their being upset, it tends to go poorly. If we are with an upset child, and we're able to contain and hold this sense of feeling our emotional reaction to them, and being present to them, the child almost always settles down. If we can accept distress, the children we are with can accept distress.

So this inner stability is particularly essential when words aren't available to us. There's a psychologist and researcher named Ed Tronick in the Boston area, and he's devised a technique, which is really quite fascinating, for studying how parents affect children, and how children affect parents. And what they'll do is they'll take two video cameras. And one of them, they'll train on a parent—often the mother. And the other one, they'll train on the child—usually a young child, around one year of age or so. And then they notice what happens between the two of them.

They run the tapes. They record what happens. And then they slow it down, so they can see what they call microcommunications. And these microcommunications occur up to 10 times a second. So, the baby gestures, the mother responds to that gesture. The baby then responds to the mother's response, and then the mother responds to the baby's response to her. And it just keeps going on like this.

Now, in the Buddhist tradition, it said that if you practice mindfulness diligently enough, you'll become aware of what are called *mind moments*. And a mind moment is the shortest period of time that the mind can be conscious of. They didn't have cesium clocks in the days of the Buddha. The way they described it is, a mind moment is one ten-thousandth of the time it takes a bubble to burst. It's very quick. Now, this is obviously much too fast to follow consciously. We can't think about being responsive to kids. We have to develop this kind of inner attunement and stability, in order to be there.

Now, you may notice as I'm talking about this, that I'm not focusing particularly on teaching mindfulness practices to kids, although we'll discuss that in a bit. I'm talking about mindfulness for caregivers, so that caregivers can provide the kind of environment that kids need to flourish, so that we can enhance connection, empathy, and love.

Now, if you would read a manual of parent guidance, virtually every manual says you have to do two things to take care of kids well: We have to support firm, consistent, and appropriate limits, to be able to say no effectively; and to be able to be empathic, connected, and loving. And if you've ever tried to take care of kids, you know that this is much easier said than done.

One of my favorite cartoons about this shows two magic markers, one obviously older than the other. And one magic marker has his cap on, but he's holding another cap. And then you see the younger magic marker is scurrying away without his cap. And the, apparently, father magic marker says, "You're not leaving this house without your cap on, young man. Don't you know that 90 percent of your moisture escapes through your head?"

Well, even if we're not magic markers, we've all been in this kind of situation where we're trying to discipline a child, trying to get them to listen, and it's not necessarily working so well. Very often, we find it frustrating. Whether the child is four years old or 14 years old, if a child isn't listening to us and we're involved in struggling, we often can make mistakes and get into trouble.

One of my favorite posters, which I recommend you print up for yourself if you have teenagers at home, and just post it on the fridge or somewhere, goes like this—it's a banner, it says, "Attention teenagers: Tired of being harassed by your stupid parents? Act now! Move out, get a job, pay your own bills—while you still know everything."

Mindfulness practices can help us to respond more appropriately to misbehavior, to not make so many of the automatic errors that get us into trouble. Another one of my favorite cartoons has a picture of two sons, one older than the other. You know, stars out there in the sky. And the younger one says, "As a matter of fact, the world does revolve around me." And the caption is, "This is the problem with raising a sun." It's very hard not to get angry and act out of anger when kids misbehave.

But mindfulness practices can help us with this. Let me give you an example. If I were to say to you, "Yesterday, I got really angry." And had you been there with me, what might have you observed? Just take a moment to think about that. When I ask audiences, they typically say, "Well, I would have seen you raise your voice, or perhaps, get red in the face, or look agitated, or say mean words."

It's actually a little bit of a trick question. Because I could have meant one of two very different things when I say, "Yesterday, I got really angry." I could have meant—and we don't even have good language in English to describe this, because we don't think this way—I could have meant, "Yesterday, I experienced anger arising in the mind and body." Or I could have meant, "Yesterday, I acted very angrily."

We're so accustomed to the emotion bringing us to action, which follows the emotion immediately, that we don't even have vocabulary for the difference between feeling anger and enacting anger. Mindfulness practices allow us a moment to take a breath. And this taking a breath can be essential for responding effectively to kids.

Now, if you've ever taken care of children, you know that children enroll adults in very sophisticated behavior modification programs. They basically train us to yell, and they train us to give in. This is how it works. Let's say, for example, you're at the supermarket and you have a five-year-old child with you, and you've just finished shopping for dinner. And as you approach the checkout counter it just so happens, for random reasons, that there's an

18-inch multicolored, absolutely gorgeous lollipop at a five-year-old level. And your child looks up and says, "Oh, oh, it's beautiful. Could I? Could I— could I have it just this once?"

And you say, in a very reasonable way, "Oh, sweetheart, I agree it's a lovely lollipop. But we've just purchased things for dinner, and in fact, remember, we just bought your favorite ice cream for dessert. So tonight wouldn't be a great time to have the lollipop. I don't want you to spoil your appetite." And then the child says, "Oh, oh, but please, please. It's so lovely. I just want— I'll just have a little of it. I promise! I promise! I promise!"

And you say, "Honey pie, as we've recently reviewed, we've purchased the ingredients we need for dinner. We have your favorite ice cream. And today would not be an appropriate day to buy the lollipop." And then, the child goes, "[Crying.] Wah! Oh, please, please. Wah! You don't love me! You know, if it were Susie, you'd get it for her! You love her better than you love me!"

And what's hard to admit to yourself, certainly not to the child, is you know, often you kind of do love Susie more than you love him, because Susie doesn't do this kind of thing. Unable to bear that, you break down and you buy the lollipop. What's going to happen the next time you come into a supermarket and the kid wants something? You know how that turns out.

They also train us to give in. And this happens in countless different forms. Let's say, it's the evening and you're going to go to your mother's house with your child. And you come in about 15 minutes prior to leaving, and say, "Oh, sweetie, please start picking up your toys, and wash up, and go to the bathroom because we're going to leave to grandma's house in 15 minutes, and we don't want to be late because she's just cooked us a lovely dinner."

So you walk out of the room, and you go tend to some things you need to do to get ready. And you come back after five minutes, and nothing's happened. You say, "Well, honey, please. Now's the time to start getting ready. You've got to put things away and wash up, because we really don't want to be late." You walk out of the room again.

You come back in, five minutes to go, and you've had it. The kid's done nothing and you start screaming. "Darn! I told you to do this! You always do this to me! You get me agitated! Now we're going to be late, and I'm upset on top of it!" And at that point, the child picks up and starts putting away the toys, and getting ready.

So what happens is we get positively reinforced every time that we give in. By buying the lollipop, the child calmed down right away, and things were fine. Going to grandma's house, we get positively reinforced for yelling, because then the kid starts picking up the toys.

Now, kids enroll in these projects quite regularly. And they have pretty big brains. They can devote about 100 percent of their resources toward training their parents. We're busy having to make dinner, having to earn a living, do these kinds of things, so that's why their behavior modification programs typically work out so much better than ours do.

Now the other thing that happens, time and again, is taking things personally. Most of our parenting mistakes occur when we take our kids' behavior personally. And they lead us into what my colleague and friend, Trudy Goodman calls, "parenting crimes." Now, parenting crimes are all the things that we do in raising children that we absolutely can't believe that we did.

I'll tell you, if you happen to be a clinical psychologist, or a clinical psychologist who has done child work, committing these parenting crimes is even more difficult to bear because we develop self-hatred thinking, "I can't believe that I did such a thing." And then, we react out of that self-hatred with even more bad behavior, basically.

In my years of working with families that had abuse within them, particularly the ones with physical abuse, almost all of the times when parents were physically abusive to their kids, it's because they felt humiliated. They couldn't bear the thought that their kid wasn't listening to them, and what that meant about the parent, and the parent's confidence, and the parent's own self-esteem. And it was out of that feeling of humiliation that then they lashed out and did something really problematic.

So mindfulness practice can help us here. Mindfulness practice can help us to begin to let go of these judgments, to just notice the feelings arising, notice the thoughts arising, and in fact, they can help us to relate to our child as we might relate to another person's child, where we weren't taking it so personally.

Let me give you an example. I moved to a town when my kids were entering the first grade. And the town is kind of nice. It has a lot of conservation land so it attracts people who really enjoy the outdoors. And I discovered that the town has community hikes. And my wife and I thought, that's wonderful, we'll go with our family on one of these community hikes. And we were involved in the hike. And we were going up the mountain, and my kids seemed to be doing pretty well at the beginning. But as time went on, it got kind of buggy, it kind of got hot and humid, and they started having more and more difficulty. In fact, they were clearly having more difficulty than the other children on the hike, their same age.

So my wife and I were somewhat disturbed about this, and we started to become less than optimally skillful in handling our kids. At which point, Katie said—she's a member of the community who had been there longer than us—she said, "It's very sweet that you have been hiking with your kids, but if you want, it's also fine—you could hike with other groups. We kind of mix it up and take care of each other kids."

And my wife and I realized, that might not be the worst idea on this occasion. So we separated. And we continued the hike, and maybe 40 minutes or 45 minutes later, we get to the top. And there are my kids, laughing and playing, and doing great—none of the meltdown problems that they were having when they were there with my wife and I. And I ask myself what had happened?

Now, of course, Katie wasn't so familiar to them, so they were probably more on their good behavior, but they were really feeling fine, as well. And I think one of the things that happened was that Katie wasn't going to take my kids' behavior personally. She knew they were the children of psychologists; she expected them to be maladjusted. She was just going to rise to the occasion and do whatever she needed to support the kids so they could make it up the mountain. And in indeed, they made it up the mountain quite well, with her tutelage.

Now so far, I've been talking about mindfulness practices for parents and other caregivers, and how they can help us to take care of kids. There are also practices that we can actually teach to children directly. And there's a wealth of these that have been developed, but you can actually invent your own. The basic principle is to think, how are kids different from adults, and how do I have to adjust the practices to meet their needs? Well, one way the kids are different, is they tend to have a shorter attention span. So in general, the mindfulness practices we're going to design for kids, are going to be shorter than the ones we would do for adults.

Another way that they are different is they tend to like more vivid stimuli. Remember we talked about either coarse stimuli, like the sensations of walking meditation or eating meditation, or more subtle ones, like the sensations of the breath in the body or the tip of the nose. Well, the kids are going to gravitate more readily to coarse ones. And this makes perfect sense. We know that when we design environments for young kids, they often have bright, primary colors, and very clear shapes. Because kids can resonate better to those than the subtle pastels and the more subtle shapes that attract adults.

So, let me give you an example of some different exercises we can do. One of them is called "the three breaths." And this is analogous to something called the "three-minute breathing space" that we'll talk about, that's part of the system called Mindfulness-Based Cognitive Therapy, which we'll discuss later in the course. And all you do is this. We're with a child and you say, "Stop whatever you're doing just for a moment and take three breaths." You can do this right now as you're listening. Just three breaths. One. Two. Three. And then you simply ask the child, "What did you notice happening in your mind and body at that time?" And this simple exercise helps to tune kids in to the current sensations, to what's happening on a body level, what thoughts are arising and passing, and the like. Because most of the times, kids never take a moment to look inside. Very simple, can be done virtually with any kids.

Then there's apple meditation. This is very much like the Eating meditation that we did with the raisin. Only we use something even more vivid than a raisin. We use a big apple. And you can also make this as an opportunity for inquiry into interbeing. And ask the child, where did the apple come from? How did it get to the store? Where did the tree come from? Assuming they know it comes from a tree. What nourished the tree? And how many people have helped the apple to arrive in your hand? And following that inquiry, you simply eat the apple as an eating meditation, paying attention to each bite and the sensations.

We can modify loving-kindness practice to work with kids. Instead of doing, May I be safe, may I be healthy, may I live with ease, or saying, may I be happy, may I be peaceful, may I be free from suffering, you ask the child, "Remember something you did that makes you feel glad inside. And then, send a smile into your whole body. And let the feeling of happiness, peace, kindness, and love, spread from your heart through your whole body." And then, much as we do with other loving kindness practices for grown-ups, we then send these feelings to other people in the family, sending them to a pet—which works well with kids—to a friend, and then perhaps to the whole class, to a neighborhood, to the country, or even the whole world.

One practice that I like to do with kids a lot is called the "bell in space meditation." Let me show you how that works. And we can do it together so you can have a feel for what it's like, basically using the bell as a vivid object of awareness.

There are a couple of different ways that we can do the bell in space meditation, and I'll try both of them. See in your own experience how they each affect you. In the first one, I'm going to ring the bell and I'm going to invite you simply to listen to the sound of the bell and let it be the object of your awareness. [Rings bell.]

In the second way, I'm going to ask you to listen to the bell again, let it be the object of your awareness, but also count the number of rings and see how that changes the experience.

So, as I mentioned, you can invent your own practices. The younger the child, the shorter the time and the more intense the stimulation, and the older the child, the more you can use practices that are like those we use for adults.

In our next lecture, we're going to begin the exploration of psychological difficulties that affect us to lesser and greater degrees and how mindfulness practices can help us to work with them effectively. We're going to start with depression. Thanks for listening.

Seeing Sadness and Depression in a New Light
Lecture 12

This lecture marks the beginning of the exploration of psychological difficulties that affect us to lesser and greater degrees and how mindfulness practices can help us work with them effectively. The focus of this lecture is on depression. In this lecture, you will learn about models for understanding depression and how to deal with depression from a mindfulness-based approach, whether you are the one experiencing depression or someone you know is.

Sadness versus Depression

- Have you ever thought about the difference between sadness and depression? We've all experienced both to some degree. How would you say that they feel differently to you? Some people say that depression lasts longer. But it's possible to be depressed for a few hours or sad for days, so that might not really be what distinguishes the two. Other people say that depression is more intense. But we can certainly have the experience of being a little depressed or very sad.

- Some people say that depression includes hopelessness, and that seems to be true. In addition, depression almost always involves a narrative about you and about your circumstances that ends with the conclusion that things are not good.

- Depression causes us to feel deadened, with very little joy or interest in the world. On the other hand, sadness is alive and vibrant. We would describe it as being poignant.

- What differentiates depression from sadness is the way it involves a kind of shutting down of the organism to try to avoid pain. This shutting is not unique to depression, but it plays a role in most of our psychological distress.

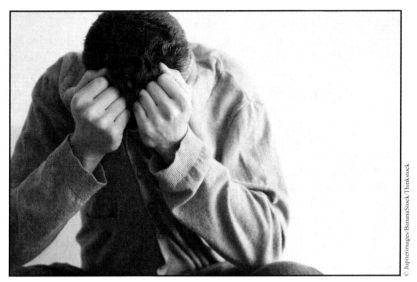

Mindfulness practice can help with depression, which involves avoiding pain, by helping you work through your thoughts about pain.

- Our tendency is to want to avoid some kind of painful experience, and in the process of avoiding it, we end up stuck in some kind of loop that keeps us trapped for a long period of time. This operates with a variety of problems, including depression, addiction, anxiety, and even psychosis.

- Experiential, or emotional, avoidance plays a role in all sorts of psychological difficulties. In all of these, it's our attempt to not feel something painful that gets us caught in the disorder. Mindfulness practice—which is, in essence, a form of experiential approach to everything—can help with all of these.

- Depression involves shutting down and turning away from pain, while mindfulness turns toward the experience at hand, and in so doing, it challenges the depressive stance. That's why mindfulness can help so much with depression.

Models for Understanding Depression

- Psychologist Martin Seligman came up with an animal model for studying depression. In his experiments, researchers constructed large rectangular cages in which they could put a dog, and the cage had the option of having a barrier put up. It had a floor that could be electrified on either side or both sides. The electrification wouldn't harm the dog in any way, but it was uncomfortable or distressing for the dog.

- They put the dog on one side of the cage, and they applied an electric shock. The dogs would always jump up and go to the other side that wasn't electrified, and they'd feel much better. But then, they put up a barrier and applied the shock to the side of the cage that the dog was in, and the dog would yelp and get upset but couldn't escape.

- After a relatively brief period of time, the dog started to look depressed. They stopped having interest in their human handlers. Their appetite and sleep became disrupted in ways that looked very much like human depression. This became the learned helplessness model of depression—the idea that we get depressed after our wishes have been thwarted just one time too many.

- The researchers thought that they could use the same model to perhaps cure depression. So, after the dogs reached a certain point, researchers would remove the barrier and then apply the shock. Initially, the dog didn't do anything. They had to physically go in and pull the dog over to the other side and, in essence, show the dog that the other side wasn't electrified before the dog would come back to normal functioning.

- This experiment became part of the evidence for the negativity bias, because it turned out that it was much easier to induce the depression-like state than it was to resolve it. You get the dog to act depressed with only a few trials, but it took many, many times showing the dog that it could have self-efficacy—that it could get up and move—before the dog would seem to recover.

- Mindfulness practice can help with this by simply redirecting attention to the present and noticing that each moment is a workable moment. Learned helplessness gets so much worse in a human than a dog because we develop a cognitive map for our circumstance that includes the idea that the situation is hopeless and it'll never get better.

- If we look at the psychoanalytic understanding of depression, this also has validity to it. We feel a lot of anger—often anger toward loved ones—but we don't feel that we can express it, so it gets turned against the self. That's why we end up being filled with all of this self-hatred, all of these negative thoughts about ourselves, when we're involved in a state of depression.

Attention to Present Emotions

- How do we work with depression when it comes up? We focus on the *what*, not the *why*. It's really about staying with what's happening right now and trying to be with, or breathe into, what's happening right now. It's very similar to a number of experiential therapies, such as focusing by Eugene Gendlin, Gestalt therapy, or Peter Levine's somatic experiencing.

- Philosopher Eugene Gendlin and psychologist Carl Rogers discovered that the pivotal sessions where people with depression really had a sense of transformation were sessions in which the patient or client closed his or her eyes, paid attention to the core of the body—not the distal parts, but the inner feelings—and talked about them.

- By helping us come into the center and notice what's happening in the body, mindfulness practices can connect us to feelings that might have been disavowed or pushed away. In that way, they can help us resolve the depression.

- Mindfulness practices help us move toward the pain by asking, what do we experience in our body? What's our relationship to the pain? Can we feel compassionate with ourselves?

- Mindfulness practices also help us get a different perspective on thought, because one of the differences between sadness and depression is that depression almost always has this narrative going through our mind. And it's almost always a narrative about how we failed, about how we're inadequate, about how nobody will love us, about how our life is hopeless.

- In cognitive behavioral therapy, the idea is to replace irrational and maladaptive thoughts with rational and adaptive ones. A mindfulness-oriented approach is different; it's about changing our relationship to all thinking. And this ultimately becomes more powerful. It's seeing that all thinking is unreliable.

Thinking about Thinking

- One conclusion we might draw from the summary of recent changes in cognitive science is that we simply cannot trust our thoughts. Our thoughts are so influenced by our culture, by our history, and by emotional biases of all sorts that our thinking is not to be trusted. Mindfulness practice helps us have this kind of perspective on thought, which is quite helpful when those thoughts are thoughts of hopelessness and self-destructive thoughts.

- One of the ways to do this is to simply think about thinking. So, when a thought arises, can we see the thought as just a thought? For example, instead of thinking that you're no good, you can instead recognize that the thought that you're no good is arising. It's not you—it's simply a neurological phenomenon generating the thought.

- Another thing that's very helpful is to practice moving below the level of thought to connect to the feelings and physical sensations that are beneath them. One way to work with this is by practicing affective, or emotional, meteorology. This is just another way of seeing the basic Buddhist principle that all things are impermanent—everything is changing.

- When feeling depressed, just simply ask yourself when in the past you did not feel depressed. Then, think about how your thought patterns were different. When we're depressed and we think about the time when we felt optimistic or positive about our lives, we think that we just didn't see how bad things are and that now we are seeing reality in the depressed state. Conversely, when we're in the state of mind where we're not feeling depressed, we remember all the depressive thoughts and think that we saw everything negatively because of the depression.

- As we're mindful of these changing thought patterns, we see how radically unreliable they are. We also see that they change over time—that everything is in constant flux. This tends to undercut the feeling that it will last forever, which tends to keep us stuck.

Entering Dark Places and Finding Meaning
- It's very important be able to enter the dark places. This is true if we're helping somebody with depression or if we're depressed ourselves. We have to be able to fully feel our despair, loneliness, and self-hate, and we have to learn not to fear these states but simply see them as transient.

- It's very important to know that it's possible to survive this despair and that we won't kill people off with it. Very often, when we're depressed, we feel toxic. We know that people don't really want to be around us in this mood. But connection is so important.

- Hope can be tricky. Often, if we try to offer premature hope—either to ourselves or to somebody struggling with depression—it feels like an empathic failure, because the hope feels to the depressed person like the other person doesn't understand. In fact, empathic connection itself offers much more hope.

- There are problems with hope. Research has shown that prisoners who are sentenced to life without parole actually adjust better and are happier than those who are sentenced with very long sentences but have the option for parole. So, we have to be careful about how much to try to offer hope to one another in these situations, versus just staying with the experience in the moment, however challenging it might be.

- It's also important to try to find meaning—to ask ourselves, what's our heart's desire? What really matters to us in life? Acceptance and commitment therapy, one of the mindfulness-based treatments, spends a lot of time on this, trying to find a way to clarify our values and find a compass for our lives. This can give us a sense of a spiritual or psychological path, and then we don't see the pain so much as an obstacle but as a developmental opportunity.

Suggested Reading

Gilbert, *Overcoming Depression.*

Martin, *The Zen Path through Depression.*

Segal, Williams, and Teasdale, *Mindfulness-Based Cognitive Therapy for Depression.*

Siegel, *The Mindfulness Solution*, chapter 6.

Williams, Teasdale, Segal, and Kabat-Zinn, *The Mindful Way through Depression.*

Questions to Consider

1. We have all experienced at least some sadness and some depression in our lives, even if these may have never reached the level of a psychiatric disorder. In your experience, how has sadness been different from depression?

2. When you (or someone you have known) have been depressed, how did this effect your (or his or her) thought processes? How would the experience of depression have been different had you (or the other person) not believed in the thoughts as fully?

Seeing Sadness and Depression in a New Light
Lecture 12—Transcript

Now we're going to begin looking at how mindfulness practices can help us with a number of everyday psychological difficulties. And we're going to begin with the exhilarating and uplifting topic of working with depression.

Have you ever thought about the difference between sadness and depression? We've all experienced both to some degree. How would you say they feel differently to you? When I ask mental health professionals this question, they typically come up with a variety of answers. Some say, well, depression lasts longer. But then it turns out that it's actually possible to be quite depressed for a few hours or quite sad for days, so that may not really be what distinguishes the two. Others will say, well, depression is more intense. But I've certainly had the experience of being a little depressed or very sad.

Some people will say depression includes hopelessness, and that one seems to hold. Depression almost always involves this narrative about me and about my circumstance that ends with the conclusion that things are not good.

The thing that we notice is that, in depression, there's a sense of deadeningness with very little joy or interest in the world. We feel as though things don't have taste to us. Things don't have meaning to us. It all feels kind of blah.

We understand, on the other hand, that sadness is quite alive, is quite vibrant. We'd describe it as being poignant. When we read Shakespeare and he says, "Parting is such sweet sorrow," we get what he means. If he were to say, "Parting is such sweet depression," we'd think this guy isn't a very good writer.

The key to depression here—what differentiates it from sadness—is the way it involves a kind of shutting down sound of the organism, closing down to try to avoid pain. Now as it turns out, this shutting down to try to avoid pain is not unique to depression, but it plays a role in most of our psychological distress. And to understand this better, I want to tell you a story. And this is a story about the men and women who finished writing recently the DSM-V—that's the *Diagnostic and Statistical Manual* of the American

Psychiatric Association—which is what we use to diagnose different kinds of psychological and psychiatric disorders.

I heard this story from Dave Barlow. He's a leading anxiety researcher. He's at Boston University. And he's been part of the committee who's writing the section of the DSM-V that deals with anxiety. And he says that, across the board, there's been this battle raging between what he calls the *lumpers* and the *splitters*. What the splitters are saying is that what was wrong with our old system with the DSM-IV is we did not yet have sufficient diagnostic categories. We were still lumping apples with oranges together. And what we really need are even more carefully subdivided psychiatric diagnostic categories so that we could separate all the subtle variations in disorders. And that would be useful so that we could develop standardized treatments and test them experimentally to treat the different sub-disorders, as well as to develop pharmaceuticals that were targeted to particular disorders.

Now when the lumpers hear this, they tend to roll their eyes and they think, "This is ridiculous." And lumpers tend to be practicing clinicians who are working with real patients. Because what the lumpers say, and what virtually all practicing clinicians say, is, "You know, I've virtually never met a patient or a client with a single DSM-IV diagnosis." Almost everybody had a little bit of this with a mixture of that. They don't fit the categories so well.

In fact, as a friend of mine put it, our diagnostic categories don't exactly carve nature at its joints. People are far more complex than this, and they have a little bit of this strength and a little bit of this weakness across so many different domains. Furthermore, the lumpers say, "I think by subdividing so much these different categories, you're missing the forest for the trees."

Now the splitters at that point quite naturally say, "What forest?" And the lumpers say, "Well, you're missing the universals in psychopathology. You're missing the universal things that cause people psychological distress." And the splitters say, "What universals? These are separate diseases. I don't understand what you're talking about." And the lumpers say, for example, "You're missing the role of experiential or emotional avoidance."

And this is our tendency to want to avoid some kind of painful experience, and in the process of avoiding it, we wind up stuck in some kind of loop that keeps us trapped for a long period of time. Let's look at how this operates with a variety of problems. I just mentioned depression. Well, in depression—we'll be exploring it in a little bit more detail—it is the shutting down of emotional experience that actually gets us into trouble.

But we can see this in other areas also. Let's look at how this works with a common problem like addiction. Many of you, like I, probably drink socially, at least occasionally. I ask you, when you drink, do you do it exclusively for the taste? I'll sometimes ask audiences this and there's often somebody who'll raise their hand—or if I'm teaching in Marin County, a lot of people raise their hand—but most of us don't drink just for the taste. In fact, I remember when I was young and first tasted alcohol and it didn't really taste so good. It was only once I had a conditioned association between the taste of alcohol and some positive feelings associated with inebriation that it started to become attractive. Rather, we drink because we want to change one feeling into another feeling.

For example, I've come home from work. I've had a hard day. I felt kind of stressed. It would be nice to have a beer or a glass of wine out on the porch before preparing dinner. Or maybe I'm going to a party. And at that party, there are going to be some people there who I don't know. Or worse, there are going to be some people there who I do know. And I think, you know, a drink or two would make this go a lot better. So most of us, when we drink, we do it because we like the experience of going from feeling some kind of tension or difficulty to feeling some kind of relaxation.

This is true with anxiety sorters as well. If I get anxious before doing public speaking or I get anxious flying in airplanes, but I speak publicly and I fly an airplane regularly, I probably don't have an anxiety disorder. Rather, I'm just a nervous guy. If, however, I start avoiding public speaking or avoiding going into airplanes in order to not feel anxious, then I'm on my way to an anxiety disorder and bigger problems.

We even see this operating in very serious problems such as psychosis. When I ask audiences of mental health professionals, what are the kinds things that they typically observe for a person who's struggling with, let's say, schizophrenia, that might push the person over from doing pretty well to doing what we call *decompensating*. Decompensating means, in essence, falling apart—falling into either a state of delusion or hearing voices or having one of these psychotic manifestations. And almost always, what the people say is, well, it's things like a change in job, or the loss of a job, or maybe the death of somebody close, or perhaps losing housing and having to move. And all of these things are events that, when they happen to people who aren't struggling with psychosis, bring up difficult feeling. But what happens with a person struggling with psychosis is instead of feeling the difficult feeling, what happens is they get these psychiatric symptoms.

So what we see is, across the board, there's experiential avoidance or emotional avoidance playing a role in all sorts of psychological difficulties. Basically, in all of these, it's our attempt to not feel something painful that actually trips us up and gets us caught in the disorder.

What we'll see is that mindfulness practice, which is, in essence, a form of experiential approach to everything, can help with all of these. There's a wonderful video that's been made. It's an animated video—you can see this online, it's on YouTube—and it has a samurai warrior, and he's sitting in meditation posture. And this fly comes along [buzzing] and lands on his face. And he starts going like this, trying to get rid of it. And then you see him reach for his sword. And he brings his sword out, and the fly goes away, and he goes wham, and he divides the fly in two. And you see these two halves of a fly.

But then what happens is the fly starts to come back to life. Crackle, crackle, crackle. It becomes a whole fly. Then you see over there, so did the other half. And now there are two flies. So he takes out his sword again and he whacks the two flies. And now he has four flies. And this just keeps going and going and going until he's just surrounded by a swarm of flies.

And it's not until he notices that it's the fighting of the fly that's causing the problem, and he's able to resume an accepting posture, that the difficulty goes away and he can release the fly and he's OK. This is what happens to us with all of these disorders. Our attempt to get rid of the symptom, to get rid of the discomfort, simply multiplies our misery.

Let's get back to depression. Do you know what happens to a sine wave—a standard S-shaped wave that you might see on an oscilloscope, or that you can see with a rope? If you move it so the bottom part doesn't dip as far below the midline, what happens is the top part comes down too. OK. It doesn't rise as far. This seems to be what's happening in depression. The mind tries, consciously or unconsciously, to avoid the bottom part of the sine wave, to get rid of the pain. And in the process, we lose the capacity for joy, for interest, for engagement. We become deadened. We lose the capacity for life.

So depression involves shutting down and turning away from pain, while mindfulness turns toward the experience at hand and, in so doing, it challenges the depressive stance. And that's why mindfulness could help us so much with depression.

We'll look at just a couple of the dominant models for understanding depression. And you can see how mindfulness can help if we understand depression in these lines. Martin Seligman was a leading psychologist, and he came up with an animal model for studying depression. And the experiment—it's a little bit cruel, but it wasn't actually harmful to the animals. What they did was they constructed these large, rectangular cages in which they could put a dog. And the cage had the option of having a barrier put up. And it had a floor that could be electrified on either side or both sides. And the electrification wouldn't harm the dog in any way, but it was uncomfortable. It was distressing for the dog.

So here's what they did. They took the dog and they put it on one side of the cage, and they applied an electric shock. And the dogs would always jump up and go to the other side that wasn't electrified at this point, and they'd feel much better. They'd be OK, and they weren't any worse for the wear. But then, what they did was they put down a barrier. And they would apply the shock to the side of the cage that the dog was in, and the dog would yelp and get upset. And it couldn't escape.

Now what they found was, after a relatively brief period of time, the dog started to look depressed. They stopped having interest in their human handlers. Their appetite was disrupted; they stopped seeming to enjoy their food or wanting to eat. Their sleep became dysregulated in ways that looked very much like human depression. And this became the learned helplessness model of depression, the idea that we get depressed after our wishes have been thwarted just one time too many.

Well, they thought they could use the same model to perhaps cure depression. So what they would do then is they would remove the barrier and they would apply the shock. And initially, what happened was the dog simply lay there. It didn't do anything. They had to physically go in and pull the dog over to the other side and, in essence, show the dog that the other side wasn't electrified before the dog would come back to normal functioning.

And this experiment actually became part of the evidence for the negativity bias because it turned out that it was much easier to induce the depression-like state than it was to resolve it. You could do it with a few trials—get the dog to act depressed—but it took many, many times showing the dog that it could have self-efficacy, that it could get up and move, before the dog would seem to recover.

Now, mindfulness practice can help us with this by simply redirecting attention to the present and noticing that each moment is a workable moment for us. Because learned helplessness gets so much worse in a human than a dog because we develop a cognitive map for our circumstance, and that cognitive map includes the idea that my situation is hopeless and it'll never get better.

If we look at the psychoanalytic understanding of depression, this also has validity to it. Freud famously said that suicide is like "murder in the 180th degree," that what happens is we feel a lot of anger—often anger toward loved ones—but we don't feel we can express it, so it gets turned against the self. And that's why we wind up being filled with all this self-hatred, all these negative thoughts about ourselves, when we're involved in a state of depression.

So I want to tell you about my experience working with depression in the context of a meditation retreat. It's actually a state of depression that drove me to do my first intensive two-week silent retreat. I'll give you the outline of the story. It was shortly after I graduated from college. There was me. There was my lovely, beautiful, warm, intelligent, caring girlfriend. And then there was her ex-boyfriend living on the west coast. To make a long and complex story short, she wound up living on the west coast, and I was not pleased.

So even though I was a meditator, I was having a rough go of it. I was performing my jobs. I was working at a psychiatric treatment center at the time. And, you know, I was functioning OK—it wasn't a serious clinical depression, but I felt mopey. I wasn't really enjoying things. Life didn't have much taste to it. And I thought, you know, mindfulness practice should help for this. It should help me to become more alive. I think I'll try going on a two-week retreat.

So I packed my bags and showed up at the meditation center. And there I learned about the structure of the day, which I've described to you before in which you basically spend the full day being with experience, doing sitting meditation, walking meditation, eating meditation. And the instruction was always pretty much the same. Once developing a certain degree of concentration, we move to open monitoring. And then whatever arises in consciousness, simply bringing one's attention to what arises in consciousness.

And I felt good. I have a plan of action. I'm going to do this. So I started with being with the breath and some concentration developed. And it was nice. There was a sense of calmness and a kind of stability. And we were practicing noble silence, so we had the experience of solitude, but surrounded by others so that it felt like a community.

And then the movie started. And I could best describe these as alternating romance and erotic films with slasher films. I would start to have images coming to my mind. I'm sitting there with my eyes closed, following the breath. And images of these delectable moments with my ex-girlfriend, complete with all sorts of physical arousal, and intense longings—how could I have lost her? How could I have her back? All of this is just coming up in waves, and I'm following the instructions. I'm simply trying to be like that Zen master who can be run through with a sword without blinking an eye and just feeling it all.

And then they would shift. They would shift into kind of slasher films where I was seeing all sorts of horrible things that might befall my ex-girlfriend and the other guy. And they would alternate like this. But then periodically, the films would stop, and I would be with that ant on the stone wall, or I'd be watching the beautiful sunset, or really feeling the shower vividly.

And my sense of the whole thing was, OK, there's a method. This is workable. And I remember, at the end of the two-week retreat, riding home in the car and first thinking, wow, an interstate is a pretty intense experience when you're really opened up to it and feeling it. Just the sounds, the sights. And then I noticed I was definitely not depressed anymore. I felt longing, I felt anger, I felt sadness, I felt the exquisite enjoyment of nature, but I was definitely not depressed—I was alive.

Here's what Bhante Gunaratana says—he's a Buddhist monk who's written about mindfulness—he says, "You become sensitive to the actual experience of living, to how things actually feel. You do not sit around developing sublime thoughts about living. You live."

So how do we work with this in our meditation practice? How do we work with depression when it comes up? Well, we don't spend a lot of time talking about the why or investigating that or doing the narrative therapy that I described before. It's really about staying with what's happening right now and trying to be with or breathe into what's happening right now. And it's very similar to a number of experiential therapies such as focusing by Eugene Gendlin, Gestalt therapy, or Peter Levine's somatic experiencing.

Let me give you an idea of how this works with Focusing just as an example. Eugene Gendlin was a philosopher. And he was quite well known as an academic philosopher who was doing well in the 1950s and the 1960s. And he came to the startling conclusion that academic philosophy is kind of abstract. And he thought, there's got to be some practical use for this. And as it just so happened, he was working at the University of Chicago at the time, as was Carl Rogers, who we've discussed before as really the pioneer in describing how to cultivate therapy relationships.

And Carl Rogers had collections of many, many audio tapes of psychotherapy sessions. So Gendlin teamed up with Rogers to try to identify which were those sessions that were most pivotal. And he found out that the pivotal sessions where people really came alive and really had a sense of transformation were sessions in which the patient or the client closed his or her eyes, went inside, paid attention to this part of the body—the core, not the distal parts like we were using for going for safety, but the inner feelings—and talked about them.

Let me see if I can demonstrate that right now. So I'm just going to be with the breath for a breath or two. And I can feel a little bit of pressure here, a little bit of pressure in the eyes. Maybe there's a little sadness. In times when I've done this recently, an image of my parents is coming up. My parents happen to be elderly and having a rough go of it on the west coast.

I could go deeper. But for our purposes, it's just a matter of noticing—now, call me a bad son, but I hadn't actually been thinking of my parents so far in recording this lecture. But all I need to do is connect in here, and it's back. So mindfulness practices, by helping us to come into the center and notice what's happening in the body, can actually connect us to feelings that might have been disavowed or pushed away. And in that way, they can help us to resolve the depression.

So they help us to move toward the pain, with the idea of asking, what do we experience in our body? What's our relationship to the pain? And can we feel compassionate with ourselves? Can we notice that this is painful, but—as we discussed earlier with self-compassion exercises—to put our hand over our heart and comfort ourselves as we experience the pain?

Now mindfulness practices also help us to get a different perspective on thought because, as we mentioned, one of the differences between sadness and depression is depression almost always has this narrative going through our mind. And it's almost always a narrative about how we've failed, about how we're inadequate, about how nobody will love us, about how our life is hopeless. And this can sometimes lead to very absurd discussions in therapy. I've found myself doing this as a therapist before, and my colleagues report the same thing, where a patient or client is basically laying out their depressive thought, and we're starting to argue with them and point out that, well, you know, that's not really necessary true. There are these options, there are those options. And our patient is becoming an even better debater.

It's as though they were in a high school or college speech and debate club, and they're refuting every one of our arguments, convincing themselves with even greater certainty that their life is basically over.

Now we discussed before how, in cognitive behavior therapy, the idea is to replace irrational and maladaptive thoughts with rational and adaptive ones. A mindfulness-oriented approach is different from that. It's about changing our relationship to all thinking. And this ultimately becomes more powerful. It's seeing that all thinking is unreliable. We can think of this as cognitive behavior therapy on steroids.

You know, one of the ways to look at the summary of changes in cognitive science that have occurred in the last 15 years or so—the big take-home point is we really can't trust our thoughts. Our thoughts are so influenced by our culture, by our history, by emotional biases of all sorts that our thinking is really not to be trusted. And mindfulness practice helps us to have this kind of perspective on thought, which is quite helpful when those thoughts are thoughts of hopelessness and self-destructive thoughts.

One of the ways to do this is to simply think about thinking. So when a thought arises, can we see the thought as just a thought? For example, instead of saying to ourselves, "I'm no good," can we say, "Oh, there's the thought arising that I'm no good." It's a subtle difference, but it makes all the world of difference in how seriously we take the thoughts, because when we see, oh, there it is again, as though the mind is a kind of "it," a kind of neurological phenomenon generating the thought.

The other thing that's very helpful is to practice moving below the level of thought to connect to the feelings and physical sensations that are beneath them. One way to work with this is by practicing what we might call affective, or emotional, meteorology. And this is really just another way of seeing the basic Buddhist principle that all things are impermanent. Everything is changing. It's all constant flux.

And here's the exercise you can do. When feeling depressed, just simply inquire, when in the past did you not feel depressed? Most of us can remember a time like that. And then how were our thought patterns different?

This is very interesting. When we're depressed and we think about the time when we felt optimistic or positive about our lives, in the depressed state, we think, oh, I was just fooling myself. I didn't see how bad things are. Now I see reality. And conversely, when we're in the state of mind where we're not feeling so depressed, we remember all the depressive thoughts and think, oh, that was just the depression talking. I saw everything negatively because of the depression.

As we're mindful of these changing thought patterns, we see how radically unreliable they are. We see also that they change over time—that thoughts, mood, everything is in constant flux. And this tends to undercut the feeling that it will last forever, which tends to keep us stuck.

Now it's very important be able to enter the dark places. And this is true if we're helping somebody with depression or if we're depressed ourselves. We have to be able to fully feel our despair, our loneliness, our sense of un-lovability, and our self-hate. And we have to learn not to fear these states, but simply see them as transient effects. If you'll recall the discussion we had earlier about being with my patient in the rather dilapidated room at Cambridge Hospital, she only started to feel better when I could really be with her in her despair.

I have a favorite poster about this. It shows a dimly lit nature scene. And the caption is, "Despair: It's always darkest just before it goes pitch black." Because that's how it feels when we're depressed—it feels as though there's no darkest before the dawn. It's simply going downhill.

So it's very important to know that it's possible to survive this despair. And it's also important to know that we won't kill people off with it. Very often, when we're depressed, we feel toxic. We know people don't really want to be around us in this mood. The writer Andrew Solomon was author of a memoir called *Noonday Demon*. And it was really a memoir of depression. And here's what he said: "You cannot draw a depressed person out of his misery with love … you can, sometimes, manage to join someone in the place where he resides."

And this is this idea that connection is so important. It's interesting. When helping adolescents, for example, who are suicidal, one of the rituals I used to like to do—and other people do this as well—is to simply have the parents go around with the child around the house and collect those items that might be dangerous, that they might use to harm themselves. Because simply the act of doing that, the ritual, makes the child feel much more connected with his or her parents.

I want to say a few words about hope because hope can be tricky. Oftentimes, if we try to offer premature hope—either to ourselves or to somebody struggling with depression—it feels like an empathic failure because the hope feels to the depressed person like the other person doesn't understand. In fact, empathic connection itself offers much more hope.

There are problems with hope. There have been a few studies that illustrate this. In one of them, they studied people who had had colostomies. And colostomies are where they're removing elements of the colon because it's been diseased in some way. But sometimes, they don't actually remove anything. They simply redirect things so that your waste products are going into a bag.

So there are two kinds. There's the irreversible ones where they've removed a lot of the colon, or the potentially reversible ones where they're hoping that, once the colon heals, they'll be able to connect the person up normally again. Guess which group of people feels better a month or two after the surgery? It's the people with the irreversible ones. Because the people with the reversible ones are everyday waking up and thinking, oh gosh, I hope my colon feels better. I hope I'm going to recover. I hope I'm going to be able to get rid of this bag.

Something similar is found among prisoners. Those who are sentenced to life without parole actually adjust better and are happier than those who are sentenced with very long sentences but have the option for parole. So we've got to be careful about this, about how much to try to offer hope to one another in these situations versus just staying with the experience in the moment, however challenging it might be.

It's also important to try to find meaning, to ask ourselves, what's our heart's desire? What really matters to us in life? Acceptance and Commitment Therapy—or ACT—one of the mindfulness-based treatments, spends a lot of time on this, trying to find a way to clarify our values and find a compass for our lives. And this can give us a sense of a spiritual or psychological path. And then we don't see the pain so much as an obstacle but as a developmental opportunity. This is really what happened to me when I was sitting on the retreat and I saw the pain as something to work with as part of a larger path to wellbeing rather than just a problem.

So I'd like to just say a word or two about medication. Because you may be thinking—you're probably aware that medications are very often given to try to reduce depressive symptoms. And if the goal in treatment is not experiential avoidance but to increase our capacity to be able to feel our feelings, then what might the role of the medication be? It does have a role.

The diagnostic question to my mind is, is the person caught in a downward spiral? Is the depressed affect, the depressed emotion, leading to behavior which itself is resulting in more depression? Now this happens. You'll find somebody gets depressed and they start not calling their friends or not showing up at work or not studying for the test at school. And soon they're going to have a circumstance of being alone or failing out of school or getting fired, which itself is going to be depressive and depressing. So we want to, whenever possible, if somebody's involved in one of these downward spirals, to use anything that's going to help pull the person out, including medication.

The goal here is to find the optimal level of challenge—not to dull feeling so much that we can't work with it, but not to be so overwhelmed that we get caught in this downward spiral. Now nowadays in the United States, primary care physicians and other non-psychiatric health care providers prescribe over 80 percent of the antidepressants that are given. And they typically, on average, spend about 4 and 1/2 minutes before prescribing. It's not their fault. They're just very busy.

So automatically just going to take the antidepressant because we happen to be depressed and a doctor's suggesting it might not always be the best course of action. It probably makes the most sense to give this some thought, including to have some time to consult with a mental health professional to weigh out the pros and cons of this, and to see how mindfulness practice might be used as an alternative or as a supplement.

I'd like to end with a poem. This comes from Rumi, the Islamic poet from the 13th century who I mentioned earlier. And it really speaks to an attitude that we can have toward depression, which is a mindful attitude that can help bring us through it. It's called "The Guest House."

> This being human is a guest house.
> Every morning a new arrival.
>
> A joy, a depression, a meanness,
> some momentary awareness comes
> as an unexpected visitor.
>
> Welcome and entertain them all!
> Even if they are a crowd of sorrows,
> who violently sweep your house
> empty of its furniture,
> still, treat each guest honorably.
> He may be clearing you out
> for some new delight.
>
> The dark thought, the shame, the malice.
> Meet them at the door laughing and invite them in.
>
> Be grateful for whatever comes,
> because each has been sent
> as a guide from beyond.

So in our next lecture, we're going to look at a close relative of depression that affects almost everybody to some degree, and that's worry and anxiety. Thanks for listening.

Befriending Fear, Worry, and Anxiety
Lecture 13

I n this lecture, you are going to learn about a close relative of depression that affects almost everybody to some degree: anxiety. People with anxiety disorders are often more accurate at appraising risk than people without anxiety problems. People with anxiety disorders actually notice that life is fragile and that it is pretty dangerous to be alive—that at any moment bad things can happen very readily to good people. This lecture will teach you how anxiety arises and how to deal with it.

Anxiety
- Researchers and clinicians have identified three basic components of anxiety. First, there is a physiological arousal, or what happens in our body when adrenaline starts pumping. Second, there is a cognitive and emotional part. There is all the future-oriented thinking and fear and the accurate and inaccurate risk appraisal. Finally, perhaps most importantly, there are the behavioral aspects—the avoidance and rituals (the things we do in order to try to not feel anxious).

- A fundamental challenge in working with anxiety is figuring out whether the anxiety is signal or noise. Sometimes, fear indicates genuine danger that needs our attention, but other times, the arousal does not actually require action. It is just noise. And we need to be able to differentiate cognitively between the two. This is difficult, because we have a negativity bias, which is a propensity toward false-positive errors.

- With mindfulness practice, we discover that there is almost always some baseline of anxiety happening in the body and in the mind. Sometimes it is little fears, and sometimes it is big ones. With mindfulness practice, we also notice that we are constantly thinking about the future, looking forward to pleasure, and dreading pain.

- There are some people who spend more time looking back, and those people tend to experience depression more than anxiety. But those who are more anxious look forward quite a bit. Neither of these is in the present. The mind leaves the experience of the present moment and goes off into these fantasies about the future.

- All anxiety is anticipatory. Even people who are in terrible present situations are worried about the future. Emergency medical technicians say that when they are extracting somebody from an accident, even if the person is bleeding and is in very bad shape, that person is worried about the future. The person will think, will I be able to walk? Will my loved ones be okay?

- Why do we do this? Sometimes we get positively reinforced. Sometimes we will get into our worry loop, and we will come up with a novel solution to the problem. But most of the time, we do not. There is just something about going through the thinking process that gives us the illusion that it is somehow going to keep us safe, help us to cope, and prepare us for what may come.

Avoiding the Risk of Fear or Pain

- There are a lot of techniques that we do to try to avoid the risk of fear or pain. This is because we find anxiety to be very unpleasant. One set of these we might call the "diver Dan" approach to life. This involves phobic avoidance and constriction. There are the things that we do in order to avoid any circumstance that might bring on fear or discomfort, and then there are the things that we do directly to tackle anxiety when it comes up.

- An awful lot of people medicate anxiety. Sometimes this is with prescription drugs that are prescribed by a doctor, but very often it is simply having a drink or using other drugs. Probably what we do more than anything else is try to distract ourselves—by watching TV or shopping, for example.

- The problem with these different forms of distraction is that we develop what is called stimulation tolerance. We end up needing

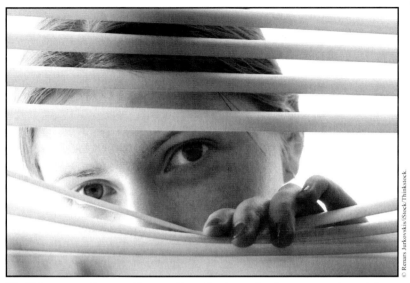

Mindfulness practice provides an alternative to medicating a person's anxiety.

higher and higher doses in order to distract ourselves from unpleasant thoughts and feelings, including anxiety. When we try to use distraction, we need more and more of it to bring ourselves away from our fears.

How Do Anxiety Disorders Develop?

- Most anxiety disorders develop through what is called escape-avoidance learning. The following is how you can create an anxiety disorder in just a few simple steps. First, you have to enter a situation. Then, anxiety arises. We find anxiety unpleasant, so most of us try to take steps to get rid of it. So, we leave the situation, and the anxiety abates.

- This reduction in anxiety is called negative reinforcement, which is a principle in learning theory about the reinforcement that comes from removing an unpleasant experience. Once your behavior is negatively reinforced, the next time you are in a similar situation, you are going to decide to leave it right away—or avoid it altogether—because you have learned that you can avoid having anxiety if you're not put in a particular situation.

- For example, agoraphobia is fear of going out into the world. But even if it does not get to that state, most of us develop these patterns, in little ways, around things that we are afraid of and we start to avoid.

- The general treatment for anxiety in modern psychology is exposure and response prevention. In these cases, the fear response becomes extinguished because people experience that nothing terrible happens when they are exposed to the cause of their anxiety. For example, someone who is afraid of snakes is exposed to one, and when nothing bad happens to them, they start to release their anxiety about snakes.

- When people come into therapy for anxiety problems, they are not actually interested in handling the snake—or whatever the equivalent might be. People want to eliminate the anxious feeling.

- Instead, in a mindfulness-oriented approach, we are going to increase their capacity to bear it, changing their relationship to the experience. During mindfulness practices, or whatever the person is doing, he or she focuses on trying not to scratch the itch. He or she does not adjust to make the pain go away but, rather, simply stay with the experience until it transforms by itself.

- Basically, what we are trying to do is learn how to face our fears. The idea that facing our fears is what can free us turns out to be true both in classical behavioral treatment and in mindfulness-oriented treatment.

Relief from Narcissistic Threats

- Many of our anxieties are actually about what we might think of as narcissistic threats. They are threats to ourselves or our loved ones. A lot of our anxieties are about threats to our self-image, health, and wealth. Broadly, it is about anticipating that we might lose pleasure or experience pain.

- We have some existential problems that we have to face. The reality of old age, illness, and death can produce a lot of anxiety, and mindfulness practices can help us with these. In part, the focus on the present moment is antithetical to the anticipatory anxiety. We can take an attitude of not knowing.

- We can take refuge in the present moment. When we are having anxious thoughts about what is going to happen in the future, often it is because we cannot stand the uncertainty. We have a lot of difficulty tolerating the fact that we really do not know what is going to happen in the next moment. Mindfulness practice can help us live without knowing by bringing us back to the present moment.

- There is also a safety that comes from identifying with the universe larger than us so that we do not have to be so worried about various narcissistic threats.

- Unwanted feelings also scare us a lot. Much anxiety is fear of our own emotions and impulses. We might be afraid of our anger, sadness, repressed or suppressed memories, or unacceptable thoughts of all kinds. When these things start to arise, we find ourselves getting anxious. Doing mindfulness practice regularly allows opportunities for these feelings and impulses to be accepted and integrated so that we no longer fear and resist them. Then, the source of anxiety abates.

- If you are particularly anxious, it can be difficult to just sit and do something like the breath meditation. So, in those situations, it is usually best to do more active practice, such as walking meditation, eating meditation, or even hatha yoga, which is a form of very gentle stretching that can be done in a mindful way. All of these things dissipate the anxiety a little bit, making it easier to work with.

Suggested Reading

Forsyth and Eifert, *The Mindfulness and Acceptance Workbook for Anxiety*.

Orsillo and Roemer, *The Mindful Way through Anxiety*.

Roemer and Orsillo, "Mindfulness and Acceptance-Based Treatment of Anxiety."

Siegel, *Mindfulness for Anxiety*.

————, *The Mindfulness Solution*, chapter 5.

Questions to Consider

1. What is the principal distinction between feeling anxiety and having an anxiety disorder?

2. What is the central goal of a mindfulness-oriented approach to working with anxiety?

Mindfulness Practice

stepping into fear: A brief exercise to practice experiential approach, rather than avoidance, when struggling with anxiety.

Befriending Fear, Worry, and Anxiety
Lecture 13—Transcript

There is a little known fact about anxiety problems, and that is that people with anxiety disorders are often more accurate at appraising risk than people without anxiety problems. Let me explain—give you an example of how this works.

A person with an anxiety disorder might be driving down the highway and a thought might occur to them. Hm. I am hurtling through space at 60 or 70 miles an hour in a tin can. This is an inherently risky position. One moment's inattention on my part, on the part of another driver, on the part of my mechanic, or even the highway crew, and I am going to be killed or maimed. You know, this feels scary. I think I will take the side roads.

Now, a person without anxiety problems gets into a car and thinks, I am in a well engineered automobile. I am certain that the designers and engineers at the manufacturing company were thinking about my safety at every juncture and not letting concerns about profit or loss or expense get involved in their decisions about design features.

And that fellow over there in the next lane screaming red-faced into his cell phone, he's paying attention. He's thinking about my welfare. My mechanic, I trust fully, and that sweet, pungent, smoky aroma that I get must be some kind of incense that he burns in the garage that helps him to pay better attention. Furthermore, I know from my own experience, as well as talking to others, that substance abuse is extremely rare in my culture, so it would be very unlikely that any other drivers might be impaired at this moment. I'm enjoying my drive.

Do you see the problem here? The problem is that people with anxiety disorders actually notice that life is fragile and it's pretty dangerous to be alive, that at any moment bad things can happen very readily to good people. This becomes an issue actually in psychotherapy, because often what happens is a psychotherapist will hear a person with anxiety talking about their difficulties and the therapist, being well-meaning, will try to talk the person out of it, will try to point out that, well you shouldn't really worry about this. It is a low-probability event and you should be OK. The person with the anxiety disorder, if they have a good relationship with the therapist, they think, oh my therapist is a nice man or lady. Obviously, he or she is in denial. I will just go along until we can change the topic and talk about something more interesting and useful to me.

I actually find these findings to be very reassuring. Temperamentally, I happen to be a somewhat anxious person, so these findings do not do anything to allay my fears, but at least I can be right, and there is some satisfaction in that.

So given this, how can we possibly help people with anxiety problems? Well, we can start by examining the basic components of anxiety. And researchers and clinicians alike have identified three of these components. First, there is a physiological arousal, what happens in our body when adrenalin starts pumping around. We are going to discuss that in more detail in the next lecture, when we talk about psychophysiological disorders specifically.

Second, there is a cognitive and emotional part. There is all the future-oriented thinking and fear, and the accurate and inaccurate risk appraisal that we have just discussed. And finally, perhaps most importantly, there are the behavioral aspects. There are the avoidance and rituals, the things we do, in essence, in order to try to not feel anxious.

Now, a fundamental challenge in working with anxiety is figuring out whether the anxiety is signal or noise, because sometimes fear indicates genuine danger that needs our attention. If a patient came in and said, "You know doc, I get pretty anxious whenever I am walking on a highway in dark clothes at night and there is no shoulder." Well, naturally.

But other times, the arousal doesn't actually require action. It's noise. It's just thinking another anxious thought that's not going to be particularly useful to respond to or take action to try to avert danger. And we need to be able to differentiate cognitively between the two. And this is tough, because we have a negativity bias that we have discussed before—it's a propensity toward false positive errors.

One of my favorite cartoons has two fish underwater, and one of them is definitely looking upset. And the upset fish says, "You know, to tell you the truth, even when I'm in the water, I don't feel that comfortable." This is what we discover with mindfulness practice. We discover that there's almost always some baseline of anxiety happening in the body and in the mind. Sometimes it's little fears and sometimes it's big ones.

We also notice with mindfulness practice that we are forever toppling forward. We are thinking about the future, the future, the future—looking forward to pleasure, trying to engineer things have pleasant experiences, and dreading pain. Of course, there are some people who spend more time looking back, and those folks, I think in general, tend to experience depression more than anxiety. Those of us who are more anxious, we look forward quite a bit.

Sometimes this can reach absurd degrees. For example, have you ever been out to eat with friends, and gone to a nice restaurant where clearly the people in the kitchen have gone through a lot of trouble to prepare a lovely meal, well-presented. And you are with your friends and you start eating the meal, and the topic of conversation, before long, starts to go to other places we might like to go eat. Oh yeah, there is that great new place that opened up across town. Wouldn't that be fun to try? So what happens is the mind leaves the experience of the present moment, leaves the taste of the food, and goes off into these fantasies about the future.

It turns out that all anxiety is actually anticipatory. And even people that are in terrible present situations are worried about the future. Emergency medical technicians—EMTs, the folks in ambulances—they say that when they are extracting somebody from an accident, even if the person is bleeding and is in very bad shape, they're worried about the future. The person will think, will I be able to walk? Will my loved ones be OK? Will we survive?

You can try this yourself. Think about something that makes you anxious. Just take a moment right now. We all don't have too much trouble usually coming up with something. You got it?

Now is the thing you're thinking about something about the past, or the future? Take a moment. Usually if it's something about the past, I'm actually not worried about what I did this morning—I'm worried that I'm going to be incarcerated tonight for what I did this morning. It really always is about the future.

And then there is worry, which I have to think is a uniquely human capacity. I'm a good worrier. I happen to do a lot of traveling, giving presentations like this one, and in the Boston area, really the only practical way to get the airport from where I live is to go through a tunnel that goes under Boston Harbor.

So one day I hadn't left really very much extra time and I was driving into the tunnel. And halfway into the tunnel, I had an opportunity for taillight meditation because the traffic stopped. And then it stayed stopped. And it became one of those traffic jams where people get out of their cars to discuss the matter. And I started to worry. I started to think, what if I miss my flight? Well, there might be a later one, but this is a pretty busy travel day. There might not be any room in it. Could I drive or take the train? No, it's too far. Well, what can I do? Should I call the airline? No, that probably wouldn't help. Guess I'll just have to be here. I'll follow my breath. Rising, falling. Rising, falling.

What if I miss my flight? There might be a later one, but this is a pretty busy travel day. And the whole cycle just starts over, and over, and over. It is really quite remarkable the way this works. And usually what happens is when we get to the end of whatever the worry loop is there is a feeling like, oh gosh, what will I do?—and then a sense of helplessness, and then we go on to start worrying again.

Now, why do we do this? Now sometimes, of course, we get positively reinforced. Sometimes we'll get into our worry loop and we'll come up with a novel solution to the problem. But most of the time we don't.

There's just something about going through the thinking process that gives us the illusion that it's somehow going to keep us safe, and help us to cope, and prepare us for what may come. Indeed, when I was sitting there in the tunnel, waiting and hoping, I wasn't just passively accepting my fate—I was actively worrying.

We have a lot of techniques that we do to try to avoid the risk of fear or pain. This is because we find anxiety to be very unpleasant. One set of these we might call the Diver Dan approach to life. And this involves phobic avoidance or constriction. It's the things that we do in order to avoid any circumstance that might bring on fear or might bring on discomfort.

You know folks like this. If they're going to the airport, they head there three hours early. In fact, often they don't even go to the airport. They decide, I'd rather not travel. I'd rather stay home. Traveling makes me nervous.

And then there are the things we do directly to tackle anxiety when it comes up. An awful lot of people medicate anxiety. Now, sometimes that's with prescription drugs that are prescribed by a doctor. Very often it's not. Very often it's simply having a drink under this circumstance or that, or using other drugs.

Probably what we do more than anything else is we try to distract ourselves. Do you want to guess what the leading leisure activity is in America? What do we do more of here than anything else in our free time? If you guessed watch television, you got that right. Then think about what number two might be. A lot of times these days people will say the internet, but that is actually a subset of what number two is. Number two is shopping; it's looking to acquire new things.

I remember in the early days of the internet when it was just shifting over from being the province of the military and the province of academic institutions into becoming the World Wide Web where it would be accessible to everybody. I heard Bill Gates being interviewed, and he was saying, you know when the internet really takes hold, it's going to be fantastic. It's going to be a worldwide marketplace.

And I thought, well, a library, I could get that; a post office, I could get that; but a marketplace? Now we know why he is Bill Gates and I am Ron. It's become a marketplace. And we spend an inordinate amount of time shopping on the internet.

Now the problem with all of these different forms of distraction is we develop what's called *stimulation tolerance*. We wind up needing more and more or higher and higher doses in order to distract ourselves from unpleasant thoughts and feelings, including anxiety.

Some of you may remember *Perry Mason*. If you don't, if you're too young to remember him, *Perry Mason* was the precursor to *Law & Order*. It was a very early cop and lawyer show. And on *Perry Mason*, there used to almost always be a scene. It would look like this: You see somebody with their hand outstretched having a pistol in the hand, and boom, you would see the gun go off, and then there would be a body lying down. I don't even think there was blood shown. It was just somebody lying down. And this was the intense moment of the show. This is all happening on a 14-inch black-and-white set, but it would rivet the whole country watching this, and distract us effectively from our own personal concerns.

Nowadays, if you are watching *Law & Order* hideous event seven, or whatever they're up to, there's never just one story, because if there were just one story, we might habituate to it. We might start again thinking about our thoughts and feelings and our fears. So instead, there are always at least two stories. And in one of them, there is a doe-eyed child being ritually dismembered by some kind of satanic cult. In another, there is some kind of very attractive vixen or something involved in some weird sexual activity. And we can be watching all of this on a 50- to 60-inch flat screen, full color TV and think, there is nothing too interesting on. I think I will change the channel. So the problem is that when we try to use distraction, we need more and more of it to bring ourselves away from our fears.

Now, how do anxiety disorders actually develop? Most of them develop through what is called *escape-avoidance learning*. So here is how you can create an anxiety disorder in just a few simple steps. First, you have to enter a situation. Let's call it the supermarket, for example. And let's say that you're walking down the cereal aisle. Now the strict biological determinists or some behaviorist will say anxiety tends to arise at random. Other mental health professionals say, you know, I don't really it's so random. But I think the process is often unconscious. So let's say I am walking down the cereal aisle. And let's say something happened when I was five or six years old with my brother at the kitchen table involving Cocoa Puffs. It's long since been repressed because it was a painful experience as a young child. But here I am walking down the cereal aisle and unconsciously I just happen to spy, out of my peripheral vision, the Cocoa Puffs. And that's enough to bring up a little bit of anxiety because this is how associational memory works. It just takes a little trigger to be able to connect us back to something that has been difficult.

So anxiety is going to arise. Now, we find anxiety unpleasant, so most of us try to take steps to get rid of it. Especially if we have some kind of misattribution, if I start to think, uh-oh, maybe I'm having a cardiac problem. Or, uh-oh, I'm getting short of breath. I may have trouble breathing. Or, uh-oh, I'm going to have some kind of real anxiety episode. I'm going to want to flee the situation. And chances are I'll leave the cereal aisle. In fact, I may even leave the supermarket entirely and go out into the parking lot.

Once I get into the parking lot, ah, that's going to feel better. The anxiety is going to abate. And this reduction in anxiety is called *negative reinforcement*. Negative reinforcement is a principle in learning theory about the reinforcement that comes from removing an unpleasant experience. Like, if I'm being hit over the head with a hammer and I do a certain behavior and I stopping being hit over the head with a hammer, I'm going to be more likely to do that behavior the next time, because it feels good to have the negative experience stop.

So once this is negatively reinforced, what do you think is going to happen the next time that I enter the supermarket, even if I don't go near the cereal aisle? I am going to have a thought that goes something like, gosh. I hope I don't feel the way I did the last time I was here. And that's going to be enough to get a little bit of anxiety going in my mind and body. And once a little bit of anxiety starts going, I'm going to have another thought. I'm going to have the thought, uh-oh. It's happening again. And chances are I am going to get into the same loop, leave again, more negative reinforcement for fleeing, and after a while I might start avoiding the supermarket entirely.

And then this can extend to other things. Then I could start avoiding the post office and other locations. This can work its way into full-blown what is called the *agoraphobia*, which is fear of the marketplace, fear of going out into the world. But even if it doesn't get to that state, most of us develop these patterns, in little ways, around things that we're afraid of and we start to avoid.

So how might we treat this? What would the answer be? Well, the general answer in modern psychology is exposure and response prevention. Let me give you an example of how this works. It has been said that by the mid-1980s, there were no upperclassmen or women left at North American universities with untreated snake phobias. And this is because they had all been recruited for studies in the psychology department. And this is what the studies looked like.

They would invite the student to come into the lab, and they would sit them in an office and just talk to them. And they would tell the student that there was a snake locked in a cage down the hall. Now in the early days, they used to think that it was necessary to do something called *reciprocal inhibition*—in other words, to train the student to do something so that they should feel less anxious. So when the student starts going uh-oh, what kind of snake? They would start teaching them relaxation training and things like that. They have since learned that it's not actually necessary to teach the student relaxation training. All you have to do is stay with the experience long enough until the anxiety abates by itself. So what you do is you talk to the student, describe the snake, answer their questions, and wait it out. Wait until nothing happens and eventually the anxiety starts to abate.

Then what you do is you move the snake a little bit closer. And you tell the student, well, now it's in the next office. They get anxious again, you wait for it to calm down. The essential thing is to actually get to the point where you can bring the snake into the office. So here, you have the scene of the snake in the cage and the student sitting in front of it. The next step, which of course is the hardest, is you have to remove the lid of the cage, take out the snake, and have the student actually handle the snake. And if, as a researcher, you've had sufficient foresight as to choose a non-venomous species, if you do this a number of times, the student loses their snake phobia. Basically, the fear response becomes extinguished because they experience that nothing terrible happens.

Now when people are coming into therapy for anxiety problems, they are not actually interested in handling the snake, by and large, or whatever the equivalent might be. People want us to eliminate the anxious feeling. Instead, what we're going to do, in a mindfulness-oriented approach, is to increase their capacity to bear it, to change their relationship to the experience—very much the way we were discussing when we discussed depression earlier.

Now, this is not a new idea. Here is what the Buddha said about it 2,500 years ago. He said, "Why do I dwell always expecting fear and dread? What if I subdue that fear and dread keeping the same posture that I am in when it comes upon me? While I walked, the fear and dread came upon me; I neither stood nor sat nor lay down until I had subdued that fear and dread."

Now, you may recall that the meditation practices we have been doing are practiced typically in four different postures, sitting, standing, walking, and lying down. So what the Buddha is saying here is, whatever I am doing, I don't scratch the itch, I don't adjust to make the pain go away—the same thing we've been talking about in meditation instructions throughout the course—but rather, I simply stay with the experience until it transforms by itself.

So basically, what we're trying to do is learn how to face our fears. There is another wonderful cartoon that shows a phone booth with a fellow in it. And the phone booth is being suspended by a cable, held out by something like a fishing rod from a high window in an apartment building or an office. And the guy in the phone booth is going nuts and trying to get out. And the caption is, "Professor Gallagher and his controversial technique of simultaneously confronting the fear of snakes, heights, and the dark." I neglected to mention that there is a snake inside as well. And fear of enclosed places also, even though it is not in the caption.

So this idea that facing the fears is what can free us turns out be true both in classical behavioral treatment, and it's true in a mindfulness-oriented treatment. And what we can do is we can try together a stepping into fear exercise where we practice doing this. It is a variation on Professor Gallagher's famous study, only we don't need the high window, and we don't need the phone booth to do it. So let's try that together.

So this is stepping into fear, a variation on professor Gallagher's famous experiment. Begin by finding a comfortable and alert posture. And for this too, allow your eyes to close and find your breath to bring your attention into the present moment.

Now see if you can sense any tension or anxiety anywhere in your body. Maybe just a little bit here or there. Once you sense that, see if you can ramp it up a bit. What we want to do is increase our capacity to be with anxiety, and to do that we have to intensify it enough to be able to really feel it. So try to ramp it up a bit, to a level where you can really feel it. You may be able to do this by simply bringing you attention to the sensations of anxiety in the body, or perhaps you'll need to conjure up an image or a thought that you know can pretty reliably get you going.

Once you feel the anxiety, see if you can bring it up to a level where it feels a little bit challenging, not overwhelming, but—yeah, this is a bit uncomfortable. Once you get it up to that level, try to keep it there for a bit. Now, it's important to keep breathing as you do this, and keep your alert and dignified posture. So just breathe with the fear, breathe with the anxiety, and just accept it as another set of body sensations—just feeling exactly how it feels in the heart, in the muscles. Ah, my old friend, fear, my old friend, anxiety—I know you.

We're just going to stay with it for a little while, increasing our capacity to bear it. Should other thoughts come up that distract you from your anxiety, come back to the sensations of the anxiety. Let them be the object of your awareness. If the anxiety starts to fade, do whatever you need to do to ramp it back up. Perhaps you'll need to come up with new images. Perhaps you'll need to focus with greater intensity on the sensations in the body. Just keep breathing and keep being with the anxiety. Don't let it get away from you; otherwise, you won't have the opportunity to practice. Just be with your old pal. You know, you evolved the capacity for anxiety millions and millions of years ago. It's protected us through so many difficulties. Let's just appreciate it, honor it, and feel it.

Do whatever you need to to make sure that it doesn't slip away, to be able to keep feeling it in the body. You may not be accustomed to embracing anxiety or fear in this way; it kind of changes the experience a bit, but we learn that it's a sensation that we can invite into our life, to simply allow to be there. Just for another few moments, feel it. Then you can come back to your breath, and allow the anxiety to seek its own level. You don't have to keep it up anymore, nor do you have to chase it away. You can just allow it to be there.

Now in this exercise, we're doing this for a short period, but to really practice being with anxiety, it helps to do it for a longer period. And that's why we have included in your recordings the stepping into fear exercise as a longer practice.

Well, I hope you found that exercise interesting. And the exercise is actually much more powerful if you extend it out during a longer period of time. And that's why we have included an audio recording of the exercise in the course materials. Even though I know it seems strange, like why would I want to make myself anxious like this? I think you'll find that if you try that exercise over a longer period over time, that it can actually be quite powerful and that it can actually help to change your relationship to anxious feelings.

Now, many of our anxieties are actually about what we might think of as narcissistic threats. They are threats to us, or our loved ones, or who we think we are. A lot of our anxieties are things like threats to our self image: I'll look badly, what will people think of me? and the like. Sometimes it is about our health: What if I get this disease or that disease? A lot of anxieties have to do with wealth: What if I don't have enough money? What if I have less money than somebody else? Broadly, it's about anticipating that we might lose pleasure or experience pain.

Another great cartoon has a couple of middle-aged women sitting around and a rather hapless middle-aged man sitting there in the middle, and the caption is, "Donald is such a fatalist. He is convinced he is going to grow old and die."

We have some existential problems that we have to face. The reality of old age, of illness, of death can produce a lot of anxiety for ourselves. And mindfulness practices can of course help us with this. In part, the focus on the present moment is antithetical to the anticipatory anxiety. If my attention is here, then I'm not so focused on what is happening later. We can really take an attitude of not knowing.

We can take refuge in the present moment. Very often, when we are having anxious thoughts about what's going to happen in the future, it's because we can't stand the uncertainty. We have a lot of difficulty tolerating the fact that we really don't know what is going to happen in the next moment. And yet, we really don't know what is going to happen in the next moment.

There is a wonderful story about a meditation teacher in a Thai monastery. And he has some Western monks there and one of the Western monks comes and says to the teacher, "I just want to let you know, I won't be around the monastery tomorrow because tomorrow I have to go into Bangkok. I'm going to be there taken care of some financial matters." And the teacher says, "Maybe."

It's very hard for us to live not knowing. And yet, mindfulness practice can help us to do that more by bringing us back to the present moment. There is also a safety that comes from identifying with the universe larger than us so that I don't have to be so worried about these various narcissistic threats.

Something else that scares us a lot are unwanted feelings. Much anxiety is fear of our own emotions and impulses, fear of the tigers within. I might be afraid of my anger, or my sadness, or sexual urges that wouldn't be accepted by others or that I'd be judged for. I might be afraid of repressed or suppressed memories, or unacceptable thoughts of all sorts. When these things start to arise, we find ourselves getting anxious. And doing mindfulness practice regularly allows opportunities for these feelings and impulses to arise and be accepted, to become integrated so that we no longer fear and resist them. And then the source of anxiety abates.

This is one reason why I have been encouraging you throughout the course, and encourage you now again, to please try these practices in between the lectures because the more time we spend sitting with our experience, the more we can integrate these different contents of the mind, and the less we have to be afraid of them.

Now, if you are particularly anxious, it can be hard to just sit and do something like the breath meditation. So in those situations, it's usually best to do more active practice, to do something like walking meditation, or eating meditation, or even Hatha yoga, which is a form of very gentle stretching that can be done in a mindful way. All of these things are easier, the same way you see when somebody is waiting outside of a surgical room, for example, at the hospital—they tend to pace. It dissipates the anxiety a little bit, makes it easier to work with.

So in our next lecture, we are going to look at a set of remarkably common difficulties that are closely related to anxiety, and that have actually become an epidemic in modern societies, where mindfulness practices are particularly well-suited to help, and these are stress-related medical disorders. As you'll see, these conditions include a number of maladies that we do not always think of as being stress related. Thanks for listening.

Transforming Chronic Pain
Lecture 14

To the surprise of both doctors and patients alike, a growing body of medical research indicates that a lot of chronic pain disorders, as well as a lot of other common medical problems, are not actually caused by injuries or illness. Rather, they're the result of a complex interaction between the mind and the body. And it turns out that mindfulness practices can help us resolve them. In this lecture, you will learn about stress-related medical disorders.

Chronic Back Pain
- Research shows that chronic back pain is not usually caused by damage to the spine or surrounding muscles. Although it's often thought to be an orthopedic problem, the accumulating evidence is that, for the vast majority of sufferers, it's actually one of the more common stress-related medical conditions.

- The orthopedic story, or the explanation for why we have such enormous epidemics of chronic back pain in the modern world, is that we originally evolved to walk on all fours, but in order to use tools and get fruit and the like, we learned to stand up. And we've adopted all sorts of ergonomically unwise work postures that are giving us the trouble.

- Indeed, it does seem that there's an evolutionary accident that's responsible for our epidemics of chronic back pain, but it's one that has nothing to do with

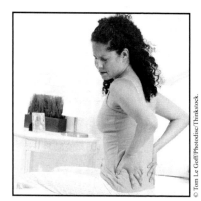

Mindfulness practice can help chronic back pain, which is a stress-related disorder.

structural damage. Instead, it has to do with the various factors and forces that predispose us toward developing chronic muscle tension.

- Research shows that most chronic back pain isn't due to damage to structures of the spine. One study showed that two-thirds of people who have never suffered from any kind of serious back pain had the same sorts of abnormal back structures that are often blamed for the pain.

- Furthermore, millions of people who suffer from chronic back pain show no abnormalities in their backs at all. Finally, there are people with abnormal back structures who still suffer from chronic back pain even after a successful surgery.

- What possibly could be going on here? "Smoking gun" studies offer some answers. Pretty much the entire industrialized and developed world has a chronic pain epidemic, while people in the developing world have much lower incidences of chronic back pain.

- Chronic back pain costs billions of dollars, so some companies have tried to study who is going to get it. In one study, Boeing analyzed thousands of their employees before they developed chronic back pain. The most robust predictor for who would develop chronic back pain over the ensuing years was job dissatisfaction.

- Finally, there are studies that look at what's the quickest way out of acute, rather than chronic, back pain. In study after study, the quickest way out is a rapid return to vigorous exercise.

- None of this would make any sense if the orthopedic story were accurate in accounting for our epidemic of chronic back pain. Instead, chronic back pain is a stress-related disorder.

Stress
- Stress involves the activation of two very important systems in the human body. One of them is the sympathetic branch of the autonomic nervous system. The autonomic nervous system

has a parasympathetic branch, which tends to calm the body, and a sympathetic branch, which tends to arouse the body. The sympathetic nervous system is activated immediately when we experience ourselves to be in danger.

- The second system that is activated is the hyopthalamic pituitary adrenal axis. This is the hormonal system that does similar things as the sympathetic nervous system, but it just comes in a little bit slower.

- Disorders of chronic overarousal or disregulation of the fight-or-flight system include back, neck, and other chronic muscle pain, gastrointestinal distress, headaches, temporomandibular joint disorder, tinnitus, bruxism, insomnia, eczema and other skin disorders, sexual dysfunctions, and panic and other anxiety disorders.

- All of these disorders can be caused either entirely by these arousal patterns, or, as is often the case, there's a medical component to it, and then the arousal component on top of that exacerbates the condition.

- In the case of chronic back pain, a cycle gets established. For example, the cycle might begin with a minor injury, such as overuse. If the person lives in a country that has a preexisting epidemic of chronic back pain, he or she may start to worry about the sensations of pain that arise in the back. When we start to worry, we start to have negative thoughts, and these thoughts bring with them fear, frustration, or even anger. And these negative emotions themselves affect the back. Tense muscles increase the sensation of back pain, which increases the negative thoughts.

- After a short period of time, almost everybody starts to give up activities, because we don't want to reinjure ourselves. Then, we tend to lose strength, endurance, and flexibility, and we get into a bad emotional funk. Sometimes this whole cycle begins with stress or tension from an event in our life that causes the tensing of the muscles and the sensation of back pain, and the problem takes off.

Pain Is Not Imaginary

- While psychological stressors of all types can contribute to chronic back pain, the pain is not imagined. Rather, it's the effect of changes in the musculature of the body.

- Conversion disorders—such as hysterical blindness or hysterical paralysis—are situations in which the body is intact, nothing is broken in terms of organ systems, but we're experiencing it as if it doesn't work. Psychophysiological disorders are not conversion disorders. These are about actual changes in all kinds of aspects of organ systems operating correctly.

- For people to get free from conversion disorders, they need to see that it's real muscle tension that's causing the problem. There are four steps that we go through to resolve these disorders. The first involves a medical evaluation. If there's an underlying medical problem that can be addressed, you certainly want to address it. The next steps involve cognitive restructuring, which is shifting our thought patterns; exposure treatment, which is what is often used for anxiety disorders; and working with negative emotions. Mindfulness practices can help with all of these steps.

- Kinesiophobia is the fear of using the body normally. Treating this fear involves resuming activities often enough to be convinced that they're not damaging. There are a few ways to do this. One that's quite radical works very effectively, and it's done in the gym. A new patient is given a plastic crate filled with weights, and they're asked to take a weight and aerobically put it on the middle shelf and the top shelf of some industrial shelving as quickly as they can.

- This is a very fast method of getting over one's kinesiophobia. The problem is that it has a great chance of dropout, because it can really scare people to start moving their backs so vigorously if they've been so cautious up until then.

- Then, there's a gradual approach, which involves simply beginning with activities that are relatively easily, that are pleasurable or rewarding, and that can be done three or more times per week. You continue until it's no longer feared and until you're convinced that it's not going to make the pain any worse.

The Role of Mindfulness

- We learn through mindfulness practice that pain can be observed as being separate from suffering. Impermanence is a gift, not just a curse. We notice that pain comes and goes. And apparently solid pain states can be observed like frames in a movie. We start to notice that they change from moment to moment.

- We learn that pain is inevitable in life, but suffering is optional. Suffering comes from resisting the pain, which includes grimacing, wincing, and bracing; all of the aversive thoughts; wishes for relief; self-punitive thoughts; and anger, fear, and depression about the condition.

- Neurobiological studies have shown that if we induce pain in a meditator, a meditator responds differently than a non-meditator. Novices showed less activity in areas associated with proprioception—feeling what's going on moment to moment inside the body—but more activity in areas associated with cognitive appraisal, with evaluating and thinking about and reacting to the sensations.

- The more experienced meditators had more activity in the proprioceptive areas. In other words, they were feeling the pain more vividly but less in the areas of cognitive appraisal. So, the experienced meditators actually felt the sensations more but evaluated and resisted them less. Experienced meditators also typically reported the pain as being at a much lower level than the novice meditators.

Cognitive Restructuring

- Mindfulness increases cognitive flexibility. This is important, because we need to believe or understand that beliefs are part of the problem. We need to understand that it's the thought, for example, that you're orthopedically damaged that is part of what's inducing your fear, and that fear is causing the pain. Mindfulness can help us be more flexible about this and notice the relationship between thinking and the body's reactions.

- We can use mindfulness to observe pain-related thoughts, and we can see that anxious thought and feeling is actually playing a big role in the disorder. We can also notice future-oriented catastrophizing, as well as budgeting activity.

- We need to develop what's called creative hopelessness in acceptance and commitment therapy. This is the central paradox in the treatment of psychophysiological disorders generally: Attachment to symptom reduction, or trying to feel better, perpetuates the disorder. In the case of chronic back pain, it's avoiding using the back normally, because we want to "heal," that actually locks us into the cycle. This applies equally in other disorders.

- Because we become subject to control addiction, we try desperately to get the problem or symptoms to go away. Through mindfulness practice—awareness of present experience as acceptance—we learn that it's useful to control our behavior. In the case of chronic back pain, it's useful to go to the gym, but we can't control the sensations. The sensations are going to come and go.

- This can be difficult given our cultural bias toward symptom relief, because we're always being offered medicine to make the symptoms go away. Instead, we're going to be increasing the capacity to bear experience rather than getting rid of experience.

Suggested Reading

Dahl, Wilson, Luciano, and Hayes, *Acceptance and Commitment Therapy for Chronic Pain*.

Shubiner and Betzold, *Unlearn Your Pain*.

Siegel, *The Mindfulness Solution*, chapter 7.

———, "Psychophysiological Disorders.".

———, Urdang, and Johnson, *Back Sense*.

Questions to Consider

1. How in the past has medicine misunderstood chronic back pain and other often stress-related pain syndromes?

2. What more broadly are psychophysiological disorders, and how are they different from the conversion disorders that Sigmund Freud studied and treated?

Transforming Chronic Pain
Lecture 14—Transcript

To the surprise of both doctors and patients alike, a growing body of medical research indicates that a lot of chronic pain disorders, as well as a lot of other common medical problems, are not actually caused by injuries or illness. Rather, they're the result of a complex interaction between the mind and the body. And it turns out that mindfulness practices can help us to resolve them.

Let's start by looking at chronic back pain, which, oddly enough, we're discovering is not usually caused by damage to the spine or surrounding muscles. Although it's often thought to be an orthopedic problem, the accumulating evidence is that, for the vast majority of sufferers, it's actually one of the more common stress-related medical conditions.

So if you have chronic back pain and show up in the orthopedist's office, typically we're shown a diagram or a photograph of the back, the spine in particular. And what we see are a series of hard bony vertebrae separated by cushioning disks. And what we're told is that these cushioning disks are kind of like jelly donuts—they have a firm outer compartment, or outer surface, and a squishy inner part. And that what happens with wear and tear over the years is that some of the squishy inner part bulges out, might break off entirely, and winds up pushing against nerves that run up against the spine, and that this is the cause of a lot of the problems.

I was actually a chronic back pain patient myself once. And I can tell you that there's nothing quite like being told that your spine consists of a series of bony vertebrae separated by jelly doughnuts to give you a sense of its robust nature, and to give you confidence that you can use your back in all sorts of different life activities.

The other thing that we're frequently told we might call "the orthopedic story." And this is the explanation for why it is that we have such enormous epidemics of chronic back pain in the modern world. And what we're told is that we originally evolved to walk on all fours, but, in order to use tools and get fruit and the like, we learned to stand up. And now we've adopted all sorts of ergonomically unwise work postures. And it's these ergonomically unwise work postures that are giving us the trouble.

Indeed, it does seem that there's an evolutionary accident that's responsible for our epidemics of chronic back pain, but it happens not to be this evolutionary accident. In fact, it's one that has nothing to do with structural damage. What it has to do with instead are the various factors and forces that predispose us toward developing chronic muscle tension.

Now when working with patients who have chronic back pain, it turns out that in order to help them begin to resolve the disorder, they have to first start changing their understanding of what's causing the disorder. Because as long as people think that the disorder is because their back is somehow damaged and that it's fragile, they're going to behave in ways that are actually going to perpetuate the other factors that maintain the problem.

So I like to present evidence to patients from the research literature about the idea that most chronic back pain isn't actually due to damage to structures of the spine. Let me give you a few examples.

One of my favorite studies involved doing MRIs up and down the spine of 99 people. And these were unusual people, because these were people who had never suffered from any kind of back pain lasting more than two days in a row. And only about 20 percent of the population fits that criteria. And what they did was they did these scans, and then they gave them to specially trained neuroradiologists to evaluate. And the neuroradiologists went to read the films, but the researchers didn't want to tip them off about what the study was about. So they took the films of these unusually healthy people and they mixed them in with people with chronic back pain, had the radiologist look at them, then looked at the results of the reads of just the subjects in the study. And they found that two-thirds of these people who had never suffered from any kind of serious back pain before had the same sorts of abnormal back structures that are often blamed for the pain.

Then there are studies that show millions of people suffer from chronic back pain, and they show no abnormalities in their backs at all. They go from doctor to doctor. They get multiple MRIs, and they all look clean. Finally, there are people who have abnormalities on their MRI. They go in for surgery. The surgery is a success. The only problem is the pain doesn't go away. And nowadays surgeons will take a look six months or a year later, do a repeat MRI, and most of the time the craftsmanship was fine. The back looks fully repaired. The only problem is that the person is still suffering.

So what possibly could be going on here? Well there are what we might call the "smoking gun studies." Would you like to guess what countries have chronic back pain epidemics? Chances are if you're watching this, the country you live in is included because it's the United States, it's Canada, it's all of Western Europe—although there something curious happened, because when the Iron Curtain was intact, East Germany had a low incidence while West Germany had a high incidence. Then the wall came down. The Berlin Wall was taken apart and the East Germans actually caught the disorder from the West Germans. Now that's curious. Looking for other areas that have this, the Pacific Rim—pretty much the entire industrialized and developed world has a chronic pain epidemic.

If we ask the question the other way, it gets even more interesting. Who doesn't have this problem? Well, it turns out that people in the developing world have way lower incidences of chronic back pain than people in the developed world. In fact, a study by the WHO showed that Nigeria had the lowest rates of any country. And within Nigeria, it was the poor rural farmers that seemed to have the least pain. Now that really doesn't make a lot of sense if we think this is due to structural damage.

I don't know if you've ever traveled in the third world, but the standard mode of transportation is usually a pickup truck with a couple of benches on the back and people go jostling over rutted roads with their spines being shocked—there usually aren't even very good springs or shock absorbers. And they might go hours a day to get to market or to get to their fields. And these folks don't seem to have chronic back pain. They also don't have ergonomically designed workstations, and they don't sleep on Sealy Posturepedic mattresses either. That's very curious.

Chronic back pain costs industry billions of dollars, so some companies have tried to study who's going to get it. And these are prospective studies. One of the best was done by the Boeing Corporation. And they analyzed thousands of their employees before they developed chronic back pain. And they looked at their psychological makeup. They looked at what their workstations were like. They looked at their health habits.

You want to guess what the most robust predictor was for who would develop chronic back pain over the ensuing years? It didn't have anything to do with whether they had to lift things in the factory floor, or sat in a seat on a truck, or were hunched over a computer—those factors weren't important. The most important factor was job dissatisfaction. People who didn't like their work tended to develop chronic back pain.

Finally, there are studies that look at what's the quickest way out of acute, rather than chronic, back pain—in other words, short-lived back pain. And the quickest way out, in study after study, is a rapid return to vigorous exercise. Now none of this would make any sense at all if the orthopedic story were accurate in accounting for our epidemic of chronic back pain. Rather, something else is afoot here.

There's a cartoon about this that has two women facing each other, and one says to the other, "Honey stress, isn't par for the course, it is the course." So these are stress-related disorders.

Now what do we mean by stress? When we're talking about stress, we're basically talking about the activation of two very important systems in the human body. One of them is the activation of the sympathetic branch of the autonomic nervous system. You may recall that the autonomic nervous system has a parasympathetic branch, which tends to calm the body, and a sympathetic branch, which tends to arouse the body.

The sympathetic nervous system is activated immediately when we experience ourselves to be in danger. Close on its heels is the activation of the HPA axis. That's the hypothalamic pituitary adrenal axis. And this is a hormonal system that pretty much does similar things to the activation of the sympathetic nervous system. It just comes in a little bit slower.

So let's look at how these systems operate in a well-adjusted individual. Unfortunately, I wasn't able to find one among *Homo sapiens*, so we're going to have to use a bunny instead. And I want you to imagine a bunny sitting in a field quietly munching on some grass. And let's just imagine that that bunny spies a fox at the corner of the field. He's going to have some very predictable psychophysiological responses.

The bunny's ears are going to perk up. He's going to actually be able to orient them toward the fox—bunnies look very cute when they do that. And his hearing will become more acute; he'll be able to hear better than he could have before getting aroused. He'll obviously look at the fox. He's likely to have the muscles at the base of the hairs all contract to make his hairs stand up. That's to make him look big and ferocious. And if you think that's silly in a bunny, that's our goose bumps. You can imagine how many lions we've warded off with our goose bumps over the years.

His heart rate is going to pick up, his respiration rate is going to pick up, his body temperature is going to go up, his blood pressure is going to go up. At the same time, his digestion is going to tend to shut down, and of particular relevance for studying back pain, is all of his skeletal muscles are going to tense, because he's getting ready to do some combination of fight, freeze, and flee.

Now bunnies aren't particularly big fighters, so he's probably getting ready primarily to freeze, and then run out of there when he gets his chance. Now if the fox leaves, all of these systems are going to reverse. The parasympathetic nervous system is going to become activated. The HPA axis is going to return to baseline. And inside of something like 20 minutes, the bunny will look the way he looked before the fox ever arrived on the scene.

But this bunny is a poor primitive creature. He has none of our capacity for abstract logic, for anticipatory thought, and for problem solving. If the bunny were sophisticated like us, he'd be able to think, I wonder where the fox went. Maybe he went back to his den to tell his friends about me. Or worse, maybe he's headed for the next field where my wife and kids are. Damn. Now if the bunny were really sophisticated like us, he'd be able to think, gee, do I still have sufficient carrots in my 401(k) to make it into retirement, and other concerns.

Now this sets the poor bunny up for what we suffer with, and this is a whole host of disorders of chronic overarousal or disregulation. This involves back, neck, and other chronic muscle pain; gastrointestinal distress of all sorts; upper GI distress of gastritis and things associated with too much stomach acid production; lower GI problems such as irritable bowel syndrome; headaches; temporomandibular joint disorder, which is a pain in this joint here; tinnitus, which is ringing of the ears; bruxism; insomnia; eczema another skin disorders; a whole host of sexual dysfunctions; and of course panic and other anxiety disorders.

Now I'm not suggesting that all of these disorders are always caused by this over activation or disregulation of the fight or flight system—they can, of course, have independent medical causes. But all of these disorders can actually be caused either entirely by these arousal patterns, or, as is often the case, there's a medical component to it, and then there's this arousal component on top that exacerbates the condition.

So let's look at how this might work in the case of chronic back pain, because a cycle gets established. And the cycle might begin with, let's say, an injury. Maybe a minor injury, such as overuse. Where I live in the northeast, this often occurs sometime in December when the white fluffy stuff starts to fall, and people begin to do this motion [shoveling] after having spent most of the year not doing that motion. And the back muscles start to hurt.

Now if the person is so unfortunate as to live in a country that has a pre-existing epidemic of chronic back pain, he or she may start to worry about the sensations of pain that arise in the back. When we start to worry, we start to have negative thoughts, and these thoughts bring with them fear. They may also bring with them a sense of frustration or even anger. And these negative emotions themselves affect the back.

I want you to join me for a moment, if you're in a situation where you can do this, in doing a little bit of acting, to see how these different emotions affect the body. We're going to begin with fear. So if you can join me in this, when I say three, I want you to enact in your body what fear feels like. You don't have to call out, because it might not be appropriate where you are, but simply show the body sensations. Ready? At three, we're going to do fear. One, two, three. OK, excellent. Now we're going to do anger. Ready? One, two, three. Great. Now we're going to move toward frustration and really join me in this, so that you can see what's happening in your body. Do frustration. One, two, three.

And then finally—this is the final exam for acting—show what it's like to have a feeling of anger, but not wanting to show it. Like perhaps you're frustrated with your doctor, or you're frustrated with your boss, or with your in-laws, or the cop that's just pulled you over and you don't think it was fair. Ready? One, two, three. OK.

Now what was happening to your skeletal muscles in all of those conditions? I think you'll notice that in all of those conditions, the skeletal muscles tense. So we have this very interesting phenomenon in human beings, which is that our chief negative emotions, the ones we have the most difficulty with, all involve the tensing of the musculature.

Now tense muscles, we know, hurt. Have you ever had these muscles tighten up on your back? Or perhaps had a charley horse on your calf muscle and felt that tighten up? Tense muscles can be extremely painful. So coming back to our cycle, tense muscles increase the sensation of back pain. This increased sensation of back pain increases the negative thoughts. Now I thought, uh-oh, it's getting worse. I've really damaged myself. And this goes off and running and becomes a whole cycle.

After a very little period of time, almost everybody starts to give up activities, because we don't want to re-injure ourselves. And then we tend to lose strength, endurance, and flexibility, and we get into a bad emotional funk. Now sometimes this whole cycle gets going without ever shoveling the snow. It just begins with stress or tension from an event in our life that causes the tensing of the muscles and causes the sensation of back pain, and the problem takes off.

Now it's very important to resolve these disorders to recognize that the pain is not imaginary. Psychological stresses of all sorts can contribute to it, but it's not all in the head. Rather, it's the effect of changes in the musculature of the body.

So to my mind, [there's] an interesting story about Freud's history and how he came up with psychoanalysis that actually pertains to this. Freud originally trained as a research neurologist, and he wanted to be an academic. Actually, he wanted to study the sexual functioning of the giant squid. Now, this wasn't because he was some kind of oddball, it was because in the giant squid there's a very large nerve that runs down the center of the squid and, in Freud's day, it was one of the only nerves that you could get electrodes into and measure.

But he happened to be Jewish, and there were very strict quotas on Jews entering the Academy. And he couldn't get a job doing research. So he decided he'll go into clinical neurology. And clinical neurology in his day was largely treating what we call *conversion disorders*. These are things like hysterical blindness, or hysterical paralysis—situations in which the body is intact, nothing's broken in terms of organ systems, but we're experiencing it as though it doesn't work. Psychophysiological disorders are not conversion disorders. They're not about the body being intact but us experiencing it as though it doesn't work. They're about actual changes, in this case, in the musculature, or, as we look at others, we'll see there are changes in the digestive system, changes in blood flow, changes in all sorts of aspects of organ systems operating correctly. For people to get free from this, they need to see that it's real muscle tension that's doing it.

So there are basically four steps that we go through to resolve these disorders. The first involves a medical evaluation. I was taught early in my training that it's very bad form for a psychologist to psychoanalyze or do behavioral treatment for a brain tumor. If there's an underlying medical problem that can be addressed, you certainly want to get that addressed. And the same is true here. If there's kidney disease, if there's an actual tumor or something like that, obviously that needs treatment.

Then the other steps are going to involve cognitive restructuring, which is shifting our thought patterns about this, exposure treatment, like we talked about with anxiety disorders, and then working with negative emotions. And as we'll see, mindfulness practices can help us to do all of these steps.

We're going to do exposure and response prevention, only instead of treating our fear of snakes, we're going to treat our fear of movement. We're going to treat what's called *kinesiophobia*, the fear of using the body normally. And the way we do this is by resuming activities often enough to be convinced that they're not damaging.

Now there are a couple of ways to do this. One that's quite radical works very effectively, and it's done in the gym. We could think of it as the weird science experiment gone awry. Here's what it looks like. There's industrial shelving—imagine this at about three feet and five feet, and imagine a gym filled with people. And what's happening is a new patient comes in, and they're given a milk crate, a plastic crate filled with weights. And they're asked to just take this weight and aerobically put it on the middle shelf and the top shelf as quickly as they can, and to ignore everything that they learned in back school—everything that they've ever been told about being careful with the back. Instead, they're told to do it as a child would do it at 10 years of age who is in a contest, who is being paid or is going to win a prize for doing it as quickly as possible. This is a very fast method of getting over one's kinesiophobia. The problem is that it has a great chance of dropout, because it can really scare people to start moving their backs so vigorously if they've been so cautious up until now.

Then there's a gradual approach, and that's where you simply begin with activities that are relatively easily, that are pleasurable or rewarding—there's no reason to start with something you hate—and that can be done three or more times a week. And the advantage of doing it three or more times a week is if the pain kicks up, and we're doing it only once a week, we might start to think, oh gosh, you see it's because I did that exercise. It's now causing me problems—and then we want to avoid the exercise. If we're doing it regularly, then the pain is going to come and go. It's going to fluctuate even as we keep up the activity. And you continue until it's no longer feared and until you're convinced that it's not going to make the pain any worse.

So now let's talk about mindfulness and the role that it plays in this. The Buddha spoke about this 2,500 years ago, and here's what he said:

> When touched with a feeling of pain, the uninstructed run-of-the-mill person sorrows, grieves, and laments, beats his breast, becomes distraught. So he feels two pains, physical and mental. Just as if they were to shoot a man with an arrow and, right afterward, were to shoot him with another one, so that he would feel the pains of two arrows.

So let's take a moment. The first arrow is the moment-to-moment pain sensations, and the second arrow is this sorrow, grieving, lamenting—basically the resistance that we have to the pain.

I was talking to a patient of mine who worked at MIT, and beginning to outline basically the Buddhist message around this, and my patient said, as people who work at MIT often do, "Hey there's a mathematical formula for that." And he suggested it's pain times resistance equals suffering. And I thought about it for a bit, and I realized he's right.

If pain is very, very intense—let's say you've literally been shot by an arrow—even if you're a very good mindfulness student, and you're practicing awareness of present experience with acceptance, unless you're really good at it, there's still going to be suffering. But oftentimes pain is in a more moderate range, and nonetheless gives us a lot of grief. And if we can shift our resistance, it transforms the experience.

Let me give you an example that's quite common where I live. In the late spring or the summertime, it's often very nice go out on the porch after work. And during that period of time when the light is just golden and it's the time of day that the artists and the photographers particularly prize, I might be sitting there with a drink or something to eat. And suddenly I might start to hear [buzzing]. And then we start the swatting, right? And it can be so bad as to drive me or whoever I'm with inside.

Now in the early days of mindfulness practices in the United States, sometimes we'd be sitting and practicing outside, let's say at a retreat. And the instruction was don't kill anything if not necessary and simply be with experience. And this was before concerns about eastern equine encephalitis, or West Nile virus, so mosquitoes in the US in those days were pretty harmless. And I remember several experiences in which I would be sitting, doing my meditation practice, rising, falling, being with the breath. And I'd start to hear [buzzing]. And you notice the moment when sound stops that the trouble starts, right?

And sometimes I could actually see where the mosquito had landed. Let's say it was on the back of my hand. And I'd see her—because it's the [female] mosquitoes that do this—[she] would be burying her little proboscis, or whatever that front part is, into my skin, injecting the anticoagulant, beginning to drink—and you could actually see the back part of the mosquito expanding and turning red—and then she would fly off to make other mosquitoes. After a few moments, the little bump would start to emerge as the anticoagulant irritated the tissues of the hand. And the whole thing was not only not aversive, it was fascinating. It was like having my own National Geographic film happening right here on my hand. And this stood in such contrast to what it would be like on other occasions.

I remember going camping at times, when I'd get into the tent with my wife, perhaps, and we'd zip it up, and we'd start to hear [buzzing]. And then the dialogue would start. "Is it in the tent? Oh god, I think it's in the tent." "Oh no, it's in the tent. We'll never sleep." Same mosquito, very different level of resistance.

So what we learn through mindfulness practice is that pain can be observed as being separate from suffering. Impermanence is a gift, not just a curse. We notice that pain comes and pain goes. And apparently solid pain states can be observed like frames in a movie—we start to notice that they change from moment to moment. So we learn that pain is inevitable in life, but suffering is optional. Suffering comes from resisting the pain. And that's the grimacing, wincing, the bracing, all the aversive thoughts, the wishes for relief—when will it stop?—the self-punitive thoughts—I never should have shoveled the snow—and the anger, fear, and depression about the condition.

Now there have been studies—neurobiological studies—that show that if we induce pain in a meditator, a meditator responds differently than a non-meditator. Novices showed less activity in areas associated with proprioception, with feeling what's going on moment to moment inside the body, but more activity in areas associated with cognitive appraisal, with evaluating and thinking about and reacting to the sensations.

The more experienced meditators had more activity in the proprioceptive areas—in other words, they were feeling the pain more vividly—but less in the areas of cognitive appraisal. So the experienced meditators actually felt the sensations more, but evaluated them and resisted them less. And when they were asked to report how was that for you, the experienced meditators typically reported the pain as being at a much lower level than the novice meditators.

So now, let's talk about cognitive restructuring. Mindfulness, as we've discussed other lectures, helps us to increase cognitive flexibility. And this is important because we need to believe or understand that beliefs are part of the problem. We need to understand that it's the thought, for example, that I'm orthopedically damaged that is part of what's inducing my fear, and that fear is causing the pain. So mindfulness can help us to be more flexible about this and to notice the relationship between thinking and the body's reactions.

We can actually use it to observe pain-related thoughts, to notice how often a frightened thought comes into the mind about the back. And we can see that anxious thought and feeling is actually playing a big role in the disorder. We can also notice future-oriented catastrophizing—"Oh no, what if I'm not able to work," et cetera—as well as the budgeting of activity—that's the thought of, "I've already sat for two hours, I better cancel dinner; It'll be too much for me."

We need to develop what's called "creative hopelessness" in Acceptance and Commitment Therapy. You know the Chinese handcuffs that we had as a kid? You put your fingers in there and you try to separate them. What happens the harder you pull on them? The tighter they grip, right? This is the central paradox in the treatment of psychophysiological disorders, generally. It's attachment to symptom reduction. Trying to feel better is what perpetuates the disorder. In the case of chronic back pain, what this is, is it's avoiding using the back normally because we want it to "heal" that actually locks us into the cycle. We'll soon see that it applies equally in other disorders.

Because we become subject to control addiction, we try desperately to try to get the problem to go away, to try to get the symptoms to stop. And what we learn through mindfulness practice, awareness of present experience with acceptance, is that it's useful to control our behavior—in the case of chronic back pain, it's useful to go to the gym—but we can't control the sensations. The sensations are going to come and go like the weather. And this can be difficult given our cultural bias toward symptom relief, because we're always being offered take this medicine, take that medicine to make the symptoms go away. Instead, as we've discussed before, we're going to be increasing the capacity to bear experience, rather than getting rid of experience.

It should be quite clear now that we're not talking about relaxation training here, we're talking about changing our attitude toward the symptoms. And we increase symptom tolerance by doing this. You can simply sit, let's say you're doing breath meditation, and pain might appear on the back, and we can simply allow the object of awareness to move from the breath to the moment-to-moment sensations of back pain. If the back pain is really hard and we're having trouble bearing it, sometimes expanding the area—in other words, paying attention to—let's say the back pain is right here. We expand the area to go everywhere from the shoulders down to the buttocks. Embracing a larger area can make it easier to tolerate it.

Now finally I want to say few words about working with negative emotions. Do you remember Spock on *Star Trek*? I think his mother was a human and his father was a Vulcan. And he was one of these guys who couldn't really talk about feelings very well. He had what we used to call *alexithymia*, which is "no words for feelings." You might just call it being a guy sometimes. When we don't have words for feeling, and we don't notice what's happening, we react with tension every time that some unwanted feeling comes up in our awareness. And this tension can actually contribute to these chronic stress disorders. Mindfulness practices, as we've seen before, can help us to notice all these different thoughts and feelings and, as a result, to deal with these tensions better and not have them accumulate.

Now while mindfulness practices can be very helpful in working with chronic pain, they of course only work if we practice them. So once again, and I'm sorry if I sound repetitive about this, but I encourage you to remember the challenge of how to get to Carnegie Hall. You have to practice and practice. And the more you practice these, the more they'll become useful tools for you to work with dealing with chronic pain, and, as we'll see shortly, other chronic medical disorders that are caused by stress.

In our next lecture, we're going to look at some of these stress-related medical problems that can be helped through mindfulness practices. And we'll also see the amazing power of placebos—how illnesses can become a doorway to psychological growth when we start to understand the effect that the mind has on the body. Thanks.

Placebos, Illness, and the Power of Belief
Lecture 15

One of the biggest challenges that people face in recovering from psychophysiological or stress-related disorders is believing that the mind could be powerful enough to cause the illness. And this is because these disorders are so disruptive to the body. One of the ways that patients can understand this is by learning about placebo studies, because in the effects of the placebos, we see just how powerfully the mind can influence our organ systems.

The Effects of Placebos

- Placebos are inactive substances—sugar or starch pills—that are given to people with some suggestion that they might help. Among placebo pills, bigger pills are more effective than smaller pills, and two pills tend to be more effective than one pill.

- The dose-response curve of most placebos is remarkably similar to aspirin, ibuprofen, or acetaminophen. It reaches maximum efficacy

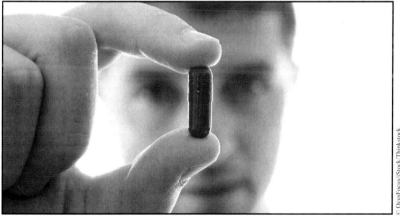

The widely studied placebo effect is the notion that a sugar pill can improve the condition of a patient in similar ways as a real pill.

in 20 to 30 minutes, and then it tends to trail off in its effectiveness after four to six hours. Active placebos are much more effective than passive placebos. An active placebo isn't just sugar or starch; it's some medicine that in some way causes some response in the body that is uncomfortable, even if that response has nothing to do with the purported effect of the placebo.

- Injections tend to be much more effective than pills. Active injections—in other words, injections of substances that change how we feel in the body—are more effective than injections of saline. And the really powerful placebos are surgical.

- An example of the remarkable power of placebos dates back to the 1970s and involves treatment for temporomandibular joint (TMJ) disorder, which is pain that occurs in the joints of the jaw muscles and the jaw joint. At that time, it was thought that the epidemic of TMJ problems were due to the deterioration of the joints, and oral surgeons were busy putting replacement disks into the joint.

- One enterprising group of dentists believed that TMJ was not about the structure of the jaw. Instead, they believed that it was about the patient's attitude toward the TMJ symptoms. They decided to try an intervention called sham tooth grinding. They created a dental instrument that was about an inch in diameter and maybe six or eight inches long that vibrated a lot.

- They told patients that they were going to realign their bite, and they would put this instrument into the patient's mouth and vibrated it for about 45 minutes, after which they told the patient that they had restructured the shape of the patient's teeth so that he or she would have a better bite, which should resolve the difficulty.

- Perhaps not surprisingly, 64 percent of the patients who had sham tooth grinding had total or significant relief a year after only one application of the procedure. Of course, this type of experimentation with patients is unethical, especially by today's standards. And for a long time, studies like this one were not conducted.

- In the year 2000, a team of enterprising surgeons and researchers at the University of Texas came up with a plan by which they could do a placebo/control surgery and get it passed by an institutional review board, because it was an ethical plan.

- They told subjects in advance that they were going to be randomly distributed to groups receiving either arthroscopic debridement, which involved making little incisions around the knee to do arthroscopic surgery and smoothing out the structures under the kneecap; arthroscopic lavage, which involved washing out the structures under the kneecap; or incisions only, which was the placebo group.

- The surgeons did the surgery, but then they never saw the patients again. But the researchers followed them in the post-operative period, and then for over the next two years. The researchers were completely blind to the condition; they had no idea who had the surgery and who had only placebo interventions. They found that everybody improved. Real surgery had no advantage of the placebo at any point during the two years following the surgery.

Using Mindfulness to Treat Disorders
- Studies of the placebo effect show that the body and mind are closely interacting with one another, and the mind is extremely powerful in the effects that it can have on our subjective experience of the body. So, how do we use these principles to treat disorders?

- Muscle tension disorders, which are remarkably similar to chronic back pain in their dynamics, include headaches; temperomandibular joint disorder; and neck, knee, foot, wrist, and shoulder pain.

- With chronic back pain, we know that the correlation between what's found in the imaging of the spine and what people experience in terms of subjective distress is very, very low. The condition of the spine only rarely actually influences whether or not people will be in pain.

- With neck, knee, wrist, and shoulder pain, we don't quite have the data—largely because we haven't done large-scale studies in which we take people without knee, shoulder, or wrist pain and assess what the body parts look like for them. The science isn't there yet, but the basic principle of treatment is the same.

- The central dynamic in a lot of sexual dysfunctions is fear of the dysfunction itself. Before Viagra and Cialis existed, we had the inventions of Masters and Johnson to treat erectile dysfunction. They were sex therapists who had some pretty effective non-pharmacological treatments. They were teaching mindfulness practice where the focus was central touch. For erectile dysfunction, they found that about 75 percent of the time, just training couples to focus on touch would resolve the disorder.

- The conventional treatment for insomnia is stimulus control, or teaching people to associate the bed with sleep; sleep hygiene, which involves waking up and going to bed at the same time each day; and relaxation training.

- An alternative is to do mindfulness treatment—to simply use the time in bed as an opportunity to be aware of present experience with acceptance. It turns out that mindfulness practice actually reduces our need for sleep. In addition, if we trust that mindfulness practice will help to be restorative for us, then we can give up the goal-orientation aspect of needing to fall sleep.

- The gastrointestinal (GI) system is remarkably sensitive to our emotional lives. Our GI system will often shut down when we're under stress, or it will suddenly become overactive. People experience all manner of GI distress, including upper and lower GI symptoms.

- Ulcers were once thought to be caused by stress, and then we discovered the role of H. pylori. You can treat an ulcer by giving an antibiotic that kills H. pylori bacteria. But then we discovered that H. pylori infections are actually endemic to large percentages of the population—so what determines whether somebody with *H. pylori* infection gets an ulcer? It turns out that stress is a critical factor in whether the stomach lining becomes broken down in a way that makes it vulnerable to the infection.

- Irritable bowel syndrome (IBS) is a very common disorder. It often consists of alternating constipation and diarrhea. The distress about the symptoms is often the stressor that keeps it going, not unlike what happens with chronic back pain. It's only when people can relax about IBS, and actually use mindfulness practices to simply ride the waves of different sensations, that they do considerably better.

- Another interesting disorder that works similarly is called hyperacusis, which is a somewhat unusual disorder where people become afraid of loud sounds. Loud sounds don't just feel uncomfortable, but they become terribly painful to people. So, naturally, these people try to avoid loud sounds, and they get into a pattern where they work so hard to avoid loud noise that then any noise becomes too intense.

- You can use mindfulness practice to try to resolve hyperacusis. The idea is to simply listen to the noise, noticing how there's the actual experience of the sound, the sensations, and then there's our reaction to the sensations. And as we notice that these could be separated, it becomes much easier to work with the symptoms.

- Another disorder is fibromyalgia. People with this disorder feel particular sensitivity to pain at certain trigger points. In fact, we've learned that people with fibromyalgia are actually sensitive to pain everywhere. This has become something of an epidemic. Fibromyalgia could be one of the stress-related disorders.

Illness Anxiety
- Illness anxiety is a component of all of these different disorders. It's unavoidable, and it's actually remarkably easy to generate. For example, people who live with people with brain tumors have a

lot more headaches than people who don't live with people with brain tumors. And people who have had chronic headaches before rivet on any sensation of pressure, and it becomes a problem, which expands into a headache.

- All it takes is bringing anxious attention to a part of our body, and we can start to feel sensations in that part of our body and start to worry about them. And these things can get amplified very easily.

- There are two basic reactions when we experience something untoward in the body. When we're younger, we might think that it's probably nothing and that you don't have to worry about it. But when we're older, we might start to think that it's probably something serious. These thoughts are now exacerbated by the Internet, because many people resort to searching their symptoms online, which leads to becoming scared of the possibilities.

- Illness anxiety itself can become the problem, and it can be very tricky to figure out which error to make. You wouldn't want to ignore a grapefruit-sized growth coming out of your neck, thinking that it's a zit. Nor do you want to rivet on, and pay attention to, every one of these different sensations when they arise, because doing that can make any of these sensations turn into one of these disorders.

- An important challenge to keep in mind when dealing with stress-related disorders is to realize that even if we're a good mindfulness student, and even if we take a good attitude toward these disorders, we can still run into trouble. Some of these disorders are resolvable, and some are not. We don't want to fall into the trap of blaming ourselves for a disorder that we can't resolve.

Suggested Reading

Harrington, *The Placebo Effect*.

Kabat-Zinn, *Full Catastrophe Living*.

Siegel, "Psychophysiological Disorders."

———, *The Mindfulness Solution*, chapter 7.

———, Urdang, and Johnson, *Back Sense*.

Questions to Consider

1. What do studies of placebo effects tell us about the power of the mind to influence pain and other symptoms?

2. How can our efforts to make unpleasant physical symptoms go away keep us stuck in those symptoms?

Placebos, Illness, and the Power of Belief
Lecture 15—Transcript

One of the biggest challenges that people face in recovering from psychophysiological or stress-related disorders is believing that the mind could be powerful enough to cause the illness. And this is because these disorders are so disruptive to the body.

One of the ways that I try to help my patients understand this is by talking to them about placebo studies. Because in the effects of the placebos, we see just how powerfully the mind can influence our organ systems.

Let me tell you a little bit about what's known about placebos. Placebos, you know, are inactive substances—usually inactive—things like sugar, or starch pills that are given to people with some suggestion that they might help. Well it turns out that among placebo pills, bigger pills are more effective than smaller pills and two pills tend to be more effective than one pill.

The dose response curve of most placebos is remarkably similar to aspirin, ibuprofen, or acetaminophen. It reaches maximum efficacy in 20 to 30 minutes and then it tends to trail off in its effectiveness after four to six hours. Now active placebos are much more effective than passive placebos. An active placebo isn't just sugar or starch, it's some medicine that in some way causes some response in the body which is uncomfortable. So it's like giving somebody niacin that will make them flush, or giving them something that will give them a dry mouth—something so that the person can feel a change in the body, even if that change in the body has nothing to do with the purported effect of the placebo.

To get really effective though, it helps to move beyond pills. Injections tend to be much more effective than pills. And active injections, in other words injections of substances that change how we feel in the body, are more effective than injections of saline. And as we'll soon see, the really powerful placebos are surgical.

Let me give you some examples of the remarkable power of placebos. One of them that dates from the '70s involved treatment for temporomandibular joint disorder, which is pain that occurs in the joints of the jaw muscles and the jaw joint. It was thought, in the 1960s and the 1970s, that the epidemic of temporomandibular joint problems that was happening at the time were probably due to the deterioration of the joints. And oral surgeons were busy putting replacement disks into the joint. They used Teflon for example, for some of them. But the problem was that the Teflon started to deteriorate, and they had big problems.

So one enterprising group of dentists who thought, you know, I don't think this is about the structure of the jaw, I think this is about the patient's attitude toward the TMJ symptoms—they decided to try an intervention called "sham tooth grinding." And what they did was they created a dental instrument that was about an inch in diameter, and maybe six or eight inches long, that vibrated a lot.

And what they did was they told patients that they were going to realign their bite. And they would put this instrument into the patient's mouth, and shake, rattle, and roll. They basically vibrated for some 40 or 45 minutes, after which they told the patient, we think we've done it. We've reconstituted or restructured the shape of your teeth so that you should have a better bite now, and this should resolve the difficulty. Sixty-four percent of the patients who had sham tooth grinding had total or significant relief a year after simply one application of the procedure.

Some studies are even more startling than that. I want you to reflect: If you were alive during the second half of the 20th century, as many of you probably were, roughly the period from 1950 to 2000, which group do you think of as having been more powerful in our societies, doctors or lawyers? Take a moment to think about that. When I ask audiences, usually most people vote for the lawyers. But I think that's actually a recency effect. I think they're remembering around the year 2000. They're not really remembering what things were like in 1950.

There was a common surgery that was done for angina pain. Angina pain, as you probably know, is pain that comes from partial or greater occlusion of blood vessels in and around the heart. And it's a kind of chest pain that comes from this. And it was found that they could do something called "mammary artery ligation" to resolve this. And what they would do is the following surgery. First, they would open up the chest. They made an incision all the way from the collar bone down most of the way to the naval. Then they would saw through the breastbone, they would retract the rib cage, and they would tie off this artery, the mammary artery, and then sew people back again. And the logic behind this was that by tying off the mammary artery, you'd induce the heart to grow collateral vessels. It was kind of like creating nature's own bypass, if you will.

And it used to work pretty well. They got 80 percent to 90 percent success rate of people recovering from angina pain with the surgery. The only fly in the ointment was that every once in awhile, somebody would subsequently die and would have an autopsy—not usually from the surgery, but die from other causes. And upon autopsy, they never found the collateral vessels. So that raised the question, what's up? What could be causing the relief from the pain? One enterprising group of doctors thought, let's test this more scientifically. And they took the next series of patients that came into their hospital, who were appropriate candidates for mammary artery ligation, and they did most of the surgery as usual.

They did the incision from the collar bone down, they sawed through the breastbone, they retracted the ribcage. But they didn't actually touch the heart. They just sewed people back up again and told them that they had had successful mammary artery ligation. They then followed these patients and saw what happened once they healed. And what did they discover? Eighty to ninety percent success rates—same success rates that they had with the real mammary artery ligation.

Now, you as a modern person may be thinking there's an ethical problem with this. And indeed, perhaps there was an ethical problem. It's a little hard to find this journal article. It just so happens that the journal article reporting on the surgery was published by a little publishing house that is literally just down the road from where I live in Massachusetts. The name of the journal, you've probably never heard of it, it's called *The New England Journal of Medicine*. And it was published there in 1959 without a single mention of ethical issues. The next year, it caused quite a stir. Another team of doctors did the exact same surgery on a new group of patients, also not telling them about it. That was published in *The American Journal of Cardiology* in 1960.

And then the lawyers got involved. They started saying, you can't do that. These are human beings. You have to give informed consent—which, while I'm very sympathetic to that argument, entered us into the Dark Ages. Because then, how are we to know going forward, when a surgical intervention seemed to be helpful to people and eliminate pain, or reduce pain, how could we know whether it was a placebo effect or the effect of the surgery? Frankly, we couldn't.

Until the year 2000, when we started coming out of the Dark Ages because of a team of enterprising surgeons and researchers at the University of Texas because they actually came up with a plan by which they could do placebo controlled surgery, and get it passed by an institutional review board, because it was an ethical plan. And here's what they did. They took subjects and they told them in advance that they were going to be randomly distributed to either arthroscopic debridement, which meant making little incisions around the knee to do arthroscopic surgery, and smoothing out the structures under the kneecap, arthroscopic lavage, which meant washing out the structures under the kneecap, or the incisions only. That was the placebo group. And they followed these folks for two years.

The study was very well done because what happened was, the surgeons did the surgery, but then they never saw the patients again. The researchers followed them in the post-operative period, and then on over the next two years. And the researchers were completely blind to the condition. They had no idea who had had the surgery, and who had not had real surgery but only had placebo interventions.

Now, because of my interest in placebo research, and because I use it clinically to help patients understand that the mind is so powerful, and its effects on the body, I was following this study very closely. And at the end of the study, it got a lot of media attention. And I was listening on National Public Radio while they interviewed one of the subjects who had been in the study.

And this subject said that he was very glad to have participated because starting about a week or so after the surgery, once the incisions healed, he had felt much better, and he'd actually been free from knee pain for the last two years. And what he said was, "I think the surgeons were top notch because clearly they cured me. But the researchers, they were very sweet, very nice supportive people, but they weren't as competent as the surgeons." The reporter said, "What makes you say that?" He said, "Well, the other day, when they finished the study, the researchers got all confused. They thought I was in the placebo group."

Everybody improved. Real surgery had no advantage over the placebo at any point during two years following surgery. This is very powerful stuff.

Let's look at acupuncture. These effects aren't simply limited to surgery. In 2005, there were two large, high quality trials in patients with headache. They found little difference between the effects of acupuncture and placebo acupuncture, but a very big difference between placebo acupuncture and no acupuncture at all. It turned out that placebo acupuncture was pretty much as good as real acupuncture.

Then in 2002, there were 131 consecutive lower back pain patients at a university in Germany who were randomly assigned to three groups, and each group received active physiotherapy across the whole study. The control group got no further treatment. There was an acupuncture group that got 20 sessions of traditional acupuncture. And then there was a sham acupuncture group that got 20 sessions of sham acupuncture. Now, sham acupuncture is an interesting procedure. They stuck in needles, but they stuck them in superficially. And they stuck them between 10 and 20 millimeters away from the true acupoints, outside of the meridians. And, the needles weren't simulated, as they often are in real acupuncture. They found significant improvement in traditional acupuncture for chronic low back pain compared to the routine care—the physical therapy—but no difference from sham acupuncture. Sham acupuncture also worked just as well.

Josephine Briggs is the doctor who's the director of the National Institute for Health, the Center for Complementary and Alternative Medicine here in the United States, and she's come to the conclusion that acupuncture is a particularly effective placebo intervention. It's so well-designed with a whole ritual, it involves breaking of the skin—which we know works so much better than simply taking pills—it requires time, and the person has a full-body experience when they go in for acupuncture.

Perhaps even more remarkably, we now know that placebo interventions will work even when people know that they're getting a placebo intervention. There's a center for placebo studies in one of the Harvard teaching hospitals, and they took 80 patients who were randomized to either open label placebo pills—in other words, they were told this. They were told placebo pills are made of an inert substance, like sugar pills, and they've been shown in clinical studies to provide significant improvement in irritable bowel syndromes through mind-body self-healing processes. And the subjects had irritable bowel syndrome. So they thought, OK, this can work. But they were told that these are sugar pills, and they were told the truth, which is that sugar pills do help with this disorder. So they either got the placebo pills, or they were in no treatment control group that got the same quality and type of interaction with the providers, but no placebos. The people with the open label placebos had significantly higher global improvement scores on their irritable bowel syndrome symptoms at both 11 day midpoint of the study, and at the 21 day end point.

What was fascinating to me, I was following this on the radio also, was that the patients, after the study, who got the placebo pills said, "This is great. Thank you. I'm glad I participated. Where can I continue to get the placebo pills?" And the researchers said, "Well, they're just inert. You could just use Tic Tacs." And the subject said, "No, no, no. I want those placebo pills. Those are what worked for me." And they're actually upset when the researchers couldn't provide them because there are various ethical and legal strictures that made it so that they wouldn't do it.

OK. So these stories are presented to you, and I present them to my patients, so that we can get an idea that, wow, the body and the mind are closely interacting with one another, and the mind is extremely powerful in the effects that it can have on our subjective experience of the body.

So how do we use these principles to treat other disorders? Let's look at other muscle tension disorders, which are remarkably similar to chronic back pain in their dynamics. And here I'm talking about headaches, temporomandibular joint disorder, a lot of neck, knee, foot, wrist, and shoulder pain. Now, we don't have quite the data we have about these disorders that we have with chronic back pain. With chronic back pain, we know that the correlation between what's found in the imaging of the spine and what people experience in terms of subjective distress is very, very low. The condition of the spine only rarely actually influences whether or not people will be in pain. It's not never—there are people for whom, yes, it's the spine that's causing the problem and yes, repair of the spine is what's called for—but in the vast majority of cases, this isn't the case.

With the case of neck, knee, wrist, shoulder pain, we don't quite have the data. Largely because we haven't done large-scale studies in which we take people without knee pain, without shoulder pain, without wrist pain, and take a look at what the body parts look like for them. The preliminary data is interesting.

For example, there's a study of knee pain that showed that a torn meniscus is very common in men over the age of 55. The majority of pain-free men have a torn meniscus. And there are studies that showed that major league baseball players who are pitching balls at nearly 100 miles an hour typically have torn rotator cuffs. And as we know, a torn meniscus or a torn rotator cuff is sometimes pointed to as the cause of the pain. So the science isn't in here yet. But the basic principle of treatment is the same. Rule out structural causes if you can, and follow the same four-step program.

Let's move on to some other areas. Let's move on, for example, to sexual dysfunctions. It's basically fear of the dysfunction that brings on the dysfunction. Let's take erectile dysfunction as an example. Before we had Viagra and Cialis, we had the inventions of Masters and Johnson—they were kind of the original sex therapists. They had some pretty effective non-pharmacological treatments and they all targeted awareness of present experience with acceptance. They taught what they called "sensei focus." And here's what the instructions were like. They would send a couple home and they would say, here's the deal. I want you to touch one another in a sensual and sexual way, only there are rules to this: You're not allowed to pet to orgasm, and you're not allowed to have intercourse. What you need to do instead is to simply bring your attention to the sensations of touching your partner (if you're the one doing the touching) or being touched by your partner (if you're the one being touched). Every time your mind wanders and goes off to other things, just gently bring your attention back to the sensations of touching or being touched and let go of any goal orientation and simply accept whatever happens.

At this point in the course, this should sound familiar to you. They were teaching mindfulness practice where the focus was sensual touch. And they found, for example, with erectile dysfunction, that about 75 percent of the time, just training couples to do this would resolve the disorder.

They also addressed other issues, such as people's attitudes toward sexuality, and the dynamics of the couple's relationship, whether people felt close or not. Nowadays, I'm sorry to say, these kinds of interventions are a little bit academic. We have Viagra and Cialis where people who don't really like each other and can't communicate can successfully have intercourse on a regular basis.

Let's look at insomnia. The conventional treatment for insomnia is stimulus control, sleep hygiene, and relaxation. And stimulus control means, we want to teach people to associate the bed with sleep. And the standard instruction is, I want you to reserve the bed for sleep and sex.

Now, if we're really being logical about this, and we want to develop a paired association between the bed and sleep, we should really reserve it for just sleep—not just not reading and not watching TV, but not having sex either. We should be saying, you should have sex in another room, but sleep in the bed. I'm afraid that researchers have been a little bit too prudish to say, "Have sex in the living room, sleep in the bed," so we include both.

The second thing we ask for is sleep hygiene. That means get up the same time each day, even if you haven't had a full night's sleep, and try to go to bed the same time each day, even if you're not tired. And thirdly, they do relaxation training.

An alternative is to do mindfulness treatment. And the way mindfulness treatment works is to simply use the time in bed as an opportunity to be aware of present experience with acceptance. This is, frankly, what I do every night when I go to sleep. I lie down, I close my eyes, and I begin following the breath as we've done in the breath awareness training. If the mind wanders to other things, I gently bring the attention back to the breath.

Now it turns out that mindfulness practice actually reduces our need for sleep. People who go on meditation retreats who are doing mindfulness practice all day long find that they need a lot less sleep. And there're two theories to this. One is that what's happening is that some of the processing of what happens, the restorative functions of sleep, is happening in mindfulness therapy, or in mindfulness practice. Well, you could think of this as what's happening in sleep is all sorts of unintegrated material is being re-integrated. We're reconnecting with thoughts and feelings and memories that might have been difficult to be with. So if some of that's happening while we're doing the mindfulness practice, we don't need as many hours of sleep to do it. The other hypothesis is that because we work through these things, we tend to sleep more deeply during the hours that we are sleeping, so that it's more efficient. Either way, what happens is if we trust that mindfulness practice will help to be restorative for us, then we can give up the goal orientation.

And we all know that it is much easier, typically, to fall asleep on a Friday night if you don't work over the weekend, then it is on a Sunday night if you work during the week. Because on Sunday night, you're thinking, gosh, I got to get to bed so I'll be well rested, otherwise tomorrow's going to be a disaster at work, whereas on Friday night, it doesn't really matter.

So when we remove the goal orientation, that helps a great deal. So the way I think of it is one of two things is going to happen: I'm either going to have the opportunity for eight uninterrupted hours of mindfulness practice—pretty good in a busy life, you don't get that opportunity that often—or I'm going to fail and I'm going to fall asleep. And that would be fine as well.

Let's look at gastrointestinal distress. Now, this system is remarkably sensitive to our emotional lives. What the stress physiologists tell us is, there's no need to digest your own lunch when you're about to become somebody else's lunch. So our GI system will often shut down when we're under stress, or it will suddenly become overactive—kind of dump its load, if you will, so we can run away. And people experience all manner of gastrointestinal distress. They experience upper GI symptoms, in which the stomach is producing too much stomach acid, and churning too much. And they experience lower GI symptoms very often that have to do with having alternating diarrhea and constipation, as we see in irritable bowel syndrome, or other kinds of disruptions.

Now ulcers were once thought to be caused by stress, and then we discovered the role of *H. pylori*. It turns out that you could treat an ulcer by giving an antibiotic that kills *H. pylori* bacteria, and often it would heal. But then we discovered that *H. pylori* infections are actually endemic to large percentages of the population. In fact, there are some countries, I know Columbia was one of them, in which the majority of people have *H. pylori* infections. So then that brings up the question, what's determining whether somebody with *H. pylori* infection gets an ulcer or not? Well we're back to the stress hypothesis. It turns out that stress is a critical factor in whether the stomach lining becomes broken down in a way that makes it vulnerable to the infection.

I mentioned irritable bowel syndrome. This is very, very common as a disorder. This is where you have this often alternating constipation and diarrhea. And here, the distress about the symptom is often the stressor that keeps it going, not unlike what we saw in chronic back pain. So a person's afraid that they're going to be caught off-guard and suddenly need the bathroom and they won't be in a place where it's convenient. Or they're afraid that they're going to get backed up, and they're going to feel terrible cramping and things, and that's going to get in the way of participating in life. It's only when people can relax about IBS, and actually use mindfulness practices to simply ride the waves of different sensations. Like OK, this is what needing to go feels like. OK, this is what being stopped up feels like. Then they do considerably better.

This is true for the upper GI symptoms as well. Very often, people start to micromanage their diets. They start to try to figure out which foods are making me feel better or worse, and then eliminating foods from their diet.

Now of course, there are genuine food allergies, and these need to be treated medically. However, for a lot of people, what happens is as they're trying to figure this out, as they're becoming a junior scientist, we can't differentiate from eating a tomato being problematic because the tomato is interacting with our stomach in a bad way, or whether the thought of eating a tomato is causing us anxiety and that anxiety is upsetting our stomach. Because as soon as we have the experience of a tomato making our stomach worse, we're locked in a pattern where all future tomatoes will make our stomach worse through the anxiety mechanism.

So, mindfulness practices can help us with this. Mindfulness practices can help us to simply ride out these changing waves of sensations. I got into treating psychophysiological disorders because I've had a lot of them. And I remember when I was applying to grad school, I had a lot of upper GI distress. And I remember asking my girlfriend at the time, "What does a normal stomach feel like?" And she said, "You know, it's hard to describe, but I'll tell you this: You just don't think about it that much."

Another interesting disorder that works similarly is something called *hyperacusis*. I've actually treated a lot of this. It's a somewhat unusual disorder where people become afraid of loud sounds. And loud sounds don't just feel uncomfortable, but they become terribly painful to people. And what people do naturally is they try to avoid loud sounds. And they get themselves into a pattern, which is like what would happen if they had photophobia, which is a disorder in which normal levels of light are too bright. We all experience this a little bit if you ever go to the eye doctor and you have your pupils dilated so that it lets in all the light. If you were to respond to that all the time by wearing dark glasses, what do you imagine it would be like to take off the dark glasses on a bright afternoon? It would be unbearable. Well, the same thing happens with hyperacusis. What happens is people become so phobic of loud noise and they work so hard to avoid loud noise that then any noise becomes too intense.

You can use mindfulness practice to try to resolve hyperacusis, and it actually works quite well. To simply listen to the noise, and notice—this is separating the two arrows that we discussed before—noticing how there's the actual experience of the sound, the sensations, and then there's our reaction to the sensations. And as we notice that these can be separated, it becomes much easier to work with the symptoms.

Now another disorder you may have heard of is fibromyalgia. And this is a bit controversial. This was identified as a disorder in 1990 in which they identified these trigger points, these spots in the body in which people with is this disorder felt particular sensitivity to pain. And it was established by the American College of Rheumatology as an official disorder back then.

What we've later learned, though, is that people with fibromyalgia are actually sensitive to pain everywhere. You could take any part of their body, even like the thumb, put it in a little vice—not something dangerous, just something used for research—squeeze the thumb, and they will report a level of pain equivalent to what a person without the disorder feels at half the amount of pressure. So, you only give a pound of pressure, and the person experiences pain that somebody else would experience as two pounds of pressure.

Doctor Frederick Wolfe, who was the one who first identified the disorder, has said, I'm afraid "we are creating an illness rather than curing one," because this has become something of an epidemic. And just to show you how this gets in the complicated political and social milieu we work in, in the United Kingdom, those psychologists and physicians who are treating fibromyalgia as a stress-related disorder have needed Scotland Yard protection because people suffering from the disease are saying, "You're just not trying hard enough to find the underlying mechanism." That may be true, but it may also be one of the stress-related disorders.

Now, illness anxiety is a component of all of these different disorders and it's unavoidable. One of the reasons why the Buddha supposedly left the palace and went out into the world to follow spiritual practices was because of illness anxiety. And illness anxiety is actually remarkably easy to generate. Let's try some right now.

Take a moment, and if you can, close your eyes. And I want you to sense whatever is happening inside your head right now. And see if you can sense a little bit of discomfort, maybe a kind of pressure that's there. Just try it.

See, can you feel any pressure in your head? And see if you can sense the kind of pressure that, if it were to get more intense, might start developing into a headache. Uh-oh, it may be happening.

We find that people who live with folks with brain tumors have a lot more headaches than people who don't live with folks with brain tumors. And folks who have had chronic headaches before rivet on any sensation of pressure, and it becomes a problem which expands into a headache.

Or consider this, imagine that you just learned that there was something wrong with your laundry. And there's been a lice outbreak, and there's some in your clothes. And just feel what's happening in your body right now and notice whether you sense any itching anywhere—maybe around the scalp, maybe somewhere else. Uh-oh, it could just be lice. Oh, I got another notice. It said it actually doesn't affect your laundry, just other people's laundry. It's important to undo hypnotic suggestion.

So you probably notice if you tried those experiments that all it takes is bringing anxious attention to a part of our body, and we can start to feel sensations in that part of our body and start to worry about them. And these things can get amplified very easily.

Now, we have two basic reactions when we experience something untoward in the body. When we're younger—and it helps if you come from certain ethnicities—you may think, it's probably nothing. You may think, oh, this is just a coming or going sensation, I don't really have to worry about it. But if you're older, you may start to think, it's probably something serious. And this happens too if you grow up in an ethnicity or a family that's very focused on medical disorders. One of my favorite cartoons about this has an anxious woman, and she's reading the *Big Book of Horrible Rare Diseases*. Near her feet is the *Merck Manual*, *A Child's Garden of Maladies*, *Lock Jaw Monthly*, and all these other reading materials—which now that we have the internet can be any of us, because we can all search online for a symptom and get some pretty scary possibilities about it. What happens is illness anxiety itself can become the problem. And it can be very tricky to figure out which error to make. You wouldn't want to ignore a grapefruit-sized growth coming out of your neck and think, it's probably a zit. But nor do we want to rivet on, and pay attention to, every one of these different sensations when they arise because doing that can make any of these sensations turn into one of these disorders.

Now, the biggest challenge—or, I shouldn't say the biggest challenge—but an important challenge to keep in mind when we're treating, for ourselves or others, these stress related disorders, is to realize that even if we're a good mindfulness student, and even if we take a good attitude toward these disorders, we can still run into trouble.

Now, no matter how good we are as a mindfulness student, we're all headed for the same place. And the bodies are going to fall apart, eventually. And some of these disorders are resolvable, and some are not—and we don't want to fall into the trap of blaming ourselves for a disorder that we can't resolve.

In our next lecture, we're going to look at another big challenge for most of us, and that's troubling habits, including the addictions. And these will look at everything from everyday behavior to those kinds of habits that can really get us into trouble. Thanks for listening.

Interrupting Addiction and Troublesome Habits
Lecture 16

Almost all of us have some habits that we'd like to change. Some are relatively harmless, like overeating from time to time, checking our smartphones a bit too often, or perhaps procrastinating a bit on work. But others can be quite destructive, including alcoholism and other forms of substance abuse, sexual addictions, and compulsive gambling. In this lecture, you will learn about a range of addictions and how mindfulness practices can help control them.

Addictions

- All addictions—from everyday habits to the kinds of habits that are more damaging—involve the principle that it's our hardwired impulse to seek pleasure and avoid pain. Ironically, we can break free from being enslaved by our habits, but first we have to be willing to give up some of what we might think of as our freedom.

- With mindfulness practice, we see that we're actually all addicts. We see that much of our behavior is automatic and compulsive. We don't notice this unless we pay attention. But when we're mindful, we can see that we're thinking all day about how to try to feel good and avoid feeling bad. And this can be quite subtle.

- The process begins with our hardwired, evolutionarily determined predilection to seek pleasurable experiences and avoid painful ones. Then, it's exacerbated by our thinking disease, because we're able to anticipate the future, recall the past, and make plans to maximize future pleasure and minimize future pain. It's great for survival, but when we're successful, our efforts are actually positively reinforced, and that can become quite addictive.

- In traditional Buddhist language, the tendency to hold on to the pleasant, avoid the unpleasant, and ignore neutral experiences are called greed, hatred, and delusion. They are referred to as poisons,

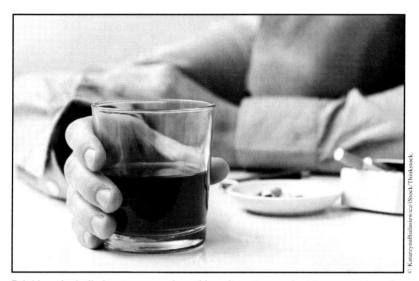

Drinking alcoholic beverages and smoking cigarettes are just two examples of activities that people can become compulsively attached to.

unwholesome roots, or fires that control our behavior. And it's these hardwired tendencies that lead to a remarkable range of addictions, including ingesting substances like alcohol and other drugs like nicotine or caffeine, and we become easily imprisoned by compulsion toward any of these.

- There are other compulsive activities, such as over- or under-eating; sex, love, or abusive relationships; gambling; shopping; work; religious activity, including meditation practices; Internet surfing, texting, and video games. There are all kinds of things that we can become compulsively attached to.

How Do We Get Hooked?

- There are many models that try to explain why we get hooked on things in our lives. A popular one was put forth by psychiatrist Edward Khantzian, who said that when we're doing addictive habits, we're actually medicating underlying psychiatric conditions, such as anxiety or depression. In fact, certain activities tend to treat certain underlying problems.

- We also have evidence that some of us have genetic predispositions toward becoming addicted to certain substances, for example. But most experts in addiction these days say that whatever else might be going on, we learn to be addicts through predictable mechanisms of positive and negative reinforcement.

- One particularly clear model comes from Dr. Judson Brewer, whose model talks about associative learning addictive loops. Smoking, drinking, or another addictive behavior becomes associated with positive and negative feelings through positive and negative reinforcement.

- Positive reinforcement refers to a pleasurable experience that follows a behavior, such as ingesting a substance, and makes it more likely that we'll repeat the behavior as a result—because it felt good. Negative reinforcement, such as fleeing a situation when we're anxious, refers to the removal of a painful experience that comes from an addictive behavior, which also makes it more likely that we'll do it again in the future.

- Some examples of positive reinforcement can be feeling high when we have a drink, having fun, being funny, having sex, or connecting with friends—any good feeling that comes from the addictive behavior. Negative reinforcement usually involves reductions in anxiety, worry, sadness, anger, boredom, or some other unpleasant emotion.

- Once we've had some experience with our addictive behavior, then we get triggered by cues. Positive cues include seeing the cigarette, beer, candy bar, or gambling casino, and this makes us desire it again. Negative cues include feeling stressed out, lonely, anxious, depressed, and this triggers a cue-induced craving to get rid of the negative feeling.

- Following this urge, we typically enact the addictive behavior by smoking, drinking, eating, or going to the casino. This makes the unpleasant feeling go away temporarily, or it brings on a good feeling for a little while. This creates more positive or negative reinforcement, increasing the likelihood that we'll reenact the problematic behavior. Through repetition, this process becomes automated over time.

Conventional Treatments versus Mindfulness

- Conventional treatments don't dismantle this addictive loop. Many conventional treatments either target the avoidance of positive and negative cues, or they target learning to enact substitute behaviors so that we don't do the addictive behavior. The avoidance of cues includes staying away from bars and liquor stores, casinos, and bakeries. This dampens the input into the addictive loop.

- While substitute behaviors, such as calling a friend when you're tempted to drink or gamble, circumvents the addictive behavior for a little while, it doesn't do anything with our underlying craving. So, the alternative is to try to change our relationship to craving. And mindfulness practice can help us to do just that.

- Traditionally, many religious and philosophic traditions have tried asceticism to try to kill off cravings. In that way, they try to get us away from the pain of unfulfilled desires as well as to interrupt unwholesome habits.

- Mindfulness practices can help us transform our desires and cravings by giving us a way to forge a new relationship with craving. We learn to accept the changing experience, instead of compulsively chasing pleasure and avoiding pain. In addition, we learn not to take our relapses so personally. The times we slip stop being such a big issue about how we failed and start being new opportunities to start fresh.

- How do we use mindfulness practices to cultivate acceptance of changing experience, rather than acting compulsively to try to obtain pleasure or get rid of discomfort? It begins by just noticing whatever sensation is happening right now in the mind and in the body. Then, it's noticing the impulse to fix or escape it. These impulses wax and wane, and we become conscious of their constantly changing nature.

- Most compulsive behaviors occur because we believe that we can't tolerate the experience and, therefore, must act to change it, or we have the mistaken belief that unpleasant experiences will last forever if we don't take action to interrupt them. Mindfulness practice helps us to see that neither of these beliefs is actually true.

- Mindfulness practices help to increase our capacity to bear experience. Because compulsive behaviors are designed to reduce the intensity of unpleasant experiences, or to ensure a pleasant one, if we can ride the waves of pleasant and unpleasant feelings, we're not going to be driven so hard toward our compulsive behaviors. And if we don't reenact them, then they won't be continually positively and negatively reinforced.

- A model for working with troublesome behaviors generally is called motivational interviewing, which is based on the idea that people have different levels of motivation for change at any given moment. The therapist asks the person questions about his or her addiction: What do you enjoy about it? How does it improve your life? What might you lose if you gave it up? This method is often called motivational interviewing, and it is related to some scientific work on change that began with smoking cessation done by James Prochaska and Carlo DiClemente.

- When working with habits in this way, we first do this assessment so that we can address it in a kind of stage-based way, because we need different approaches depending on our relationship to the addiction. What stage we are determines what we're ready to do. Prochaska and DiClemente came up with six habit change stages.

- The first stage is precontemplation, which is when we don't have any awareness that life could be improved by changing our behavior. The next stage is contemplation, where we see that it's a problem, and we're not really ready to do much about it, but we are gathering a little bit of information about what might help. Then, people move on to preparation, which is where you start to really think about the pros and cons of taking action.

- Then, we move into action. Once we've taken the action, we've actually started changing the behavior. The next stage is maintenance, which is consolidating the changes. The last stage is termination, because at the end we get to a point where we no longer miss the habit. Sometimes we get to that point, and sometimes we don't, depending on what the habit is.

- There are number of programs that explicitly use mindfulness practice to change our relationship to craving. These programs offer us techniques that any of us can use in working with our own troublesome habits. One of them is mindfulness-based relapse prevention, which helps people who become free from a habit not to fall back into it. The main thrust is giving us a new relationship to craving.

Suggested Reading

Bays, *Mindful Eating: A Guide to Rediscovering a Healthy and Joyful Relationship with Food.*

Bien and Bien, *Mindful Recovery: A Spiritual Path to Healing from Addiction.*

Brewer, "Breaking the Addiction Loop."

Peltz, *The Mindful Path to Addiction Recovery: A Practical Guide to Regaining Control over Your Life.*

Siegel, *The Mindfulness Solution*, chapter 9.

1. What are a few of your addictive behaviors or habits?

2. How might you use mindfulness practice generally, and urge surfing in particular, to exercise greater choice around these behaviors?

Mindfulness Practice

mindful intoxication: An exercise designed to increase our awareness of our use of intoxicants. This is not recommended if you've already learned that you have difficulty with an intoxicating substance and are trying to be abstinent.

urge surfing: An exercise developed as part of the mindfulness-based relapse program designed to help us ride out urges toward unwanted behaviors, such as excessive drinking, overeating, gambling, or speaking unskillfully.

Interrupting Addiction and Troublesome Habits
Lecture 16—Transcript

I'd like to tell you another story about my first intensive meditation retreat. As an American kid, I grew up with the notion of external freedom and choice being very deeply ingrained. I felt I shouldn't have dress codes at school, and traditional sexual mores didn't seem very necessary. The freedom to choose what I want to do when I want to do it seemed most important. The strict schedule with no talking and no freedom to choose of the retreat seemed antithetical to freedom.

But I discovered that, within the context of that strictness, real freedom became possible. How was that? Well it turns out that mindfulness opens up a gap between sensation (an emotion or other bodily experience), the urge or impulse to do something about it, and then the movement that flows from that urge (our behavior). In non-mindful daily life, we rarely notice this gap.

The realization that I could learn to simply be with rather than fix experiences was remarkably liberating. I found I could actually choose whether or not to act on my desires, even little desires like scratching an inch or moving when my leg hurt from sitting for a long time, or seeking entertainment by reading, talking, or the things I'd do outside the retreat like visiting the fridge or turning on the TV. And when I chose not to pursue some of them, I found that I felt freer than ever before.

Years later, when I became a clinical psychologist, I realized that the same principle could help to free us from a remarkably wide range of common problems. And this is nowhere more obvious than in dealing with addictions.

Now almost all of us have some habits that we'd like to change. Some are relatively harmless, like overeating from time to time, checking our smartphones a bit too often, watching TV more than we should, or perhaps procrastinating a bit on chores or work. But others can be quite destructive, including alcoholism and other forms of substance abuse, sexual addictions, compulsive gambling—there's quite a list.

All of these addictions involve a principle which we've discussed before in the course: It's our hard-wired impulse to seek pleasure and avoid pain. Ironically, just as I saw in retreat, we can break free from being enslaved by our habits, but first we have to be willing to give up some of what we might think of as our freedom.

With mindfulness practice, we see that we're actually all addicts. We see that much of our behavior is automatic and compulsive. We don't notice this unless we pay attention. But when we're mindful, we can see that we're thinking all day about how to try to feel good and avoid feeling bad. And this can really be quite subtle.

The process begins with our hard-wired evolutionarily determined predilection to seek pleasurable experiences and avoid painful ones. And then it's exacerbated by our thinking disease, because we're able to anticipate the future, recall the past, and make plans to maximize future pleasure and minimize future pain. It's great for survival, but when we're successful with this, our efforts are actually positively reinforced, and that can become quite addictive.

In traditional Buddhist language, the tendency to hold onto the pleasant, avoid the unpleasant, and ignore neutral experiences are called greed, hatred, and delusion. They're referred to as poisons, or unwholesome roots, or fires that control our behavior. And it's these hard-wired tendencies that lead to a remarkable range of addictions.

There are so many possibilities. We can ingest substances like alcohol, other drugs like nicotine or caffeine, and we become easily imprisoned by compulsions toward any of these. There are other compulsive activities like over- or under-eating. Sex, love, or abusive relationships. We can get addicted to gambling, to shopping, to work. We can even get addicted to religious activity, including meditation practices. And in the modern age, we have the options for internet surfing, texting, video games—all sorts of things that we can become compulsively attached to.

So how do we get hooked? Well there are many models out there. When I was in training, a popular one was put forth by a psychiatrist named Edward

Khantzian, who's actually at the Cambridge hospital where I worked. And he said when we're doing these addictive habits, we're actually medicating underlying psychiatric conditions, such as anxiety or depression. And in fact, he had a whole system for looking at what our compulsive behaviors were and kind of reverse-engineering it to figure out what probably was the underlying difficulty. The idea was that certain activities tend to treat certain underlying problems.

We also have evidence that some of us have genetic predispositions toward becoming addicted to certain substances, for example. But most experts in addiction these days say that whatever else might be going on, we learn to be addicts through predictable mechanisms of positive and negative reinforcement.

One particularly clear model comes from Dr. Judson Brewer, a friend and colleague of mine, at the University of Massachusetts Medical School. His model talks about associative learning addictive loops. Smoking, drinking, or whatever the other addictive behavior is becomes associated with positive and negative feelings through positive and negative reinforcement.

Now positive reinforcement refers to a pleasurable experience that follows a behavior, like ingesting a substance, and makes it more likely that we'll repeat the behavior as a result because it felt good. Negative reinforcement, which we talked about before in terms of anxiety problems—like fleeing the supermarket when we're anxious—that refers to the removal of a painful experience that comes from an addictive behavior. In other words, the addictive behavior removes the painful experience, and that makes it more likely that we'll do it again in the future.

Some examples of positive reinforcement can be feeling high when we have a drink, having fun, being funny, having sex, connecting with friends—really any good feeling that comes from the addictive behavior. Negative reinforcement usually involves reductions in anxiety, worry, sadness, anger, boredom, or some other unpleasant emotion. Once we've had some experience with our addictive behavior, once we've done it a number of times, then we get triggered by cues. Positive cues like seeing the cigarette, the beer, the candy bar, the gambling casino, gets us jazzed up and makes us desire it again. And negative cues, like feeling stressed out, lonely, anxious, depressed, that triggers a cue-induced craving to get rid of the negative feeling.

After the urge, we typically do the addictive behavior. We have the smoke or the drink, eat the cake, or go to the casino. And this makes the unpleasant feeling go away temporarily, or it brings on a good feeling for a little while. And that creates more positive or negative reinforcement, increasing the likelihood that we'll reenact the problematic behavior. And this just goes on and on, and, through repetition, the process becomes quite automated over time.

Now conventional treatments don't actually dismantle this addictive loop. Many conventional treatments either target the avoidance of positive and negative cues, or they target learning to enact substitute behaviors so we don't do the addictive behavior. The avoidance of cues is things like, well, stay away from bars and liquor stores. Stay away from casinos and bakeries. And that dampens the input into the addictive loop.

While substitute behaviors, things like calling a friend when you're tempted to drink or gamble, or eating carrot sticks when you're tempted to eat the chocolate cake, that circumvents the addictive behavior for a little while, but it doesn't do anything with our underlying craving. So the alternative is to try to change our relationship to craving. And this is where mindfulness practice comes in, because it can help us to do just that.

Now traditionally, many religious and philosophic traditions have tried asceticism to actually kill off cravings. And in that way, they try to get us away from the pain of unfulfilled desires, and they use them to interrupt unwholesome habits. We can see this in the store the Buddha's life when he tried to do the same thing during his ascetic period. And the Buddha was very good at what he did, so he took it to the max. Here's what the traditional description is of how he was as an ascetic.

> He tried various plans such as abstaining from rice meal and living on fruits which dropped from trees, then on fruits which dropped from the tree under which he sat, then living on [only] one fruit, one

sesame seed, or one grain of rice a day. By this lack of nourishment his body was reduced to skin and bones and lost its golden color and became dry and black.

And if you travel to Buddhist cultures, you'll see various kinds of artwork that depict this totally emaciated, half-dead Buddha during his ascetic period. But the Buddha found that this didn't actually provide a path to psychological freedom. He was still constantly wrestling with his desires. And the failure of his ascetic strategy is actually what led him to develop mindfulness practices, the same sorts of mindfulness practices that we're discussing this course.

So how did mindfulness practices help the Buddha? And how can it help us to work differently or transform our desires and cravings? It's because they give us a way to forge a new relationship with craving. We learn to accept the changing experience, instead of compulsively chasing pleasure and avoiding pain. We basically learn how to ride it out. The other thing we learn from mindfulness practice is not to take our relapses so seriously. The times we slip, the times we go and have the chocolate cake, or have the drink stop being such a big issue about how we failed, but they start being new opportunities to starting fresh.

Let's examine the first approach, how we change the relationship to cravings. What we're going to learn how to do is to be with feelings rather than act compulsively to try to get rid of them. This begins by just noticing whatever sensation is happening right now in the mind and in the body. Then it's noticing the impulse to fix or escape it. And what we get to see is that these impulses wax and wane, and we become conscious of their constantly changing nature.

Most compulsive behaviors occur because we believe that we can't tolerate the experience, and therefore must act to change it. Or we have the mistaken belief that unpleasant experiences will last forever if we don't take action to interrupt them. And mindfulness practice helps us to see that neither of these beliefs is actually true.

We've discussed before how mindfulness practices help to increase our capacity to bear experience. Remember the Zen master who could be run through with a sword without blinking an eye? This is what I saw develop— to an admittedly lesser degree—on my first retreat, where giving up one kind of freedom yielded a much more valuable one.

Now since compulsive behaviors are designed to reduce the intensity of unpleasant experiences, or to ensure pleasant ones, if we can ride the waves of pleasant and unpleasant feelings, we're not going to be driven so hard toward our compulsive behaviors. And if we don't reenact them, then they won't be continually positively and negatively reinforced, so we won't have the learning loop that gets us so trapped in them.

Now what might motivate a person to take this approach? To move toward what's unpleasant and away from what's pleasant, or to give up the freedom to satisfy immediate desires? In the old days, when I was first in training, psychotherapists used to demand abstinence from people who had addictions before agreeing to treat them in psychotherapy. So if an alcoholic came to see us, the idea was well, you have to go over to AA, you have to become dry, and then we'll do psychotherapy. But in later years, some people working with the addiction said this a little bit like having somebody come into your office who's depressed and saying go home, cheer up, and when you come back feeling better, we'll do some work together.

So now, we take a different, somewhat more investigative approach. Somebody comes in with an addictive behavior, and typically a therapist will ask well, what do you enjoy about it? How does it improve your life? What might you lose if you gave it up? This method is often called "motivational interviewing," and it's based on the idea that people have different levels of motivation for change at any given moment. And it's related to some scientific work on change that began with smoking cessation. This was done by James Prochaska and Carlo DiClemmente back in the early 1980s, and it's become a model for working with troublesome behaviors generally.

You can try this for yourself now. Think of a habit that you have at least some wish to alter. Come up with one. Think of one in your mind first so you can follow along. You got it? What feels good about the habit? Whether it's drinking, smoking cigarettes, eating a lot, eating junk food, surfing the net, checking your smartphone, whatever it is. What feels good about the habit? What benefits does it offer you? And then what might you lose if you were to give it up, even if you just relinquished it sometimes?

Now after getting a sense of the behavior's benefits, look at its drawbacks. Does the habit cause you any difficulties? Do you imagine it might some day? Does it create any risks—not immediate difficulties, but things that could go wrong in the future? And then finally, on balance, does it enrich your life or detract from it? Have you ever tried to stop or cut back? And if so, what happened?

So in working with habits in this way, we first do this assessment so that we can address it in a kind of stage-based way, because we need different approaches depending on our relationship to the addiction. What stage we are determines what we're ready to do. Prochaska and DiClemmente came up with six habit-change stages, and most people working in habit-change fields talk to their clients or patients about these.

The first is *precontemplation*. That's when we don't have any awareness that life could be improved by changing our behavior. It's not even on the table. And then there's *contemplation*, where we see it's a problem, but we're not really ready to do much about it. But we are gathering a little bit of information about what might help. Then people move on to what's called *preparation*. And this is where you start to really think about the pros and cons of doing this, and think, maybe I really should take some action. And then finally we move into action. We actually start attending AA, take up a mindfulness practice, go to the exercise class.

Once we've taken the action and we've actually started changing the behavior, then there are other stages of maintenance, which is consolidating the changes, and finally termination, because at the end we get to a point where we no longer miss the habit. You don't even think smoking a cigarette would be at all pleasurable anymore. Sometimes we get to that point. Sometimes we don't, depending on what the habit is.

Now there are number of programs that explicitly use mindfulness practice to change our relationship to craving. And these programs actually offer us techniques that any of us can use in working with our own troublesome habits. One of them is mindfulness based relapse prevention. And this was started by Alan Marlatt and his colleagues at the University of Washington in Seattle. And the idea was to help people who had become free from a habit not to fall back into it. And the main thrust is giving us a new relationship to craving.

First what we do in this program is to simply develop mindfulness and watch every time we seem to go on automatic pilot and every time that a craving occurs. And then we start to develop mindfulness of the positive cues—the bars, the liquor stores—noticing what kinds of things in our environment bring up this feeling of yes, I want to do the behavior. And then it gets interesting. We start practicing mindfulness—being with the breath, doing walking meditation—in high-risk situations to identify where they are, and practice entering the situation and being mindful there. This could include walking into a bar, sitting down, and doing mindfulness practice, and just noticing everything that comes up.

One of the best and most important innovations of the mindfulness based relapse prevention program is the idea of working with abstinence violation effects. Now, abstinence violation effects are what happens when we fall off the wagon. And we all fall off the wagon when we're trying to change a habit. We're dieting and then suddenly we go out to dinner and overdo it. We've been trying not to drink for a long time, a social situation comes up, and we start drinking again—many, many different examples of this.

Usually what happens, when we fall off the wagon, is we feel so terrible about having just screwed up that we then want to self-soothe. And what we do to self-soothe? We go and eat more, or we go and have the drink. So we get caught in a loop in which a little slip becomes the entrée to a whole pathway of being addicted once again to the problematic behavior. Just noticing this, and noticing that it's an impersonal process, and using mindfulness practice to notice the upwelling of negative feeling that comes after a slip, can help us to not act compulsively on it and not go back to the substance.

Another very useful contribution of this program is the practice of urge surfing. And this helps us to be mindful of cravings in a different way. Let me give you a little example of urge surfing, because we've all done it in one particular circumstance. It's a little indelicate, but this is the best one I know for illustrating this. Have you ever been a situation—like on an airplane and the "fasten your seatbelt" sign is on—where you needed to go to the bathroom and you weren't able to? Or perhaps you were on a bus, and it wasn't going to stop for a while. That's an example in which all of us have had experience in urge surfing.

It goes something like this. Oh gosh, I think I got to go. Oh yeah, I got to go. Well, I can hold it for a little while. It'll be OK. Oh gosh, I really got to go. I've really got to go. How long is this going to be? I really got to go. All right, just breathe a little bit. Don't relax too much, but it'll be OK. I really, really got to go. I really got to go. You've been there right?

What happens is the urge comes, reaches a kind of crescendo, and then settles down. It comes, and reaches a kind of crescendo, and settles down. It's interesting. When we have to go the bathroom, it usually feels just when we finally get to the bathroom, like, thank god I definitely could not have held this for another moment, even though we probably could have held it longer.

So let's try a little urge surfing right now. Se if you can locate some kind of urge or craving right now in your experience. Maybe even something like you want a drink of water, you're a little hungry, maybe you need the bathroom a little bit. Try visualizing the urge or craving as an ocean wave. It begins as a small wavelet, then it builds into a cresting wave. And what we do in urge surfing is to use the breath as a kind of surfboard to ride the wave. So just breathe as you feel the urge. And the goal is to surf the urge by allowing it first to rise up and decline without being wiped out by giving in to the urge.

In urge surfing, we treat urges as conditioned responses that are triggered by environmental cues and emotional reactivity. And we see our conditioned responses to these grow in intensity—the craving—until it reaches a peak level, and then fall off. Every time we surf the urge and don't actually enact the behavior, the reinforcement pattern is weakened. Basically, what happens is as we learn to be with difficult experience and surf our cravings rather than act on them, our conditioned responses—the poisons or fires in but Buddhist psychology—are extinguished. So then we needn't be so careful anymore to avoid positive or negative cues, nor do we have to find alternative behaviors. We can just be mindful of our changing experience, and in that way, grow free from our addiction.

Now there's an unusual form of mindfulness practice that you can try to understand more clearly your relationship to potentially addictive intoxicants in particular. Things like alcohol or other mind-altering drugs. And this exercise wouldn't be helpful if you already know you have a problem with drinking or some other substance, and you know you're trying to be abstinent. But for many of us, we drink alcohol, or maybe even use other drugs sometimes, perhaps after work or with dinner at social gatherings, and we may not have noticed that they have a deleterious effect, but it could be helpful to see more clearly how they affect us. This exercise can help us to do just that. So if you're not needing to abstain, you might try this little exercise in mindful intoxication the next time you ordinarily would drink or use another substance.

This is an exercise in mindful intoxication. Once again, don't try this if you know that drinking or using another substance isn't a good idea for you, if you know you've got a problem with it. Use it, though, if you want to investigate the matter. I'm going to use alcohol as an example, but we can use the same exercise with any mind-altering substance.

You'll start with a few minutes of sitting meditation practice. Settle into your seat, notice your breathing, and try to follow the breath for complete cycles. I'd advise that you take 10 or 20 minutes of breath meditation before moving onto the next step of imbibing.

Notice all the thoughts and feelings that arise as you meditate, both the pleasant ones, such as anticipation of what you're about to do, and perhaps the unpleasant ones, things you'd rather escape that maybe the drink is going to make you feel better about.

Once your mind has settled a bit and you've had a chance to attend to your breath, have a drink. Take just enough to bring about some changes in your awareness, but not so much as to seriously interfere with your ability to pay attention. Once you've had your drink, go back to following your breath. Notice what you experience in your body. Notice the thoughts and feelings that arise in the mind. Let yourself be aware of aspects of alcohol that are pleasant and those that are unpleasant.

If urges to drink more come up, just watch them arise, reach a crescendo, and perhaps diminish again. After a few minutes of being with intoxicated experience, drink some more and observe what happens. Simply continue alternating between drinking a little more and meditating on the effects until you reach a point that seems like enough to you.

After the exercise, ask yourself, what did you discover being mindful of your substance use in this way? How did you determine your stopping point? And see if you can carry some of this awareness into normal circumstances in which you drink alcohol or use other substances.

Now troublesome eating habits can be particularly tricky, because, unlike intoxicants, abstinence here isn't an option. There are programs like Overeaters Anonymous, where we abstain from particularly addictive foods, like simple carbohydrates, but in general, you have to eat.

Now one mindfulness program that tries to deal with the challenge is called MB-EAT, Mindfulness Based Eating Awareness Training. This was developed by Jean Kristeller at Indiana State University. It uses a number of techniques that anyone working with an eating habit problem can use.

They start with simply learning mindfulness meditation, and then they do a very slow eating exercise, such as the raisin exercise. And then they move on to mindfully eating something bigger, like cheese and crackers. And they use the body scan, which is a form of mindfulness practice in which you start at one end of the body, either the head or the feet, and systematically feel all the different areas of the body to notice the effects of food on the body.

Then they have some other techniques, which are really quite interesting. They do hunger meditation, which involves paying attention to the sense of hunger, and trying to differentiate physical hunger from emotional hunger. And then they do taste satiety meditation, and this is noticing the craving for sensations of food in the mouth and learning to be with the sensation, just noticing how it feels to really want it in the mouth. And this is different from stomach satiety meditation, where we notice whether we feel full or not in the stomach. So we really start to see what's hunger about, and what does fullness feel like, and what are the different ways that we might feel hungry or full. They also work with abstinence violation effects, and do forgiveness meditation, loving-kindness practices to help when we're in pain in this way.

Here's a little meditation that you could try on your own. It usually works best after doing some breath or walking meditation. Begin by doing the raisin-eating meditation, like we did earlier in the course. Or if you don't like raisin, choose any other small piece of dried fruit or similarly healthy morsel. And then try doing the same deliberate eating meditation with a food like chocolate, fudge, potato chips, ice cream, or whatever other food you find seductive, but is kind of unhealthy.

I often find that after awhile, I habituate to the unhealthy food, and the oh-goody excitement about eating it tends to drop away and it's not so satisfying. In fact, I find foods that are engineered to be addictive, things like potato chips or extremely sweet and other fatty snacks, tend to feel too intense. Their lack of nutrients, or the lack of more subtle flavor variations becomes apparent.

Another practice that you might try is buffet meditation. Here you go to a party or buffet with the intention of practicing mindful eating. See if you can notice when hunger plays a role versus when your eyes are bigger than your stomach. And pay particular attention to the sensations of fullness. The trick is to eat slowly enough so your digestive system has enough time to signal your brain when you've had enough. And then once you feel full, you practice saying "No, thank you" to people who offer you more. And then you can notice all of the thoughts and feelings that arise eating in this setting.

I actually find that the only times that I'm not at all eating-disordered are when I'm on an intensive meditation retreat. All the rest of the time, I'm eating to some degree to self-soothe, to some degree to distract myself. And when I sit in intensive meditation retreat, my food intake starts to drop lower, and lower, and lower.

The first few times that I'm having a meal, well it's a big entertainment—the meal during a retreat—so I tend to fill the plate up rather full. But then I find that I can't get through it because I actually notice the feelings of fullness, and that makes me want to stop sooner. You don't want to be a waster, so each time I go back for food at another sitting at the meditation retreat, at another meal, I wind up taking less and less. And it takes several times before I realize that I only need much less food than I normally would take when I'm eating mindfully.

Now, often people find that the excitement of eating all we want in a buffet setting or at a party is actually more of the draw than the actual central experience of eating it. And when mindfully eating in that kind of setting, the feeling of fullness makes us want to stop much earlier than we otherwise might.

I'd like to share with you an example of mindfulness in action and how it can help with an addiction. This is a story of one of my patients with the details of his life disguised a bit to protect his confidentiality. He's a successful businessman. He grew up as a sensitive guy who was pretty emotional. He felt feelings a lot. And that wasn't such a great fit for his family, where he had some very rough brothers and a father who was very dismissive of emotions. So he grew up with a lot of inadequacy feelings. And on top of this, he had been small as a kid. And the early rejections that he had as a child really stung and they really stuck with him.

He discovered drugs and alcohol as an adolescent and instantly had a social group. He was tremendously relieved, both because he had a social group and because the drugs and alcohol made his feelings of inadequacy go away. He also really enjoyed getting high. He felt like he could have fun, play, be successful, be the man of the party. So he had both positive and negative reinforcement of his conditioned drug-taking and drinking behavior. As often happens, after a while, almost all of his social connections involved drugs and alcohol. So any time he'd get together with friends, it would be about getting high.

After being in treatment with me for a while, he had a dream. And in the dream, he arrives at the intersection of a maze. The path to the left goes up a hill, and it's full of obstacles, and dangers, and difficulties. That path to the right looks much easier. It slopes downward, and it's wide open. The problem is the path to the right, ultimately, when he'd go down it, leads to a sewer with no exit. And the only choice when you get down to the sewer is to come back up to the intersection again. Again and again in the dream, he comes to the same intersection, goes down to the right, takes the easier path, only to discover that he's got to come back up and be stuck at the same intersection.

The dream is a wonderful metaphor for how troublesome habits work. They seem to provide an easy path, but ultimately they lead us to some very unsatisfying places. Now I taught my patient mindfulness practice to notice that he can actually bear the feelings—even feelings of inadequacy, of rejection, of smallness, of failure—and if he stays with them as moment-to-moment experiences in the body, they actually change by themselves. He needn't do anything to fix the problem.

And this was really a revelation because, since adolescence, he had treated all discomfort as a kind of crisis—something that needed to be handled with drugs or alcohol. And he was very good at mixing and selecting just those drugs and alcohol products to make the feeling go away. But he had simply never noticed that physical and emotional pain is usually self-limiting. Using mindfulness practice, he could see another pathway through them.

His work these days is to reorient his whole goals from feeling good, which had been the goal, to simply being present to what is. It's not always easy— sometimes the feelings are overwhelming, and he needs support from other people. But when he's able to have freedom as his goal, rather than orchestrating a pleasant state and avoiding emotional pain as his goal, he's much, much happier.

Overcoming Traumas Large and Small
Lecture 17

Any event that brings up reactions that are stronger than our felt capacity to experience them can become traumatic. Often, we push the feelings out of awareness. We either repress or suppress them. Then, they show up as symptoms. There are many studies that show promise for using mindfulness practice to work through the effects of trauma. Given the number of people who have been afflicted by trauma, both large and small, it's nice to know that mindfulness practices can give us an effective way to work with them.

Traumatic Experiences

- Many psychiatric interventions for trauma are designed to make us feel better by reducing the intensity of unpleasant experiences. Mindfulness practices instead increase our capacity to bear experience rather than decreasing the intensity of the experience. They prepare us to better handle whatever good or bad fortune may come our way.

- Joyful and fulfilling aspects of life are inextricably intertwined with experiences of pain and loss. Some people's adversities are especially hurtful and destabilizing. Many children have been abused, unloved, or abandoned. Many adults have endured disasters, war, assaults, torture, or traumatic deaths of loved ones. The incidence of these adverse events is much higher than most people imagine.

- A large study of patients at Kaiser Permanente, a health maintenance organization, was designed to assess childhood exposure to multiple types of adverse events, including abuse, neglect, domestic violence, and serious household dysfunction (such as substance abuse). They derived an adverse childhood event (ACE) score, with one point for each major category of abuse. Two-thirds of the patients reported at least one ACE, with 26 percent experiencing one event, 16 percent experiencing two events, and 27 percent experiencing three or more events.

- And that doesn't include traumas that happen after childhood. They found that trauma has a huge impact on well-being, with higher ACE scores corresponding to more life problems. Compared to persons with an ACE score of 0, those with an ACE score of 4 or more were twice as likely to be smokers, 12 times more likely to have attempted suicide, 7 times more likely to be alcoholic, and 10 times more likely to have injected street drugs.

- What exactly makes these events traumatic? When a painful event or loss is of sufficient magnitude, it pushes us into an emergency state and activates our fight-freeze-or-flight system, which we experience as great anxiety. This usually narrows our awareness to immediate survival.

- Memories are formed, carrying with them emotions, cognitions, and sensations that become associated with the event. These can be triggered and relived as flashbacks, intrusive thoughts, painful feelings, and other aspects of posttraumatic stress. Sometimes these memories are continuously activated, leading to chronic anxiety, depression, or anger.

- These events can also change the assumptions most of us carry about ourselves, our safety, the future, and even the goodness of other people. This sort of trauma can completely upend our world. A rape, heart attack, or traumatic loss can leave us feeling entirely alone, irrevocably changed, and flooded with awareness of the fragility of life and well-being.

- When faced with such difficult experiences, most of us, consciously or unconsciously, try to avoid thoughts, feelings, and memories about what happened. So, we try to suppress these. We might engage in addictive behaviors or even engage in harmful acts toward ourselves or others.

- Of course, during a crisis, it can be very useful to block out feelings in order to cope with immediate challenges and demands. But in the long run, this tends to makes matters worse, both by causing all sorts of distressing symptoms and also robbing us of the opportunity to integrate the painful experience.

- Research shows that trauma survivors who use drugs or alcohol, dissociate, externalize, or engage in denial or suppression of upsetting thoughts are more likely to develop intrusive and chronic posttraumatic problems and syndromes. It appears that what's happening is that avoided material can't be processed and resolved. And others' reactions, including cultural assumptions of those around us, often make matters worse.

Trauma Large and Small

- Sometimes we block out feelings connected not only to major adverse events, but also feelings connected to smaller emotionally painful experiences. In fact, much of what we call "stress" is the tension that comes from trying to push little emotional hurts out of awareness. Whether or not an event is experienced as "traumatic" depends on the ratio between our capacity to handle pain when it occurs and the intensity of that pain.

- Many cultural messages encourage us to bury painful thoughts, feelings, and memories. They teach us to deal with emotional pain and uncomfortable states through behaviors that distract, suppress, or numb. Other people may say after a while to "just get over it," "put your past behind you," or "move on already."

- Endless ads promote pain relievers or other medications to fix simple discomfort. We're encouraged to buy things to feel better or get rid of feelings of inadequacy or dissatisfaction. The message we hear over and over is that pain, distress, and dissatisfaction are bad things that should be removed, medicated, or distracted from. We come to expect that once we've done things to stop feeling bad, we will, by definition, feel good.

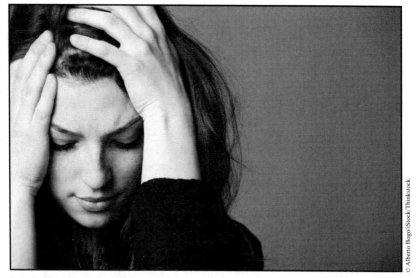

Painful thoughts that result from a traumatic experience can be alleviated by engaging in mindfulness practice.

- The problem is that the mind doesn't actually work this way. Research shows that in general, those who are able to more directly experience distress—whether through mindfulness, psychotherapy, or other ways of "being with" traumatic memory—are likely to experience less distress over time.

- It seems that "being with" non-overwhelming psychological pain allows the mind to integrate traumatic or upsetting material, until it no longer needs to intrude on consciousness. So, when in distress, to the extent possible, we should consider doing the exact opposite of what we or others may want us to do—that is, to directly feel painful states and/or think painful thoughts. We should avoid, in a sense, avoidance.

- Mindfulness practices increase our ability to stay with discomfort, both by practicing not scratching the itch and by seeing emotions as impersonal events arising in the mind and body.

Using Mindfulness Practices to Engage in Therapeutic Exposure

- "Being with" experience in mindfulness practice desensitizes us to difficult material and decreases its power to overwhelm us. By experiencing traumatic memories with less judgment and with more awareness of present experience with acceptance, their effects are less likely to be exacerbated by catastrophizing, shame, or guilt.

- Less disturbing memories require less avoidance and, therefore, increase exposure and psychological processing. A virtuous cycle gets set up that eventually helps us integrate the traumatic event. Again, we're learning to see thoughts as just thoughts.

- As we see intrusive thoughts as merely words, images, and body sensations, we have less to be afraid of or angry about. And as we come to view triggered thoughts and memories as "old tapes" or "just trauma talking," avoidance strategies such as withdrawing from activities or substance abuse become less necessary.

- There are two sources of distress associated with traumatic experience: just discussing the event itself and the pain it produces, along with the pain that persists if we resist processing the feelings associated with the event; and the suffering associated with attempts to maintain previous models of self, others, and the basis for happiness, in the face of intruding reality.

- Mindfulness practices can help with the second difficulty as well. Mindfulness practices, by helping us notice how all phenomena are in constant flux, can lead us to recognize more clearly the inevitability of illness, aging, change, and death so that we're not so shocked to learn about them. We're then less likely to be traumatized by life's misfortunes.

Processing Trauma

- People find it much easier to integrate trauma from natural disasters than trauma caused by other people. With a natural disaster, there's nobody else to blame and no shame, and it's not a personal event.

- This leads to appreciation of what is called, in Buddhist terms, "dependent origination," which describes the fact that all things come from causes and conditions. Every event happens because other events caused it to happen. This can help us see all trauma, even trauma perpetuated by others, as a more impersonal event. This has a way of transforming the trauma quite radically.

- From this perspective, there are four steps to working with trauma: open to the painful emotions and memories, explore the facts of the trauma, see it through the lens of dependent origination, and develop compassion toward ourselves and the others who are involved.

- The first two steps are actually more on the level of relative truth, the way we think about life in general. We're simply going to open to the painful emotions and explore the facts of the trauma. The third and fourth steps are really about absolute truth. Can we step back and look at things—not from a personal perspective, but from the perspective of impersonal factors and forces unfolding in the world?

- In doing this work, timing is vitally important, because you can't rush things. In treating trauma, you always have to start with safety. Until a person feels safe in their current situation, then trying to reintegrate the split-off feelings and look at them in a new light is useless. You have to be able to feel that you can manage your feelings before delving into them.

- Whether we're using mindfulness practices to develop more safety or to integrate thoughts, feelings, and images that we may push out of awareness, continued practice is key. Unless we have the regular practice to draw upon, it's very difficult to use mindfulness practices to deal with these difficult circumstances.

- Our ultimate goal is integration. We can, in fact, think of integration psychologically as health—when memories are no longer split off or suppressed, when the feelings and cognitions are all connected, and when mind and body are connected. With integration, we become comfortable with ourselves. We become comfortable with our mammalian nature, with our sexuality, with our aggression, with all of our body functions, with all of our instincts, and with all of our emotional responses to what has happened to us.

- This ultimately leads to a kind of spiritual development, an integration between who we think we are, other people, and the wider world. But we can only do this work when a person is ready for it. The reason we split off feelings is because the feelings were too difficult to bear at the time.

- An important caveat is that we need safety first. You need to have a stable life first. You may want to try a simple integration exercise that goes by the acronym RAIN: recognize, allow, investigate, non-identification. You can use this with any trauma-related difficulty, whether a large one or a small one. It's a technique that is taught by many different meditation teachers.

Suggested Reading

Briere, "Mindfulness, Insight, and Trauma Therapy."

Briere and Scott, *Principles of Trauma Therapy: A Guide to Symptoms, Evaluation, and Treatment.*

Herman, *Trauma and Recovery.*

Levine and Frederick, *Waking the Tiger: Healing Trauma, the Innate Capacity to Transform Overwhelming Experiences.*

Questions to Consider

1. What makes an experience traumatic? Name a few experiences, whether seemingly serious or not, that you have personally found to be traumatic.

2. During what times in your life have you needed more safety and stability to deal with challenging events? When might you have benefitted more from turning toward the sharp points to integrate previously split-off mental contents?

R-A-I-N: A brief practice designed to help us "be with" and investigate challenging emotional or physical states.

Overcoming Traumas Large and Small
Lecture 17—Transcript

I want you to imagine two very different days. On the first day, you've had a bad cold. You haven't been sleeping well. Because you felt crummy, you've been eating bad foods to kind of self-soothe. You haven't been working out and you haven't been meditating.

You wake up in the morning exhausted again. You didn't sleep very well because your nose was all stuffed up. You look out the window and it's 33 degrees and raining. You managed to drag yourself out of bed. And if you live with somebody, you go into the kitchen and you have one of those five-minute interactions with a friend or a loved one that can ruin your whole day. You know, the kind where you get off really on the wrong foot.

And you take a look at your appointment book and you realize that you're meeting with way too many people, and a lot of them aren't your favorites. And it's with this as a backdrop that you drag yourself out to your car and you start driving to work.

On the way to work, you're driving. And very subtly at first, you hear and feel thump, thump, thump. But as time goes on, it starts to become [faster] thump, thump, thump. And you realize you have a flat tire. And you just have this overwhelming feeling of, I can't believe it. Not today. I just can't take it.

Now, I'd like you to imagine a completely different day. You've been healthy. You've been working out. You've been meditating regularly. You wake up in the morning quite refreshed after a long and deep sleep because this time you had the wisdom to go to bed early enough. You look out the window and it's 68 degrees and the sun is shining. And if you live with somebody, you go into the kitchen and you have one of those five-minute interactions with a friend or a loved one that just makes you so happy to have somebody else in your life, to have connections, to have other people.

And you look at your appointment book and it's a Goldilocks day for whatever kind of work or recreational activity you're involved in—not so many activities that you're going to be exhausted, not few that you're going to starve or feel bored.

And as you look at names of some of the people you're going to be with that day, you realize that a lot of them, if they're not already your close personal friends, if you're working with them professionally, you'd like to have them as your close personal friends. And it's with this as a backdrop that you go on and get into your car and start heading for work.

And on the way to work, you're enjoying the day. You're being very mindful. And you stop at a red light. And suddenly, you feel—bam. And you realize you've been hit from behind. You take a moment and you realize, oh, I seem to be OK. You look over, the other driver's already pulling their car over. They seem to be OK. And you just have this profound sense of, thank god. It's just going to be metal and plastic and some money, but it'll all be all right.

Now on the first day, the intensity of the experience was relatively moderate. It's down here. It was a flat tire on a rainy day. But your capacity to bear experience was lower still, so you felt overwhelmed. On the second day, the intensity of the experience was considerably higher than that. It was an automobile accident. But your capacity to bear experience was higher still, so the net result was you felt it was OK. It was no big deal.

Any event that brings up reactions that are stronger than our felt capacity to experience them can become traumatic. Often, when the experience is too intense, we push feelings out of our awareness. We either repress or suppress them, and then they show up as symptoms.

Now, many of our psychiatric interventions are actually designed to make us feel better by reducing the intensity of unpleasant experiences. Mindfulness practices instead increase our capacity to bear experience rather than decreasing the intensity of the experience. They prepare us to be able to better handle whatever good or bad fortune may come our way. Let's step back and look a little bit at what happens during traumas, both small traumas and the larger ones.

Joyful and fulfilling aspects of life are inextricably intertwined with experiences of pain and loss. Some peoples' adversities are especially hurtful and destabilizing. Many children have been abused, unloved, or abandoned. Many adults have endured disasters, war, assaults, torture, or traumatic deaths of loved ones. The incidence of these adverse events is much higher than most people imagine.

A large study of patients at Kaiser Permanente, which is a health maintenance organization, was designed to assess childhood exposure to multiple types of adverse events—to abuse, to neglect, to domestic violence, and serious household dysfunction, such as substance abuse. The researchers derived what they called an ACE score, an Adverse Childhood Event, or A-C-E score. And they gave one point for each major category of abuse, neglect, or other difficulty somebody had experienced. They found in this normal population of adults, just regular folks signed up at a health center, two-thirds of the population report at least one adverse childhood event. Actually, 26 percent had one event, 16 percent had two events, and 27 percent had three or more of these serious events, and this doesn't even include the traumas that happen after childhood.

They also found that these adverse childhood events had a huge impact on well-being with higher ACE scores corresponding to more of life's problems. Compared to people with an ACE score of zero, those with a score of four or more were twice as likely to be smokers, 12 times more likely to have attempted suicide, 7 times more likely to be alcoholic, and 10 times more likely to have injected street drugs. Childhood trauma sets us up for trouble later on.

But what exactly makes these events traumatic? Why do they so negatively affect our well being, even years after the adverse event? When a painful event or loss is of significant and sufficient magnitude, it pushes us into an emergency state. It activates our fight, freeze, or flight system, which we then experience as great anxiety. And it usually narrows our awareness to immediate survival. We just think, how am I going to get through this?

Memories are formed. And these memories carry with them all sorts of emotions, thoughts, and sensations that become associated with the event.

And then these memories can be triggered and relived as flashbacks, as intrusive thoughts, or simply as painful feelings and other aspects of post-traumatic stress. Sometimes, these memories are continuously activated, leading to chronic anxiety, depression, or chronic anger. And these events can also change the assumptions most of us carry about ourselves, about our safety, about the future, and often, about the goodness of other people.

Trauma can completely upend our world. A rape, a heart attack, or a traumatic loss can leave us feeling entirely alone, irrevocably changed, and flooded with an awareness of the fragility of life and how hard well-being can be to obtain. When we're faced with such difficult experiences, most of us, either consciously or unconsciously, try to avoid the thoughts, feelings, and memories about what happened. So we try to suppress them. We might and often do engage in addictive behaviors like the ones we discussed in the last lecture, or even engage in harmful acts toward ourselves or others.

Now, of course, during a crisis it can be very useful to block out feelings in order to cope with immediate challenges and demands of the situation—to do what needs to be done. But in the long run, this tends to make matters worse both by causing all sorts of distressing symptoms and also by robbing us of the opportunity to integrate the painful experience.

A good deal of research shows that trauma survivors who use drugs or alcohol, who dissociate (which means basically to space out), externalize (see problems as out there), or engage in denial or suppression of upsetting thoughts are more likely to develop intrusive and chronic post-traumatic problems and syndromes. It appears that what's happening is that the avoided material can't be processed and resolved.

As one Zen teacher and psychologist put it, "What we cannot hold, we cannot process. What we cannot process, we cannot transform. What we cannot transform haunts us." Or a bit more succinctly, as one of my patients once said, "When we bury feelings, we bury them alive."

Now, other people's reactions, including all sorts of cultural assumptions about how to handle things, often makes things worse. As a mental health professional, I hear stories about this all the time. Like the Iraqi woman who couldn't mention her rape and kept it secret from her husband and other family members for decades because it was so shameful in her culture. Or the divorced Cambodian woman who couldn't find refuge in her community. Apparently, the word for divorcée in Cambodian is something like refuse, like garbage. She both felt and was treated like garbage, and had no family or friends to turn to.

Now, sometimes we block out feelings connected not only to major adverse events, but also feelings connected to smaller emotionally painful experiences. In fact, most of what we call stress is actually the tension that comes from trying to push little traumas out of awareness, little feelings that were a little bit too much to bear at the time and that we distracted from or withdrew from in the moment.

Now, whether or not an event is experienced as traumatic depends on the ratio between our capacity to handle the pain when it occurs and the intensity of the pain—Just what I was talking about with the flat tire or the automobile accident. If our capacity to handle it is very high, even if the pain is pretty high, we're OK. But if our capacity to handle it is low, we become overwhelmed, we push it out of awareness, and it becomes a trauma.

Now, we all receive many messages that encourage us to bury painful thoughts, feelings, and memories. They teach us to deal with emotional pain, uncomfortable states through behaviors that distract, or suppress, or numb us. Other people may say after a while to just get over it, put your past behind you, or move on already. And there're certainly endless ads promoting pain relievers and all sorts of medications to fix simple discomfort. We're even encouraged to buy all sorts of consumer products to feel better or to get rid of feelings of inadequacy or dissatisfaction.

The message we hear over and over in all sorts of forms is that pain, distress, and dissatisfaction are bad things that we should get rid of, medicate, or distract ourselves from. And we come to expect that if only we would do that, get rid of those things, stop feeling bad, we would, by definition, feel good. The problem is that the mind doesn't actually work this way. As my friend and colleague, the psychologist John Briere at the University of Southern California says, the way the mind actually works is a "pain paradox."

Research shows us that in general, those who are able to more directly experience their distress, whether through mindfulness practice, through psychotherapy, or other ways of being with traumatic memory, are likely to experience less distress over time. It seems that being with non-overwhelming psychological pain allows the mind to integrate traumatic or upsetting material until it no longer needs to intrude into consciousness.

So when we're in distress, to the best extent possible, we should consider doing the exact opposite of what we and others may want us to do. That is, we should consider directly feeling the painful states and/or even thinking the painful thoughts. I know this sounds odd, but we should avoid avoidance. Or as a Zen master said, "Invite your fear to tea."

You may notice we're back again to the story of the Zen master who can be run through with the sword without blinking an eye. It's about using mindfulness practice to increase our ability to stay with discomfort—both by practicing not scratching the itch or adjusting to fix the ache when we're doing our meditation practice, and by seeing emotions as impersonal events that arise and pass in the mind and body.

This is also like we discussed in treating the snake phobia—we use mindfulness practices to engage in a form of therapeutic exposure and response prevention. Practicing being with experiences in mindfulness practices desensitizes us to the difficult material and decreases its capacity to overwhelm us.

By experiencing our traumatic memories with less judgment and with more, simply, awareness of present experience with acceptance, their effects are less likely to be exacerbated by catastrophizing, by shame, by guilt, by all the stories we add on top of it. And the less disturbing memories then require less avoidance and they increase psychological exposure and processing. A kind of virtuous cycle gets set up that eventually helps us to integrate the traumatic event.

Here again, we're learning to see thoughts as just thoughts, developing what cognitive behavior theorists call *metacognitive awareness*—the ability to simply see thinking as it is. And as we see these intrusive thoughts as just words, images, and body sensations, we have less to be afraid or angry about. We start to see the triggered thoughts as old tapes or just trauma talking. And we see the avoidance strategies, like withdrawing from activities of substance abuse, as far less appealing and necessary.

Now, there are actually two pretty independent sources of distress that are associated with traumatic experience. The first is the one we've just been discussing, the memories of the event itself and the pain that's associated with it. The second is the suffering that's associated with our attempts to maintain our previous models or views of our self, of others, of the world, of our basis for happiness. And mindfulness practice can also help us with the second difficulty as well.

Imagine, for example, what might happen after a heart attack. Now, a heart attack may involve great physical pain, but it also tends to challenge our beliefs and expectations about our health, about our immortality. And perhaps later, when we're recovering, all of our assumptions about autonomy and being able to be independent, assumptions about financial security, our future generally, and the idea of having a life without pain or illness all get challenged. The psychological shock of these realities may be at least as hard to deal with as the pain and terror associated with the physically injured heart.

Mindfulness practices, by helping us to notice how all phenomena are in constant flux, can help us to recognize more clearly the inevitability of things like illness, aging, change, and even death so we're not so shocked to learn about them. We're then less likely to be traumatized by life's misfortunes.

Now, the processing of trauma is quite different depending on its source. There have been many studies that show that people find it far easier to integrate traumatic experiences that come from natural disasters than those that are caused by other people—those that are perpetrated by other people's misdeeds. When it's a natural disaster, assuming the problem wasn't that humans didn't respond adequately, then there's no one else to blame. There's no shame involved. It's not a personal event. It's experienced as an impersonal event. And it usually affected not just us, but a wide number of people.

This leads to appreciation of, what in Buddhist terms, is called *dependent origination*. And this is a term to describe the fact that all things come from causes and conditions. Every event that happens happens because other events caused it to happen. It's very easy to see in meteorology. The hurricane happened because of the various forces in the world at the moment, and it really wasn't anybody's fault. But what's interesting is the same view of dependent origination can even apply to traumas that are caused by other people, and that has a way of transforming them quite radically.

So from this perspective, there are four steps to working with trauma. The first is to open to the painful emotions and memories. The second is to explore the facts of the trauma. The third is going to be to see it through the lens of dependent origination, and I'll explain that in some detail in a moment. And then finally, to develop compassion toward ourselves and the others who are involved.

The first two are actually more on the level of what I called earlier *relative truth*, the way we think about life in general. We're simply going to open to the painful emotions and explore the facts of the trauma. The second, or the third and the fourth are really about absolute truth. Can we step back and look at things, not from a personal perspective but from the perspective of impersonal factors and forces unfolding in the world?

Let's look at these in some detail through the experience of one of my patients who had a very traumatic childhood experience. And this childhood experience, ironically, was brought about by his own actions. But as we'll see, his own actions were brought about, in many ways, by his situation.

This, in disguised form, is Tom's story. Now, Tom was raised by a very neglectful aunt. And he turned to his sister for comfort. His sister was only about a year younger. And this turning to one another for comfort eventually morphed into having some sexual encounters.

Now, one day, his older cousin with whom he lived walked in on him with his sister. Didn't say word, but from then on the cousin tormented him throughout his adolescence. The cousin was like a big man on campus in high school, and he made sure that Tom was rejected by everybody.

Eventually, Tom found himself completely ostracized by the family in which he had grown up.

So how to work with this from this mindful perspective? Well, we begin by working with opening to painful emotions, to simply gradually process the thoughts and feelings with acceptance to the degree that which we can of all of the feelings of distress. And the way we do that is by revisiting the painful event and noticing exactly what comes up in the heart and mind.

We notice in this process that the bad feelings are not bad in the sense of unuseful; they're simply painful, even though it's normal and healthy for them to come up. And it's very important when doing this not to push for any kind of premature closure or forgiveness or anything. It's really about just staying with the hard feelings, including feelings of hatred, disgust, shame, desires for retribution, whatever comes up because these are all perfectly understandable human reactions to trauma.

What happened to Tom was he noticed that he felt like a freak, like a pariah, and he spent his entire life vulnerable to being found out, afraid that people would discover what he had done with his sister.

The second step is to really explore the facts, and to explore them objectively—kind of like if you remember the old show *Dragnet*, the way Friday used to speak: "Just the facts, ma'am." You want to really try to remember what happened, and then look at whatever conclusions we might have formed about ourselves and about others who were involved at the time of the event, including all of the self-blaming conclusions. And the goal is to really see things as they are.

For Tom, this involved recalling that his sister was actually a willing and active participant their times together, and recalling his own desperation and loneliness, how he had nowhere to turn to.

The next stage—and this is where we get more directly into mindfulness practice and the implication of Buddhist psychology—is we try to look at the event through the lens of dependent origination. This has to do with our whole notions of blame, and even of good and evil. Let me explain.

At what age would you start blaming another person for his or her behavior? If a six-month-old baby starts carrying on crying or acting upset or keeping us up at night, we don't usually think that the baby's doing it willfully or the baby's a bad person. We think, well, they must be wet, or they're sick, or maybe teething early. We try to figure out, what are the factors and forces causing this?

By the time the baby is six years old, well, we might go back and forth between thinking, if they're misbehaving, they're doing it willfully—rotten kid—or we might be thinking, what's making my child do this?

By 16, if somebody's behaving badly, it's quite easy to start blaming them and judging them for it. This is actually connected to the very idea of evil, because evil is predicated on the idea that if we had the exact same genetics and the exact same environmental history as the other person, we'd somehow behave differently. And yet, scientific psychologists trying to understand human behavior see human behavior as the result of genetics interacting with environment over the course of a life. So the idea of evil suggests there's something other than this going on.

When we start looking at things through the lens of dependent origination, we realize, no, all behavior really is the result of these things. I remember seeing the head of Bridgewater State Hospital being interviewed on TV when he was retiring. And that was the hospital that treats the criminally insane in Massachusetts. And he said in his 25 years running this institution, he never once met an inmate who had done something heinous who hadn't him or herself—I guess it was all guys there—hadn't himself been abused.

So we start to consider the whys of the event. Why did we come to the conclusions we did? Why did the perpetrator do what he or she did? In fact, were there reasons? We're not talking about justifications, but simply reasons why this happened, or was the perpetrator intrinsically evil? It gets us to think about why people do what they do.

And this may lead to a slow transition from seeing ourselves as having deserved or caused the event and seeing the perpetrator as evil to seeing all of what unfolded as a natural consequence of some very difficult factors, forces, and conditions. We start to see the perpetrator as someone whose behavior arose from his own predispositions, difficulties, and adverse history.

For Tom, this was very important, because Tom was the victim and the perpetrator here. So for Tom, it was recalling that the aunt was either absent or critical throughout his whole childhood. There was no love or safety to be found, and it makes sense that they would turn to one another.

Now, the fourth stage, and the trickiest, involves developing compassion. And this means growing a sense of caring for oneself, and maybe even perhaps an appreciation for the suffering of the perpetrator. And compassion rests on the notion that we humans are all in the same predicament and that we're all struggling the best we can given the hand we've been dealt.

Ultimately then, awareness of dependent origination can reduce our emotional responses associated with seeing the perpetrator as intrinsically bad. For Tom, this was realizing that what he did was actually a natural consequence of the situation. I remember giving him at one point a book written for clinicians about children who have sexual contact with other children that's inappropriate. And the book was quite clear, all of the research said, virtually all of these kids who do this do it because they're in dire straits emotionally and they're in adverse environments. He also came to see his cousin's sadistic reaction as a natural response to being in that same environment, and even began to view the aunt's neglect of the kids as coming out of her own history of neglect.

Now in doing this work, timing is vitally important because you can't rush things. And if we try to move from what a person's actually feeling into these more advanced stages of letting go, or even for that matter moving into remembering the situation vividly when we're not ready to do that, we can become quite overwhelmed. We discussed this earlier in talking about modifying the practices to suit our own needs.

In treating trauma, you always have to start with safety. Until a person feels safe in their current situation, then trying to re-integrate the split-off feelings and look at them in a new light is really counter-indicated. And this means having a decent living environment, maybe enough economic security, and some support of friends, family, perhaps a therapist, or a therapy group. You have to be able to feel that you can manage your feelings before delving into them.

Of course, whether we're using mindfulness practices to develop more safety or to integrate thoughts, feelings, and images that we may have pushed out of awareness, continued practice is key. And that's why I've been reminding you throughout the course to regularly engage in both informal practice and formal meditation practice between the lectures because unless we have the regular practice to draw upon, it's very hard to use the mindfulness practices to deal with these difficult circumstances.

So just to review quickly, the things that help us establish safety are usually things that have an outer focus—walking meditation, listening meditation, nature meditation, eating meditation, and open-eyed practices generally. They're actually called "grounding activities" in the trauma field, and they can be used whenever we're in crisis, or just to strengthen the sense of safety in the present moment. We can also do things like the mountain meditation, which is included as an audio recording with the course. Or *mettā*, or loving-kindness practices, which are also available there.

We only want to turn toward the sharp points when we're really ready. And that's moving toward the trauma-related experience, perhaps following those four steps that I outlined earlier. And as we're doing that, we always focus on how whatever we're investigating is felt right now in the body—the pain, the fear, the sadness, or the anger, the traumatic images or memories.

Our ultimate goal is integration. We can, in fact, think of integration psychologically as health—when memories are no longer split off or suppressed, when the heart and the head, the feelings and cognitions are all connected, and when mind and body are connected. And with integration, we become comfortable with ourselves. We become comfortable with our mammalian nature, with our sexuality, with our aggression, with all of our body functions, with all of our instincts, as well as with all of our emotional responses to what's happened to us.

This ultimately leads to a kind of spiritual development, an integration between who we think we are and other people and the wider universe or the wider world. But again, we can only do this work when a person is ready for it. The reason we split off feelings, why we disintegrate, is because the feelings were too hard to bear at the time. They were too difficult to integrate. So we always have to do this in a thoughtful way, sensing what somebody's ready for or not ready for.

Now, keeping in mind this important caveat—that we need safety first, you need to have a stable life first—you may want to try a simple integration exercise that goes by the acronym RAIN, R-A-I-N. And you can use this with any trauma-related difficulty, whether a big one or a small one. It's actually taught by many different meditation teachers.

So this is the R-A-I-N, or RAIN practice. The R stands for Recognize what's happening. So just take a few moments to experience your breath. And whatever feeling or sensation that's around which is difficult to be with, simply recognize it. Notice what it is. And be with it for a few moments. Just breathe with whatever the experience is.

And then we can move on to the A, which is to Allow. Allow life and experience to be just as it is. So once we recognize what's happening, we practice allowing it to be there—not trying to change it or fix it or solve it in any way, just allowing the feeling to be there.

I stands for Investigate. And it's about investigating the inner experience with kindness. So once you've recognized and allowed the experience, have an attitude of curiosity to feel exactly what it's about, what's happening here and now. Be curious.

And then finally, N is Non-identification, or Natural awareness. To simply see whatever's happening in the mind and body as the impersonal phenomena that it is. Simply allow it to be. So we recognize what's happening, allow it to be just as it is. Then investigating it with kindness and then not identifying with it, just resting in natural awareness.

There are a lot of studies showing promise for using mindfulness practice to work through the effects of trauma. A number have been done recently with veterans with PTSD that have some very promising findings. Given the number of people who have been afflicted by trauma, both large and small, it's really nice to know that mindfulness practices can give us an effective way to work with them.

In our next lecture, we're going to look at some mindfulness-based programs that have been shown to help people with a wide variety of behavioral and psychological problems. Understanding the components of these pioneering approaches will help us see different ways that we might use mindfulness practices to work with the difficulties we encounter in our own lives. Thanks for listening.

Groundbreaking Mindfulness Programs
Lecture 18

In this lecture, you will learn about various mindfulness-based programs that have been shown to help people with a wide variety of behavioral and psychological problems. Specifically, you will learn about mindfulness-based stress reduction, mindfulness-based cognitive therapy, dialectical behavior therapy, and acceptance and commitment therapy. Understanding the components of these pioneering approaches will help you see different ways that you might use mindfulness practices to work with the difficulties you encounter in your own life.

Mindfulness-Based Stress Reduction

- There are several pioneering multicomponent mindfulness-based programs that have been designed to help with a wide variety of difficulties, each of which has good research support. And each of these programs offers additional techniques that any of us can use to deepen our mindfulness practice.

- Mindfulness-based stress reduction (MBSR) was the first of these. It was started by Jon Kabat-Zinn in 1979 to treat pain and stress-related disorders. His pioneering efforts are responsible for the wide-scale adoption of mindfulness practices into so many different health-care settings. It's been the most widely studied and adopted approach, and it's the independent variable in most studies.

- MBSR has several components to it. Mostly, it teaches mindfulness meditation. It encourages informal practice and teaches a number of different formal practices. It uses the breath meditation and mountain meditation. It also uses body scan and hatha yoga.

- When John developed MBSR, he wanted to know how much practice to ask participants to do. He chose to require more to make the effects tangible. He asked people to do 45 minutes to an hour a day, six days per week, of mixed formal and informal practice. There is also a six- to eight-hour intensive, or retreat, at week six, and people attend eight weekly two- to three-hour group sessions.

- MBSR has been studied more than any other treatment intervention, and many studies document its efficacy for various disorders. The early studies were typically not large in scale or well controlled. Because of this, it wasn't easy to tell whether the results were due to participating in the group, learning instructions, or actually practicing mindfulness. Increasingly, the studies use active control, which allows scientific conclusions to be drawn from them.

- MBSR has shown significant improvement in ratings of pain, other medical symptoms, and general psychological symptoms. In addition, it has shown significant improvement in generalized anxiety and panic disorder. There have been improvements in binge eating disorder and in fibromyalgia symptoms. Even psoriasis patients had quicker skin clearing. Cancer patients reported reduced mood disturbance and stress levels during their treatment.

Mindfulness-Based Cognitive Therapy

- One of the programs that grew out of MBSR is mindfulness-based cognitive therapy (MBCT), which is one of what we now call the third wave of behavior therapies. Behavior therapy began with the work of Pavlov and his dogs, in which he discovered that if you paired an unconditional stimulus with some other behavior, over time, people would respond to the other behavior as they had responded to the unconditioned stimulus. His dogs learned to salivate to the ringing of a bell in the same way that they had salivated to meat powder.

- The second part of behavior therapy came out of the work of B. F. Skinner, called operant conditioning, or behavior modification. This is the idea that by rewarding certain behaviors and not rewarding others, we can change people's behavior patterns.

- Psychotherapists using behavioral principles discovered that if humans are a different from animals in that we think a lot, then maybe it would make more sense to start changing our thought patterns and use behavioral learning principles to change those thought patterns. And that ushered in the whole world of cognitive behavior therapy. There are all sorts of different programs that are designed to change irrational, maladaptive thoughts into rational, adaptive ones.

- The innovation of this third wave of behavior therapies, and MBCT in particular, comes back to the teachings of Carl Rogers, who said that acceptance is a precondition of change. And they realized that trying to change thoughts and behaviors doesn't work as well as first developing profound acceptance of experience. So, all of the mindfulness- and acceptance-based treatments start with developing this profound acceptance of treatment.

- The founders of MBCT hypothesized that mindfulness might prevent relapse of major depression episodes. They discovered that people who get seriously depressed are different from ordinary people when they're faced with sadness, disappointment, or discouraging news. Ordinary people just feel sad or discouraged, but people who have been through serious bouts of depression bring with them thoughts that they had the last time they were depressed. This is an example of cue-dependent memory.

- The founders of MBCT said that with depressed people, the feeling of sadness or discouragement—the very mood—is what brings back the flood of all of the old memories and thoughts. So, instead of just feeling sad, people feel worthless, unlovable, rejected, and hopeless.

- The MBCT founders thought that mindfulness practice could help people see all of these thoughts as simply thoughts arising and passing in the mind so that they wouldn't get so stuck in depression. They taught these people formal practice, such as MBSR, and all sorts of informal practices, such as mindfulness of everyday activity.

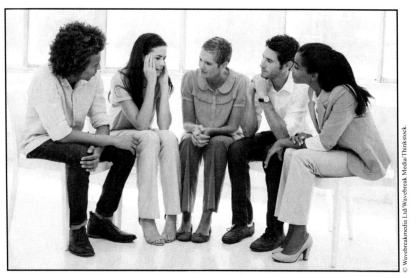

Therapies that involve group sessions help individuals cope with their issues by relating to other members of a group.

- The structure of MBCT is similar to MBSR, only it's done in groups of up to 12 recovered depressed patients over the course of eight weeks. They also give daily homework assignments that help people both do their mindfulness practice and help them notice what their thought patterns are about.

- MBCT uses a mindfulness- and acceptance-based approach. Instead of trying to replace irrational or maladaptive thoughts with rational ones, we try to see all thoughts as coming and going and not to be trusted.

- Mindfulness-based cognitive therapy was one of the first clinical interventions to have a really dramatic outcome. In a study of this approach, after one year, two-thirds of the people who had participated in at least four sessions of MBCT remained depression-free, while only one-third of the people who had the usual treatment remained depression-free.

Dialectical Behavior Therapy

- Another form of treatment is called dialectical behavior therapy (DBT). It was developed by Marsha Linehan to treat borderline personality disorder, which involves emotional disregulation. People with borderline personality disorder have very widely fluctuating moods and interpersonal relationships. They also have a very high incidence of suicide, substance abuse, and other kinds of problems.

- DBT combines mindfulness practice, particularly in the Zen tradition, and cognitive behavior therapy in order to help people with emotional disregulation. The central dialectic in dialectical behavior therapy is the tension between acceptance and change—realizing that at every moment in our life when we confront a difficulty, we have to be able to change what we can change and accept what we can't change. It's basically what's often known as the serenity prayer.

- People with borderline personality disorders, who struggle with emotional disregulation, have a heightened sensitivity to all their emotions. This increased emotional intensity takes a long time to return to baseline. They often feel that their environment is invalidating, because people with this disorder are a bit difficult, and other people are often criticizing them. So, they're used to being rejected a lot. Their emotional displays are met in different ways. Sometimes people respond to them; other times people just reject them.

- DBT is a system of helping people to realize that they can accept themselves, their history, and their current situation, but they can work to change the behaviors that create such difficulty in their environment. Mindfulness practices actually help a lot in doing this.

- The structure of DBT is different from MBSR or MBCT. The structure is usually part of an intensive individual psychotherapy, and mindfulness is also taught in year-long, two-and-a-half-hour weekly groups. The frequency and intensity of mindfulness practice is tailored by the individual therapist.

- Many of the techniques that are used can be useful for any of us. A lot of them are Zen techniques, including those of Thich Nhat Hanh. They can be helpful additions to any of our mindfulness practices, even if we're not struggling with some kind of very difficult emotional circumstance.

- There have been many, many studies showing positive outcomes from DBT. There are improvements in the frequency and the medical risk of parasuicidal behavior. Self-injurious behaviors decrease, and people stay in treatment longer when they practice DBT than when they don't. In addition, things like illicit drug use and binge eating improve.

Acceptance and Commitment Therapy

- Another form of treatment is called acceptance and commitment therapy (ACT), which was developed by Steve Hayes and his colleagues in the 1980s and into the late 1990s. He used a number of Eastern meditative traditions to develop a mindfulness-, acceptance-, and value-based psychotherapy. Many of the elements in ACT seem to come from Erhard Seminars Training, which is an organization that packages meditative techniques in a way that is accessible to Western audiences.

- ACT has several components. The first is creative hopelessness, which is about realizing the futility of current efforts to feel better. The second component is cognitive defusion, or deliteralization, which means realizing that thoughts are really just thoughts, not reality. The third component is acceptance, or just allowing experience to be just as it is.

- The fourth component is self as context, which is about identifying with the observer of the thoughts, not the thinker. The last component pays attention to what is called valuing, which involves redirecting one's life to what gives it meaning. This final component is something that is pretty much unique to ACT among the mindfulness-based interventions.

- The structure of ACT is usually part of individual psychotherapy, although increasingly it's been done as a group format as well. It teaches specific ACT skills, of which there are over 100. Many are based on images or metaphors. They teach insights that you can also derive from mindfulness practice.

- The outcomes of ACT have been very, very promising. They have reduced rehospitalization of psychotic people, social anxiety, and disability due to pain. It beat nicotine replacement for quitting smoking and reduced high-risk adolescent sexual behavior.

Suggested Reading

Harris and Hayes, *ACT Made Simple: An Easy-to-Read Primer on Acceptance and Commitment Therapy*.

Kabat-Zinn, *Full Catastrophe Living*.

Linehan, *Cognitive-Behavioral Treatment of Borderline Personality Disorder*.

Segal, Williams, and Teasdale, *Mindfulness-Based Cognitive Therapy for Depression*.

Questions to Consider

1. What are the four original empirically supported mindfulness-based treatments that were developed to ameliorate medical and psychological disorders?

2. How might you use one or more techniques from these approaches to work with difficulties in your life or help someone else with his or her distress?

Mindfulness Practice

three-minute breathing space: Developed as part of mindfulness-based cognitive therapy, this exercise can help us step out of the thought stream and bring our attention back to the sensations of the present moment at any time during the day. It's particularly useful when we're feeling stressed or overwhelmed.

Groundbreaking Mindfulness Programs
Lecture 18—Transcript

There are several pioneering multi-component mindfulness-based programs that have been designed to help with a wide variety of difficulties, each of which has good research support. And each of these programs offers additional techniques that any of us can use to deepen our mindfulness practice.

Mindfulness-based stress reduction was the first of these. And that was started by Jon Kabat-Zinn back in 1979 to treat pain- and stress-related disorders. He was a scientist working at the University of Massachusetts Medical School who had had a personal mindfulness practice and thought, these things could really help with such a wide range of physical disorders. Why don't we try to get them into medicine? And it's really his pioneering efforts that are responsible for the wide-scale adoption of mindfulness practices into so many different health-care settings.

It's been the most widely-studied and adopted approach, and it's the independent variable in most studies. You've heard me say throughout the course that people were assigned to an eight-week mindfulness training course. More often than not, that training course was simply MBSR, or mindfulness-based stress reduction.

It has several components to it, most of which will be familiar to you at this point. Mostly, it teaches mindfulness meditation. It encourages informal practice and teaches a number of different formal practices. They use the breath meditation, as we have done, the mountain meditation. They also use the body scan, which I mentioned before, where you start at one end of the body and simply use, successively, other parts of the body as the object of your awareness, until you get all the way up to the head and out to the ends of the arms.

They also use Hatha yoga, which is a kind of gentle stretching that can be done mindfully, in which you breathe into the stretch. And you simply pay attention mindfully, bring your attention to the sensations of the stretch, and every time the mind wanders, bring it back to the feelings of stretching.

Now when John developed MBSR, he had an interesting question: how much practice to ask the participants to do. What he decided on was to ask them to do a fair amount of practice. He asked folks to do 45 minutes to an hour a day, six days per week, of mixed formal and informal practice. There are also a six- to eight-hour intensive, a little retreat at week six, and people attend eight weekly two- to three-hour group sessions.

Now, the advantage of making people do or asking people to do more intensive practice is it's more likely that people can actually notice that these practices radically transform the heart, and the mind, and our everyday experience of living. It's one of the reasons I've been encouraging you to practice throughout the course, because unless you do enough practice to see that these things work, you probably won't get in the habit of doing them regularly.

Now, MBSR has been studied more than any other treatment intervention. And many studies document its efficacy for various disorders. The early studies were typically not large-scaled or well-controlled so they'd have people on a wait-list. So, as I've mentioned before, you couldn't tell whether the results were due to participating in the group, or learning instructions, or actually practicing mindfulness. Increasingly, the studies use active controls, and they have good scientific basis to them.

MBSR has shown significant improvement in ratings of pain, other medical symptoms, also to general psychological symptoms. Good improvement in generalized anxiety and panic disorder; binge-eating disorder improved; improvements in fibromyalgia symptoms; even psoriasis patients had quicker skin clearing; and cancer patients reported reduced mood disturbance and stress levels during their treatment.

Now, one of the programs that grew out of MBSR is Mindfulness-Based Cognitive Therapy. And this is one of what we now call the "third wave" of behavior therapies. Let me explain.

Behavior therapy began with the work of Pavlov and his dogs—you probably remember that from intro psych—in which he discovered that if you paired an unconditioned stimulus with some other behavior, what would happen is, over time, people would respond to the other behavior as they had responded to the unconditioned stimulus. In other words, you recall the story of the dogs learning to salivate to the ringing of a bell in the same way that they had salivated to meat powder.

The second part of behavior therapy in the early days was the work of B. F. Skinner, and this was operant conditioning, or what we call colloquially, "behavior modification." And this is the idea that by rewarding certain behaviors and not rewarding others, we can change people's behavior patterns.

What psychotherapists using behavioral principles discovered was, if humans are a little different from animals in that we think a lot, then maybe it would make more sense to start changing our thought patterns and use behavioral learning principles to change those thought patterns. And that ushered in the whole world of cognitive behavior therapy. And there are all sorts of different programs that are designed to basically change irrational, maladaptive thoughts into rational, adaptive ones.

The innovation of these third wave of behavior therapies, and MBCT in particular, comes back to the teachings of Carl Rogers, who said, "acceptance is [the] precondition of change." And they realized that trying to change thoughts, trying to change behaviors, actually doesn't work as well as first developing profound acceptance of experience. So all of the mindfulness and acceptance-based treatments start with developing this profound acceptance of treatment.

The founders of MBCT hypothesized that mindfulness might prevent relapse of major depression episodes. And these folks were cognitive scientists who were studying the thought patterns of people who get seriously depressed.

What they discovered was that people who get seriously depressed are different from ordinary people when they're faced with sadness, disappointment, or discouraging news. Ordinary people just feel sad, just feel discouraged, when that happens. But folks who've been through serious bouts of depression bring with that all sorts of thoughts, thoughts that they had the last time they were depressed.

This is actually an example of something which is called *cue-dependent memory*. There's some very clever studies where they took scuba divers and taught them various tasks, things like associating numbers with words. And they taught it to them underwater and on the beach. And depending on where they taught it, people were better able to recall the information if they were back in that setting. So if they were taught underwater, they recalled it better underwater the next time than on the beach. Or if they were taught on the beach, they recalled it better on the beach than underwater.

We all know this experience from our own simple life events. If you've ever gone back to your old neighborhood where you grew up, or perhaps your college, or your high school, or your elementary school, suddenly we're flooded with all sorts of memories of that period of our life.

Well, the founders of MBCT said, this is what's going on with depressed folks, except instead of going underwater or on the beach or back to the old neighborhood, the very mood, the feeling of sadness or discouragement, is what brings back the flood of all of the old memories and all the old thoughts. So instead of just feeling sad, people feel worthless. They feel unlovable. They feel rejected. They feel hopeless.

What the MBCT founders thought was, if we can help people to see all of these thoughts as simply thoughts arising and passing in the mind, they won't get so stuck in depression. So they taught them formal practice, like in MBSR, and all sorts of informal practices, like mindfulness of everyday activity.

They invented one—which is really quite nice for us even if we're in a difficult period, like a depression period—that's called the "three-minute breathing space." And we can do a brief version of that right now.

So this is how we do the three-minute breathing space. We start with awareness. Simply bring yourself into the present moment by deliberately adopting an erect and dignified posture. And if possible, close your eyes. And then ask, what is my experience right now? What's happening in thoughts, in feelings, and in body sensations? What's happening in this moment? And acknowledge and register your experience, even if it's something unwanted.

The second step is gathering. Gently redirect your full attention to the breathing, to each in-breath and to each out-breath, as they follow one after the other. Your breath can function as a kind of anchor to bring you into the present and help you tune in to a state of awareness and stillness.

Then we move into expanding. Expand your feel of awareness around you, around your breathing, so that it includes a sense of the body as a whole, your posture, your facial expression.

The breathing space provides a way to step out of automatic-pilot mode and reconnect with the present moment briefly, no matter what you might be doing.

The structure of Mindfulness-Based Cognitive Therapy is similar to MBSR, only it's done in groups of up to 12 recovered depressed patients over the course of eight weeks. They also give daily homework assignments that help people both do their mindfulness practice and to notice what their thought patterns are about. And it uses a mindfulness- and acceptance-based approach. Instead of trying to replace irrational or maladaptive thoughts with rational ones, we try to see all thoughts as coming and going and not to be trusted.

Mindfulness-Based Cognitive Therapy was one of the first clinical interventions to have a really dramatic outcome. And it's really what put things on the map in terms of being able to apply to major funding organizations like the National Institute of Health or the Institutes for Behavioral Health, and to be able to apply for a grant for mindfulness treatment itself. When they first wrote the grant for Mindfulness-Based Cognitive Therapy, it was a grant for attentional control training. After these results, you could write a grant for mindfulness practice.

So here's what they found. They followed people over the course of a year. And they found, after one year, that two-thirds of the people who had participated in at least four sessions of Mindfulness-Based Cognitive Therapy had managed not to relapse. They were depression-free. While the folks who had had treatment as usual, only one-third of them remained depression-free.

Now, there aren't that many interventions in mental health that'll cut the incidence of something bad, like having a relapse of major depressive disorder, in half. The fact that this could do that made quite a splash and really opened the door to widespread research into the use of mindfulness practices to treat a whole range of different disorders.

Now, another form of treatment is called Dialectical Behavior Therapy (DBT). And this was developed by Marsha Linehan to treat what's called borderline personality disorder. And borderline personality disorder involves a kind of emotional disregulation, where our moods tend to fluctuate a lot. And in particular, our evaluations of other people fluctuate a lot, so that one day we see people as kind or benevolent, the next day we may see those same people as malevolent, difficult, as our enemy. People with this kind of difficulty have very widely fluctuating moods and very fluctuating interpersonal relationships. And they also have a very high incidence of suicide, substance abuse, and other sorts of problems.

There's an interesting story about Marsha Linehan's work. She's widely known as the founder of Dialectical Behavior Therapy. And one day, she approached the Institute of Living in Hartford, which is a private psychiatric hospital, and offered to give a talk for them. She's very famous; DBT is well-known. And they thought, yes, absolutely, and they scheduled the event.

When she got to the Institute and gave her talk, she explained how, when she was an adolescent, she had been hospitalized there for 26 months, essentially with emotional disregulation difficulties. And what they had tried to do for her didn't really help. And it was because of this that she went on to develop Dialectical Behavior Therapy.

She had to find her own way. And what she discovered was mindfulness practice, particularly in the Zen tradition, and cognitive behavior therapy. And she melded these in order to help people with emotional disregulation.

The central dialectic in Dialectical Behavior Therapy is the tension between acceptance and change, realizing that at every moment in our life when we confront a difficulty, we have to be able to change what we can change and accept that which we can't change. It's basically what's often known as the Serenity Prayer.

People with borderline personality disorders, folks who struggle with this kind of emotional disregulation, have a heightened sensitivity to all their emotions. And this increased emotional intensity takes a long time to return to baseline. And they often feel their environment, other people, are invalidating, because frankly, these folks are a bit difficult and other people are often criticizing them and asking them to please cut it out already. So they're used to being rejected a lot. And their emotional displays are met in different ways. Sometimes people respond to them, and other times people just reject them.

What Marsha invented was a system of helping people to realize that they could accept themselves, their history, and their current situation, but they could work to change the behaviors that create such difficulty in their environment. And mindfulness practices actually help a lot in doing this.

The structure is different from MBSR or MBCT. The structure is usually part of an intensive individual psychotherapy. And mindfulness is also taught in year-long, two-and-a-half-hour weekly groups. And the frequency and intensity of everybody's mindfulness practice is tailored by the individual therapist. The decisions we've talked about before, about moving toward safety, or moving toward integrating difficult material, are helped along by the therapist giving advice.

Now, many of the techniques that are used can be useful for any of us. A lot of them are Zen techniques a Thích Nhất Hạnh uses. They can be helpful additions to any of our mindfulness practices, even if we're not struggling with some kind of very difficult emotional circumstance.

One of them involves the conveyor belt. It's simply sitting in meditation practice and imagining the mind as a conveyor belt with objects moving along—ca-chink, ca-chink, ca-chink, clunk, ca-chink, ca-chink, ca-chink, clunk—noticing just how impersonal all of these different thoughts are.

Another is to see the mind as like a big sky with thoughts passing like clouds and to actually visualize it that way.

One that I find particularly helpful is coordinating the breath with the footsteps. And this helps because, in order to coordinate your breath with your footsteps, you have to actually pay attention. So it makes it easier to bring thoughts out of the thought stream and to bring attention into the sensations of walking. Let me demonstrate.

I'll narrate what I'm doing, even though normally as we do this, it's done silently. So I'm going to breathe in, out, in, out, in, out, in, out. And what I'm doing as I do that is I'm paying attention both to the sensations of the breath and noticing the sensations of the feet touching the ground.

Yet another technique often done in Zen practice involves counting the breaths. And there are a number of different ways we can do this. We can simply count all of the in-breaths or count the out-breaths. You can count to 10 and then begin again. One of my favorite practices is to make it into a little bit of a game. Have you ever been volleying with tennis—or perhaps playing catch with another person—and made a game out of it, in which you see how many times you can do it before you drop the ball, before the ball goes out of bounds?

You can do the same thing with the breath, only what you do is you count the breaths until you get to the point where the mind has wandered off and left the breath entirely. And then you have to go back to zero again. It can be a little disconcerting at first, because you might only get up to two or three, but after a while, the count gets a little bit higher. Again, it's a practice that helps us to focus more when the mind is a little bit more agitated.

Another one of her techniques, which I think is very, very interesting, is called "willing hands." OK, here's how this works. Start with your hands—and you can do this with me now—in a fist. And close your eyes and breathe a little bit. And squeeze them really tight, and feel what that feels like. Feel whatever emotion is associated with that.

And now imagine holding that fist and being really angry at somebody. Feel that anger. Then reverse your hands, and open them with the palms upward. And see what happens to the feeling and what happens to the anger.

You can try one more posture, which is to reach the hands out in front of you, as though you're going to hug somebody or reach out for help, and see what that feels like.

These different postures are what are called, in yoga traditions, *mudras*, different postures that bring out different feelings in the body. And by practicing these, we can see that we can transform stuck feelings into other sorts of feelings. This is one of the reasons when we do loving-kindness practice—if you've had a chance to do it in the lecture, or hopefully do it also following the audio recordings—we put the hand over the heart. This also changes mood in this way.

Another mudra we can try that also comes from Dialectical Behavior Therapy is adopting a serene half-smile. Try this right now. Just allow yourself to smile a bit, and breathe. And notice what you feel inside as you smile. It doesn't take very much to shift our inner experience, just the movement of a few facial muscles.

Dialectical Behavior Therapy also does everyday mindfulness, like cleaning the house, making tea, or bathing, or practicing what Marsha calls "Teflon-mind," allowing things to come and slide right off the mind.

There have been many, many studies showing positive outcomes from DBT. There are improvements in the frequency and the medical risk of parasuicidal behavior. Self-injurious behaviors go down. And treatment retention—people stay in treatment longer when they practice DBT than when they don't. And their illicit drug use, binge eating—all sorts of things—improve.

Now, another form of treatment is called Acceptance and Commitment Therapy, or ACT. I had mentioned this before. This was developed by Steve Hayes and his colleagues, starting in the 1980s into the late 1990s. And he likes to call it ACT rather than A-C-T, because he wants to get across the idea that this is an action-oriented approach.

Now, Steve started out as a socially anxious guy. And he's happy to say this. He does it whenever he's giving an introductory talk about ACT. He realized that even though he was highly skilled and schooled in all different forms of behavior therapy, they weren't really working for his social anxiety. He was still having a lot of trouble just meeting new people and talking to them.

He decided something else was needed, and he pretty much worked this out on his own. But he wasn't starting from scratch. It's likely that he had been exposed to a number of Eastern meditative traditions. And he used these to develop a mindfulness, acceptance, and value-based psychotherapy.

Many of the elements in ACT, or Acceptance and Commitment Therapy, seem to come from EST. You may recall that that was Erhard Seminars Training, where a guy named Werner Erhard came up with ways to package a lot of meditative techniques in a way that would be very accessible to Western audiences.

Now ACT has several components, many of which we've seen in our own efforts to develop mindfulness. The first is creative hopelessness. And that's about realizing the futility of current efforts to feel better. It also means realizing that the mind simply evolved to create difficulty for itself and accepting that that's the state we're coming in with. It also provides a kind of motivation to try to do something about it.

The second component he calls *cognitive defusion*, or *deliteralization*. It's his word for realizing that thoughts are really just thoughts, not reality. And people undergoing ACT treatment are constantly reminded in different ways not to trust our thoughts.

The third component is acceptance, just allowing experience to be just as it is. And we've seen that throughout the course. The next is self as context, and this about identifying with the observer of the thoughts, not the thinker.

If you had the chance to try the mountain meditation—and I hope that you did that—what happens is we're sitting there as the mountain, and we're watching the seasons come and go and all these things change. Instead of identifying with the contents, with the animals coming and going and the snows coming and leaving, we start to identify with the very process of awareness, with being in awareness and having all of these events happening. That really shifts our relationship to the contents of our mind, to make it much easier to take them lightly.

Finally—and this is pretty much unique to ACT among the mindfulness-based interventions—he pays attention to what he calls "valuing." And that involves redirecting one's life to what gives its meaning. And this last one is really interesting. We can try it right now.

Remember days in the college dorm room, perhaps, sitting around asking the question, what is the meaning of life? Many people do that when they're adolescents and they kind of give it up when they get busy with earning a living, perhaps having a marriage or raising children. But it's actually a useful question. What matters to you? What is important? What does it feel like is the meaning for being here? Take a moment to actually answer the question.

As you come up with an answer, now we ask the question, what's standing in the way of you living your life as though that's what really matters? Because most of us notice, when we identify something that we feel is really meaningful, that we're not actually doing what's really meaningful much of the time. So it becomes a very interesting inquiry that can help to move us in the direction of acting in ways that are consistent with what matters to us.

Now, the structure of ACT is usually part of individual psychotherapy, although increasingly it's been done as a group format, as well. And it teaches specific ACT skills. There are over a hundred of them. And they are mainly based on images or metaphors. They teach insights that you can also derive from mindfulness practice.

Remember when we were talking about pain and other kinds of disorders, the idea of the Chinese handcuffs that, when you put your fingers in there, the harder you pull, the tighter they get? That's the kind of image that's used in ACT treatment, and it can be a very helpful reminder not to keep doing the Chinese handcuffs.

The outcomes have been very, very promising. ACT is spreading all over the world. You see a lot of it in Europe and Australia. They've reduced rehospitalization of psychotic folks, reduced social anxiety, reduced disability due to pain. It actually beat nicotine replacement for quitting smoking, and reduced high-risks adolescent sexual behavior—pretty much everything under the sun.

Now, we talked before, in talking about neurobiology, about generalized anxiety disorder. That's the problem in which we are not just anxious about a specific thing, like snakes, or public speaking, or going in airplanes, but we're generally frightened. We know that exposure and response prevention is what works, generally, for a phobia. You recall the treatment of stake phobia in the psychology department. So what do you do if a person is anxious about everything?

This is where a treatment called ABBT, Acceptance-Based Behavior Therapy, used for generalized anxiety disorder, was developed by a couple of friends of mine, Liz Roemer and Sue Orsillo, in the Boston area. And what they do is basically teach mindfulness practice to the patients and ask them to expose themselves to everything that's frightening. Because if you think about it, mindfulness practice is actually experiential approach—it's about embracing whatever comes into consciousness.

Now, often when I'm teaching mental health professionals about mindfulness practices, somebody will raise their hand and say, "Well, what about attention deficit disorder or attention deficit hyperactivity disorder?" You're probably familiar with this. This is a relatively recent label, given often to children, to describe kids who have trouble sitting still and have trouble following what's going on in math class.

I was actually at a meeting once where Jon Kabat-Zinn was addressing a large audience of psychotherapists. And somebody came up to the microphone and said, "You know, it seems to me that mindfulness practice is kind of the exact opposite of attention deficit disorder. So might mindfulness practice be useful for treating this?" And John replied, somewhat uncharitably, "Duh," and went on to say, "Precisely, what we're doing is cultivating the opposite of attention deficit disorder."

Now, people who tend to be more ADD, who tend to have more difficulty with concentration, will sometimes say, "Well, I find mindfulness practice to be difficult because my mind wanders so much." And here's a way to understand that if that happens to be your situation.

If I'm a generally anxious guy and I take a benzodiazepine, something like Ativan, or Xanax, or Valium, I'll become somewhat less anxious. If I'm already a not-so-anxious person and I take one of those tranquilizers, I'll become less anxious still. If I start out as a mellow person and I take one of them, I'll become very mellow.

The same is true for mindfulness practices. If we start out with a particularly frisky mind that jumps from thing to thing, and we do a little mindfulness practice, we'll wind up with a somewhat less frisky mind. If we start out with a medium-level mind, we'll wind up with a more focused one. And if we start out with a more focused one, we'll wind up with an even more focused mind at the end.

There are studies doing this. One's called the Mindful Awareness Practices for ADHD, or MAP, and that's Lidia Zylowska and Susan Smalley at UCLA. And they're doing this with children and adolescents and gathering data indicating that this can be quite helpful.

And I mentioned earlier when we talked about self-compassion that there's a mindful self-compassion program that's been evolved by Kristen Neff and Chris Germer. And what they've done is evolved an eight-week program which teaches mindfulness, but the main focus is on loving-kindness practices, on *tonglen* practices, on all of these practices designed to help people to be able to accept and be loving toward oneself when we ourselves are going through some sort of pain.

So in our next lecture, we're going to return to exploring the neurobiological effects of mindfulness meditation, including what we're learning about what happens in the brain when we experience our sense of self, and how mindfulness practices can affect that process. Thanks.

The Neurobiology of Self-Preoccupation
Lecture 19

In this lecture, you will explore the neurobiological effects of mindfulness meditation, including what happens in the brain when we experience our sense of self and how mindfulness practices can affect that process. Neurobiologists are discovering that mindfulness meditation practices seem to train the brain in the direction encouraged by the world's great wisdom traditions. The practices help us shift from focusing on thoughts of improving things for "me" and instead open to the present moment with acceptance. And mindfulness practice makes us happier and better able to deal with pain in the process.

The Default Mode Network

- Researchers have found that the default mode of our brains appears to be that of mind wandering. This correlates with unhappiness and with activation in a network of brain areas associated with self-referential processing—with thinking about "me."

- While our brains evolved primarily to seek opportunities and avoid threats, or to sleep, it turns out that when we're not doing either, our brains are still quite active. That's when areas of the brain that have been called the default mode network come online.

- The circuits of the default mode network include the medial prefrontal cortex and the posterior cingulate cortex. It turns out that mindfulness practice can dramatically affect the activity of these areas.

- Dr. Judson Brewer and his colleagues investigated brain activity in experienced meditators and matched meditation-naive controls as they performed meditations focused on three skills: concentration (refocused attention), open monitoring (choiceless awareness), and loving-kindness practice (which cultivates acceptance).

- They found that the main nodes of the default mode network were relatively deactivated in experienced meditators across all three meditation types. They believe that the reason for this is that the "task" common to all three meditation techniques is the training of attention away from self-reference and mind wandering and toward one's immediate, moment-to moment sensory experience. It would appear that, in this way, mindfulness meditation interrupts selfing.

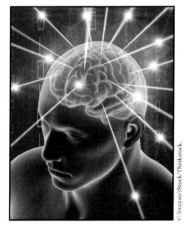

Studies of experienced meditators and non-meditators show significant differences in brain activity.

- They also observed meditation-specific regional differences in activation patterns. For example, during loving-kindness practice, there was deactivation in the amygdala, which is the brain structure that's activated when we experience ourselves as being in danger.

- This makes sense, because loving-kindness meditation is designed to soothe and comfort. We might expect that this would help us respond neurobiologically as though we're not under threat.

- Inspired by these findings, Dr. Brewer and colleagues programmed a computer to analyze in real time brain activation recorded by an fMRI machine. They had the computer focus on a particular area of the default mode network called the posterior cingulate cortex (PCC), which appears to be most activated by self-referential thinking. The PCC has been shown generally to be deactivated during meditation. It's a central hub of the default mode network.

- Dr. Brewer and his colleagues programmed the computer to draw red upward spikes on a moving graph whenever the PCC was active and blue downward spikes whenever it was quiet. He then put experienced and novice meditators in an fMRI machine so that the researchers could see this real-time feedback on a video screen.

- Remarkably, subjects were able to see a close correlation between what they were experiencing in consciousness and what the moving graph was showing. Experienced meditators could very quickly quiet the PCC, while novice meditators had to struggle more to learn how to do it.

- Subjects were amazed at just how closely the graph tracked whether or not they were involved in self-referential, judging thinking. Every time the subject got excited—and thought, in some way, that the computer was really tracking his or her mind—a red spike, indicating activation of the PCC, appeared.

- For a novice meditator, as opposed to an experienced one, the graph of the first trial contains almost all red upward spikes. The second trial has a little blue surrounded by red. In the third trial, the subject started to get the hang of mindfulness practice, and the graph shows mostly red upward spikes but with several blue downward spikes interspersed. By the fourth trial, there were all blue downward lines.

- For an experienced meditator, the first trial is almost all long blue downward lines, with just one tiny red vertical line. The second run is still mostly blue lines, but not as long, with a few more red ones. Then, in the third run, we see an occasional red line. There were many instances in the study where we can see subjects learning how to step out of self-referential thinking.

- Initially, beginning meditators approach the practice as *thinking about* the breath, because they're so accustomed to being in the thought stream. Later, they realize that it's about simply *feeling* the breath moment by moment.

- In normal, non-meditating life, the default mode network is particularly active during times of rest. Its self-referential processing plays a central role in creating our sense of self and identity. Studies have demonstrated that long-term meditators have increased connectivity between regions of the default mode network.

- Several of the studies with experienced meditators have also demonstrated that activity within the default mode network is more tightly coupled to other networks during rest, in particular to networks associated with attention and executive control. Researchers believe that this reflects experienced meditators' enhanced ability to maintain attention, disengage from distraction, and spend less time mind wandering—even when not meditating.

- These findings are the opposite of what is seen in Alzheimer's disease or autism, in which decreased connectivity within the default mode network has been reported. In these illnesses, the differences in connectivity are related to clinical symptoms that include great difficulty focusing.

- The fact that meditation experience is associated with changes of similar magnitude but of opposite direction to Alzheimer's or autism has implications for the profound nature of changes that may be occurring with meditation practice.

Research on Meditation
- These neurobiological findings point in the same direction as ancient Buddhist philosophy. The neurobiology of selfing, or creating a sense of separate self, is seen as central to our suffering. Cognitive researchers identify two different modes of self-reference—two ways of experiencing the self.

- The first is narrative focus, which is what we're engaged in most of the time, particularly if we're not trained in meditation practice. Narrative focus is talking to ourselves about ourselves. Experiential focus, on the other hand, is about momentary experience—simply experiencing the mind-body in action.

- The experiential sense of self appears to be neurally distinct from narrative self-reference and is derived from neural markers of transient body states. In particular, this happens with activation of parts of the insula.

- Experiential self-reference, the nonnarrative self-reference, relies on moment-to-moment proprioception—on feeling what's happening, inside, in each minute.

- The medial prefrontal cortex (MPFC) is part of the default mode network, and it functions by linking subjective experiences over time. It holds memory of self-traits, traits of similar others, reflected self-knowledge, and future aspirations.

- Researchers at the University of Toronto found that in novices, or non-meditators, experiential focus reduced self-referential activity in the MPFC. In MBSR graduates, or people who had learned meditation practice, the experiential focus resulted in a more marked and pervasive reduction of activity in the MPFC.

- The interpretation is that mindfulness practice teaches us how to decouple from the thought stream and how to be able to shift between narrative mode and experiential mode voluntarily.

- They also found that trait mindfulness is measured by self-report. Together they suggest that mindfulness yields improved regulation of our emotional responses and helps meditators to have more equanimity.

- There are obvious implications for therapy. Not believing in self-narrative is perhaps the most important arena in which not believing in our thoughts can lead to psychological freedom.

- There is a fundamental neural dissociation between two forms of self-awareness: the self across time, accompanied by narratives about "me"; and the unfolding of moment-to-moment experience of the mind/body. Mindfulness practice enables us to see these as separate—to see how the self is created out of a narrative.

- With mindfulness practice, we learn to differentiate previously inseparable streams in the flow of information in the mind. This ability may help in "objectifying" the mind, a process in which we are able to disidentify from mental activities as being the totality of who we are.

- Abnormal amygdala function has been consistently demonstrated across several stress-related psychopathologies. Exciting studies of short-term (one to eight weeks) meditation training found decreases in amygdala activity in response to a variety of affective stimuli.

- Another exciting area of neurobiological research involves the effect of mindfulness meditation on the experience of pain. Several of the findings that have come out of this research have practical implications for how mindfulness meditation can help us deal with all sorts of pain.

- First, experienced meditators report that they perceive painful stimuli as less unpleasant than inexperienced controls, with the extent of meditation experience being inversely correlated to subjects' unpleasantness ratings. So, subjectively, the same heat or shock feels less unpleasant to the meditators than the non-meditators.

- Second, experienced meditators report higher tendencies to observe and be nonreactive to pain sensations than inexperienced controls. This means that the experienced meditators could simply feel the pain sensations as moment-to-moment sensations, without getting particularly upset about them.

- Third, open-monitoring practice results in a significant reduction of pain unpleasantness among experienced meditators, but not novices. This implies that it takes some practice with mindfulness meditation for it to have the benefit of reducing the subjective discomfort of pain.

- Fourth, research shows that experienced meditators, but not inexperienced controls, have significant decreases in anticipatory pain anxiety when in a mindful state, meaning that the experienced people don't tense up in anticipation of future pain. This is important because a lot of research shows that this tensing up plays a huge role in what makes pain difficult to bear.

- One of the ways that mindfulness meditation seems to help with pain is by reducing this anticipatory pain anxiety. There's also a lot of research showing that in the short run, distraction reduces the experience of pain. In general, the more extensive a subject's meditation experience, the greatest benefit in dealing with pain.

- By accepting pain sensations—rather than resisting, fearing, or trying to avoid them—we are able to tolerate greater pain stimulation with less distress, whether the pain is caused by a medical condition or induced in the laboratory.

- Mindfulness practice decreases suffering and pain-related anxiety through increased processing of the pain sensations themselves. This is coupled with cognitive disengagement that involves letting go of attempts to control the sensations.

- We're seeing on a neurobiological level how experienced meditators open to pain sensations and apparently feel the pain more vividly, while letting go of attempts to control them, and consequently experience less distress or suffering. On the other hand, when novices tried to practice mindfulness meditation in the presence of a painful stimulus, they had increased activity in the lateral prefrontal cortex, suggesting that they were struggling to control the pain.

Suggested Reading

Brewer, et al, "Meditation Experience Is Associated with Differences in Default Mode Network Activity and Connectivity."

Brown and Jones, "Meditation Experience Predicts Less Negative Appraisal of Pain."

Gard, et al, "Pain Attenuation through Mindfulness Is Associated with Decreased Cognitive Control and Increased Sensory Processing in the Brain."

Garrison, et al, "Real-Time fMRI Links Subjective Experience with Brain Activity during Focused Attention."

Questions to Consider

1. What is the default network, and what are its implications for understanding how we construct our sense of self?

2. What have neurobiologists learned about how experienced meditators experience and react to pain when compared to inexperienced meditators?

The Neurobiology of Self-Preoccupation
Lecture 19—Transcript

I'd like to share with you a story I heard from my friend and colleague, Dr. Judson Brewer, the research director at the Center for Mindfulness at the University of Massachusetts Medical School. It's about the American hurdler Lolo Jones. She was favored to win the gold at the 2008 Beijing Olympics. She was in the lead at the ninth of 10 hurdles. And suddenly she got in her own way. She became caught up in her own thinking and the result wasn't pretty. Here's what she said afterwards. She said,

> I was just in an amazing rhythm … and then I knew at one point I was winning the race. It wasn't like, Oh, I'm winning the Olympic gold medal. It just seemed like another race. And then there was a point after that where … I was telling myself to make sure my legs were snapping out. So I overtried. That's when I hit the hurdle.

Instead of letting her body do what it had trained to do for years, to be perfect for this shining moment in history, she tripped herself up, literally. She tripped on the ninth of 10 hurdles and finished seventh.

Mindfulness meditation can help us to get out of our own way. Dr. Brewer and his colleagues have done a number of fascinating studies about changes in self-focus during mindfulness meditation. To understand them, we'll need a little bit of background.

Many different researchers have found that the default mode of our brain appears to be a certain kind of mind wandering. And this mind wandering correlates with unhappiness and with activation of a network in the brain that's associated with self-referential processing—with thinking about me.

While our brains evolved primarily to seek opportunity and avoid threats, or to rejuvenate themselves with sleep, it turns out that when we're not doing any of these things our brains are still quite active. That's when the areas of the brain that have been called the *default mode network* come online. The circuits of the default mode network include the medial prefrontal cortex and the posterior cingulate cortex, or the PCC. And it turns out that mindfulness practice can dramatically affect the activity of both of these areas.

Let me share with you a pioneering study that reveals a bit about how this works. Dr. Brewer and his colleagues investigated brain activity in experienced meditators and matched meditation naive controls (newcomers) as they perform meditations focused on the three skills we've been discussing throughout the course—concentration, refocused attention, open monitoring or choice-less awareness, and loving-kindness practice, which as you know, helps to cultivate acceptance. And they found that the main nodes of the default mode network were relatively deactivated in experienced meditators across all three meditation types.

They believe that the reason for this is that the task common to all three meditation techniques is the training of attention away from self-reference—thinking about oneself, and wandering into all sorts of thoughts about my to-do list and what's going to happen next and what's going to make me happy or not—and instead toward one's immediate moment-to-moment sensory experience, to what's happening in the here and now. It would appear that in this way, mindfulness meditation neurobiologically interrupts the process of selfing.

They also observed meditation-specific regional differences in activation patterns. For example, during loving-kindness practice, there was deactivation in the amygdala—you'll recall that that's the almond-shaped structure in the brain that's activated when we experience ourselves as being in danger, as [when] trying to figure out, is it a lion or a beige rock. This actually makes perfect sense. Loving-kindness meditation is designed to soothe and comfort us, so we might expect that this would help us to respond neurobiologically as though we're not under stress or under threat.

So, inspired by these findings, Dr. Brewer and his colleagues came up with a very clever idea. They programmed a computer to analyze in real time the activation recorded in a functional MRI machine. And what they had the computer focus on was a particular area of the default mode network that I mentioned before called the *posterior cingulate cortex*, or the PCC. And the PCC seems to be most activated by self-referential thinking—by thinking about me, worrying about me, and being concerned for what's going to happen to me. The posterior cingulate cortex, or the PCC, has been shown generally to be deactivated during meditation. And it's an important structure because it's the central hub of the default mode network.

Now Dr. Brewer and his colleagues programmed the computer to draw red upward spikes on a moving graph whenever the PCC was active, and blue downward spikes whenever it was quiet. He then put both experienced and novice meditators in a functional MRI machine where they could see, in real time, feedback on a video screen about what their brains were doing.

What he observed was remarkable. The subjects were able to see a really close correlation between what they were experiencing in their own consciousness and what the moving graph was showing. And experienced meditators could very quickly quiet the PCC, while novice meditators had to struggle quite a bit to learn how to do it. Let me share a few examples from the study because, at least when I saw them, I found them very striking.

First off, subjects were just amazed at how closely the graph seemed to track whether or not they were involved in self-referential, judging, me-oriented thinking. Here's what one subject reported. First, if you're looking at the graph of the subject, a big red spike appears, and the subject explains this.

So at the beginning, I caught myself. I was sort of trying to guess when the words [the instructions] were going to end and when the meditation was going to begin. So I was kind of trying to be like, "OK ready, set, go!" and then there was an additional word that popped up and I was like, "oh shoot!"

And that was when the red spike you see there appeared. So what we see was that when the person started feeling like they had blown it, they had missed it, that's when the red spike appeared. Then a series of blue spikes appeared, and the subject reported,

And then I sort of immediately settled in and I was really getting into it … and then I thought, "oh my gosh this is amazing it's describing exactly what I am saying! And then you see the red spike. ... and [then] I was like, "OK, wait don't get distracted" and then I got back into it and then it got blue again ... and [then] I was like, "oh my gosh this is unbelievable, it's doing exactly what my mind is doing." And so then [the subject laughed] it got red again. So I just find it really funny because it's a perfect map of what my mind was going through.

And this is the first finding. That the scanner combined with the computer analysis seemed to really closely track people's subjective experience, or whether or not they're involved in self-evaluative mental activity. Every time a subject got excited and thought in some way, "Oh goody, it's working, it's really tracking my mind," a red spike indicating activation of the PCC appeared.

Now let's look at what happened for novice as opposed to experienced meditators. First, we have a graph of several trials for a novice meditator— somebody who's first meditation experience was right here in the lab. Not surprisingly, the first trial contains almost all red upward spikes—almost all default mode network, PCC activation, thinking about how I'm doing, self-evaluation. The second trial had a little bit of blue mixed in, but still surrounded largely by the red. By the third trial, the subject was actually able to use the feedback to start getting the hang of mindfulness practice. To start shifting a little bit from self-referential processing and thought into being with what was going on moment to moment.

Here we still see mostly red upward spikes but with several blue downward ones starting to appear. And this subject too, said at this point, "It just looks like it tracks [what's happening] exactly." By the fourth trial there were mostly blue downward lines. And the person felt, hey, "[This] looks like exactly what I was experiencing."

The investigator then asked the subject, "So what was the difference between this fourth run that was mostly blue and the previous third run that had a lot of red in it?" And the person said, "I felt a lot more relaxed this time." "Anything else?" "I felt like it was less of a struggle to keep my mind from wandering." So we see that this feedback process actually was able to teach the person fundamental principles of mindfulness practice.

Now let's look at the graphs of three trials of an experienced meditator. The first trial is almost all long blue downward lines with just one tiny little red vertical line, suggesting that the experienced meditator, right off the bat, was able to de-connect from the default mode network and get into an experiencing of moment-to-moment experience.

Here's what the subject said about the first trial. "My focus was on the breath and in particular the feeling of interest, wonder, and joy that arises in conjunction with subtle, mindful breathing ... being curious about the draft on my hands and feet. Feeling interest and joy."

The second run of the experienced meditator was still mostly blue lines, but not quite as long with a few red ones mixed in. And here's what the subject reported. "It was smooth sailing. Having most of my awareness occupied by sensations of the breath, feeling joy and bliss, just recognizing when they were there, just working on allowing them to expand."

Then in the third run of the experienced meditator, we see an occasional red line. And the subject reports, "Definitely at the end [when there was less blue], I became less focused."

Now there are many instances in the study where we can see subjects learning how to step out of self-referential thinking. One novice meditator had very mixed red and blue for the first two trials. Then on the third, the subject had a big burst of red lines. And he reported this: "I felt like I was really concentrating on my breathing, but it looks like on the graph I had a lot of wandering thoughts." But then on the fourth trial, he had almost all blue lines. And he said, "I was able to focus on my breathing, the physical sensation, and not thinking of breathing."

The investigator caught that, and he said, "I'm sorry, did you say that you weren't thinking of breathing on the fourth trial as opposed to the third?" He said, "Yeah, I was focused more on the physical sensations instead of thinking 'in' and 'out.'"

Now we see this all the time in beginning meditators. Initially, most folks approach the practice as though they're thinking about the breath. And people use that phrase, "I was thinking about my breath." Because we're so accustomed to being in the thought stream, to being in our narration about life, that it takes a while before we realize that it's actually possible to simply feel the breath, moment to moment, and step out of the thought stream.

Finally, I'd like to share with you the report of one experienced meditator, who tried a little experiment. This person's graph looks largely blue until a big series of red lines appeared near the end of the session. And here's what they reported.

> After several minutes of blue, I wondered if this paradigm actually did measure self-referential processing so I effortfully broke the period of resting in awareness [doing mindfulness practice] and generated a sense of self by saying "X, XX, X" while trying to visualize my face and sense of myself as a subject in the scanner "doing something." This produced a large red spike at the very end of the run. And I thought, "OK, this works. Pretty interesting."

Now we have other sets of research that showed generally that reduced self-referential thinking occurs not just as a state phenomena, during the actual moments of meditation, but it actually carries over into when we're not meditating.

In normal non-meditating life, the default mode network is pretty active, and particularly active during times of rest. Its self-referential processing plays a central role in creating our sense of self and our sense of identity. In fact, studies have demonstrated that long-term meditators have increased connectivity between regions of the default mode network. And this increased connectivity seems to involve some degree of flexibility as to whether the default mode network is activated or not.

Several of the studies with experienced meditators have demonstrated that activity within the default mode network is more tightly coupled to other networks during the rest, and in particular, networks associated with attention and executive control. In other words, our capacity to direct attention seems to be stronger in meditators, and this affects the activation of the default mode network.

And researchers believe that this reflects the experienced meditators enhanced ability to maintain attention, to disengage from distraction, and spend less time mind-wandering, even when they're not meditating.

It's striking that these findings are the opposite of what's seen in Alzheimer's disease, or autism, because in those disorders, decreased connectivity within the default mode network has been reported. And in these illnesses, the differences in connectivity in the default mode network are related to clinical symptoms that we know involve a great deal of difficulty focusing. So the fact that meditation experience is associated with changes of similar magnitude but in the opposite direction of Alzheimer's or autism has pretty profound implications for the nature of the changes that are happening in meditation practice, and for their value.

Now it's striking to me that these neurobiological findings are pointing in the same direction as ancient Buddhist philosophy. Let's look more deeply into the neurobiology of selfing. As we've discussed before, in Buddhist psychology, selfing—creating a sense of separate self—is seen as central to our suffering. Now cognitive researchers identify two different modes of self-reference—two different ways in which we can experience a sense of me.

The first of these is called *narrative focus*, and that's what we're engaged in most of the time, particularly if we're not trained in meditation practice. And narrative focus is concerned about me having enduring traits. It's talking to ourselves about ourselves, which we spend an inordinate amount of time doing. Experiential focus, on the other hand, is about momentary experience—simply experiencing the mind body in action—basically, being mindful.

The experiential sense of self appears to be neurally distinct from this narrative self-referencing, and it's derived from neural markers of transient body states. In particular, we get our sense of experiential me when the insula is active.

You'll remember Sara Lazar's study that I was a participant in, in which she found that in more experienced meditators the insula didn't shrink in the way that it did an age-matched controls. And we've discussed the value of activity in the insula for developing a sense of empathy—for sensing what's going on in others—because it enhances, or it's active in proprioceptive awareness. So this experiential self-reference, the non-narrative self-reference, relies on moment-to-moment proprioception. On feeling what's happening, inside, in each minute.

Now there's a structure called the *medial prefrontal cortex*, that's the MPFC. It's part of the prefrontal cortex, and it's actually part of the default mode network. And it functions by linking subjective experiences over time. It holds our memories of self-traits—the idea that I'm smart, or I'm strong, or I'm creative, or I'm dumb, or I'm weak, or kind of a dullard. And it also holds images of other people and what their traits are. It even is involved when we have future aspirations—when we think, someday I'm going to be successful, or, someday I'm going to have love in my life.

Now researchers at the University of Toronto hypothesized that by studying activity in the medial prefrontal cortex of people trained in mindfulness meditation versus beginners, the mindfulness meditation group would show an increased capacity to disengage from narrative generation. In other words, from practicing experiential level of awareness, we'd be able to step out of the thought stream.

And the thought was that the experienced meditators should be able to activate the neural networks that support a kind of present-centered, experiential self-awareness. They really were saying that the meditators should be able to do what in Buddhist psychology we call "experiencing no self"—which isn't that there's no self, but it's that the self doesn't exist separate from its interconnectedness with all things—or the experience of interbeing, or oneness.

The idea is that absent the active and constant patter about me, we're no longer going to experience ourselves as something separate from the rest. We'll lose what Einstein called, our "optical delusion of separateness."

So here was the study. Half of the subjects were put in an eight week MBSR course and half were on a wait list. Everybody was trained in narrative focus and experiential focus modes of responding to adjectives. That meant in response to hearing about adjectives, adjectives that described the person, participants were asked to do one of two things.

In the narrative focus mode, the subjects were supposed to reflect on what the adjective meant about them as a person—thinking about themselves in relationship to it. So if the adjective was, let's say, kind, I'd be thinking, how kind am I? In what ways am I kind? In what ways am I not kind?

In the experiential focus mode, they were supposed to simply monitor their moment-to-moment experience in response to the adjective. So I might hear the word "kind" and perhaps feel a little rush of kindness or warmth arise in my heart.

The narrative focus involved all sorts of thoughts like, I'm a nice person, I'm a mean person, I'm a selfish person. And these are actually the building blocks of identity because it's stories about our traits, and what we like and don't like, that form our sense of who we are. You may recall the story of going college shopping with my twin daughters and my daughter who didn't want to go to a certain college because she didn't think of herself as emo. That's how we put together identity out of our traits.

And subjects were asked to do each approach to relate to adjectives with a narrative or experiential focus while in an fMRI machine. And here's what they found. In the novices, the non-meditators, the experiential focus reduced self-referential activity in the medial prefrontal cortex, in the MPFC. In the MBSR graduates, the people who had learned meditation practice, the experiential focus resulted in a more marked and pervasive reduction in activity in the MPFC.

So moving to experiential focus reduced activation in the medial prefrontal cortex for everybody, but it did much more so for the people who had been trained in mindfulness practice. The interpretation is that mindfulness practice teaches us how to decouple from the thought stream and how to be able to shift between narrative mode and experiential mode voluntarily.

They also found that trait mindfulness is measured by self-report—in other words, over time, how mindful people experience themselves as being correlated to decreases in activity in the amygdala during an emotion-labeling task. And we'll talk more about the amygdala shortly. Together this suggests that mindfulness yields improved regulation of our emotional responses and helps meditators to have more equanimity.

Now there are obvious implications for therapy. We're into CBT, cognitive behavior therapy, on steroids again if we don't believe our self-narrative anymore, because so many times when we're miserable, we're miserable because we're stuck in some narrative about ourselves that doesn't look so good. And if we can start to see the whole construct of self as coming and going, and fairly arbitrary, we're much less likely to suffer.

So mindfulness practice can enable us to see these different things as separate, to see how the self is created out of a narrative. And with mindfulness practice, we can learn to differentiate what were previously, without practice, inseparable streams of information. People who haven't done the practice simply don't notice thoughts about oneself as being different from the moment-to-moment experience. It also helps us to objectify the mind—to see that mental activities and objects really aren't who we are. It helps us to see the mind, as I mentioned before (or the brain, also), as an orchestra without a conductor—simply these events unfolding.

Now Buddhist monks have actually recognized this for centuries. Here's how Dogen, the 13th-century Zen master, put it:

> To study Buddhism is to study the self. To study the self is to forget the self. To forget the self is to be enlightened by all things. To be enlightened by all things is to be free from attachment to the body and mind of one's self and of others.

Let's return to talking about the troublesome amygdala. You know, it's that little area of the brain that helps us differentiate whether it's a tiger or the beige rock, and it triggers a fight-or-flight reaction. Now, abnormal amygdala function has been consistently demonstrated across all sorts of stress-related psychopathologies. It occurs in anxiety, in post-traumatic stress disorder, social phobia, depression, impulsive aggression. Two thirds of the cells of the amygdala are designed to track unpleasant experiences. We could think of it as one of the places where the negativity bias lives. It's alive and well there.

There have been exciting studies of short-term meditation training, just between one and eight weeks, finding decreases in amygdala activity in response to a variety of different kinds of challenges. And this is fascinating because we know from animal studies that the amygdala tends to grow when we're under stress. They've put rats through difficult circumstances, and if they stress the rat for 10 days, they find that they amygdala grows denser—and it doesn't recover even when the environment improves.

The human study involved 28 stressed out individuals who were put through an eight-week MBSR course. And they filled out a perceived stress scale to report on how stressful their life was. And reductions in perceived stress correlated with decreases in amygdala gray matter density. The greater reported stress reduction, the greater the decrease in the size of the amygdala. So rat amygdalae grew in response to a stressful environment, but humans have a shrinkage of their amygdalae without any change in the environment, just with a changed response to the environment—and that changed response is brought on by mindfulness practice.

Another exciting area of neurobiological research involves the effect of mindfulness meditation on the experience of pain. There have been a number of studies with experimentally induced pain with mindfulness meditators and with novices. And these studies involved putting both sorts of people into functional MRI machines and applying a painful stimulus, like a hot but harmless laser, or an electric shock to the subject's feet that are sticking out of the machine. And researchers then measured which parts of the brain are activated by the painful stimulus, and they also asked the subjects to report on their subjective experience of discomfort.

Now several of the findings that have come out of this research have practical implications for how we can use mindfulness practice to work with pain. They support the kinds of things we were talking about in an earlier lecture about using mindfulness with chronic pain disorders.

First of all, experienced meditators report that they perceive painful stimuli as less unpleasant than inexperienced controls, with the extent of meditation practice being inversely correlated to subject's unpleasantness ratings. So subjectively, the same heat or shock, as they are applying the same stimulus, feels more unpleasant to the non-meditators than to the meditators. And the people who've meditated a lot find it to be even less unpleasant than the people who have just meditated somewhat.

A second finding is that experienced meditators report higher tendencies to be able to observe and be non-reactive to pain sensations than the inexperienced controls. So this means that the experienced folks could simply feel pain sensations as moment-to-moment sensations without getting particularly upset about them.

Third, it turns out that open-monitoring practice results in a significant reduction of pain unpleasantness among experienced meditators, but not novices. So they taught novices how to do open-monitoring practice but it didn't actually reduce their ratings of pain unpleasantness. So this implies that it takes some practice with mindfulness meditation to have it give the benefit of reducing the subjective discomfort of pain.

And then fourth, research shows that experienced meditators, but not the inexperienced folks, have significant decreases in anticipatory anxiety when in a mindful state. Now you'll recall when we discussed chronic back pain that it's anticipatory anxiety, the thought that, "Uh-oh, this is going to be a crippling disorder," that feeds into the disorder and makes it worse.

So the fact that the experienced folks don't tense up in anticipation of future pain means they're much less likely to get caught in chronic back pain cycles, or other fear, pain, fear cycles. And this is particularly important because there's a lot of research showing that these fear, pain, fear, pain cycles play a huge role in what makes pain difficult and what gets people stuck in chronic pain. So one of the ways that mindfulness practices seems to help with pain is by reducing this anticipatory anxiety.

There's also a lot of research showing that in the short run, distraction reduces the experience of pain. In fact, there are a lot of pain treatments that are based on this observation. You may have heard of TENS units that people will wear that create a vibration to distract you. Or people are taught, when you're hurting, bring your attention out to something else.

So it's interesting that one study found that while concentration practice increased pain intensity for inexperienced meditators—which we'd expect, it's the opposite of distraction; we're going to focus on the pain, make it feel worse—it didn't do that for the experienced meditators. The experienced meditators were able to be with the painful stimuli without having a strong aversive reaction to it, while the novice's couldn't.

So in general, the more extensive experience a person has with meditation, the better they're skilled in dealing with pain. But you don't have to be a Tibetan monk to have a benefit. In one study, as little as three days of 20-minutes-a-day training significantly reduced the reported pain intensity and pain-related anxiety in response to experimentally induced pain. And in another, only six mindfulness training sessions were enough to increase pain tolerance to a statistically significant degree.

So what we're seeing is that the idea of the two arrows—that there's the pain itself, and then there's our resistance, fearing, and protesting against the pain—that this idea is what actually is operating and allows mindfulness practitioners, by reducing the second arrow, by not protesting and resisting the pain, to experience much higher levels of it.

Now what's going on here neurobiologically? Well, meditators practicing open monitoring while they're exposed to pain had decreased activity in another area called the *lateral prefrontal cortex*—another part of the prefrontal cortex that's associated with executive control. And they had increased activity in the posterior insula—which is involved in interoceptive and sensory processing with proprioception.

So the researchers concluded that open monitoring is a form of cognitive disengagement. It helps people to let go of trying to control. Mindfulness practices decrease suffering and pain-related anxiety by increasing our experience of the pain sensations themselves (the first arrow in the Buddhist story); we see the insula lighting up. But it's coupled with cognitive disengagement that involves letting go of attempts to control the sensations, and we see this in the decreased activity of the lateral prefrontal cortex.

So we're seeing on a neurobiological level how experienced meditators open to pain sensations can feel the pain more vividly, but they let go of their attempts to control it and consequently, they experience less distress and less suffering while the novices get themselves into trouble. When the novices tried to practice mindfulness meditation and open monitoring in the presence of a painful stimulus, they had increased activity in the prefrontal cortex, suggesting that they were struggling to control the pain. The strategy didn't work. They didn't experience less pain, in fact, they had more difficulty.

So we're finding that neurobiologists are discovering that mindfulness meditation practices seem to train the brain in the direction encouraged by the world's great wisdom traditions. The practices help us to shift from focusing on thoughts of improving things for me, and instead open to the present moment with acceptance.

And mindfulness practices make us happier and better able to deal with pain in the process. But of course, mindfulness practices only work if we take the time to do them. So let me encourage you once again to engage as regularly as you can in both formal meditation and informal mindfulness practices between our lectures. Enjoy.

Growing Up Isn't Easy—Facing Impermanence
Lecture 20

In this lecture, you will learn about how to use mindfulness practices to become more aware of impermanence and how greater well-being can result. Because most people don't like to focus on aging and death, these can be difficult topics, but facing them can also be tremendously liberating. Mindfulness practice can help us see things as they actually are, loosen our preoccupation with a separate self, and experience the richness of the moments we have while we still can.

The Challenges of Aging

- A remarkable amount of time is spent thinking about the future, imagining that the future is going to bring us some form of happiness. We think about the long-term future, including losing weight or finding our true love, and the short-term future, including looking forward to the weekend or the next week. These fantasies about what will make us happy someday become increasingly dubious as the number of possible days diminishes as we get older.

- The central legend of the Buddhist tradition speaks to this. By practicing mindfulness, the Buddha discovered that everything changes, that all things are interdependent, that our trying to hold onto changing phenomena causes endless suffering, that all we actually experience is the present moment, and that our thoughts—no matter how often they occupy our attention—are not actually reality.

- It's precisely these insights that are essential in dealing skillfully with illness and aging, because we see that it's thoughts about illness and aging more than the moment-to-moment experience of these events that distresses us so much.

- It's our thoughts about ourselves and our loved ones as separate selves that make the life cycle feel so difficult. Mindfulness practice

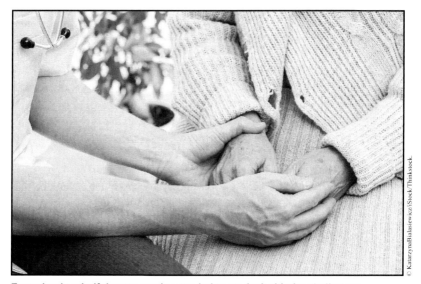

Engaging in mindfulness practice can help you deal with the challenges associated with aging and even death.

can help us loosen our identification with these thoughts. One of the practices we can do is every time a thought comes into our mind, just label it as thinking or planning. We can watch the thoughts come and go like clouds across the sky or ripples in a pond. Then, we can see how they're dependent of our feeling states, even while they help determine our feeling state. Doing this helps us see how unreliable thoughts are and how they cause unnecessary suffering.

- One way to work with illness and aging is to practice stepping out of the thought stream and participating more fully in the current moment, rather than dwelling in our fantasies of what illness and aging will be like. Of course, while stepping out of the thought stream can help us appreciate the moments of our lives, thoughts are not likely to stop entirely.

- This leaves us with two broad options to manage our awareness of impermanence. We can either use denial and distraction, which is probably most people's preferred approach, or we can practice identifying with something larger than "me" and "mine."

- The problem with denial and distraction is that it's a very unreliable solution. Reality keeps threatening to invade our consciousness. We become constantly stressed trying to keep out realization of illness and aging. How many times can we reassure ourselves—thinking, "I won't get cancer; I never smoked"?

- The alternative is to identify with something larger than "me." This is the better option. Mindfulness practices help us notice that all of these thoughts are just thoughts and that there really is only moment-to-moment experience unfolding. In addition, it helps us see the interconnected nature of all phenomena and embrace the reality of impermanence and change.

- The Buddhist tradition emphasizes facing this reality as a path to happiness. One of the exercises that is prescribed is known as five subjects for frequent reflection. Try reflecting on the following statements for a moment. In fact, you can try writing them down and posting them in a prominent place as a reminder.
  o I'm sure to become old. I cannot avoid aging.

  o I'm sure to become sick. I cannot avoid sickness.

  o I'm sure to die. I cannot avoid death.

  o All things dear and beloved to me are subject to change and separation.

  o I'm the owner of my actions. I will become the heir to my actions.

- Of course, this can be a difficult practice. While our resistance— our tendency for distraction and denial—ultimately causes greater suffering, we do it for a purpose. We tend to grasp onto these kinds of defenses because we find it difficult to be "with" these experiences. But with continued mindfulness practice, we notice that our perspective begins to shift.

- Of course, timing matters. Our defenses serve a purpose, even if they keep us unhappy, and prematurely challenging these can be destructive. We need to assess our readiness—our stability in life—prior to engaging in meditations on impermanence.

- If you're already overwhelmed by challenges in your life, it's probably not the best time to go headlong into these impermanence practices. But if you're not in a crisis at the moment, and you're feeling a bit more secure in that sense, you can try meditating on the changes associated with aging.

Facing Death
- For some people, even more difficult than facing aging is facing death. After all, all things change. The house we grew up in doesn't last forever—neither does a mountain, the course of a river, or ultimately the whole planet. But it's amazing that this surprises us.

- It is helpful to step back and get a big-picture perspective on this. The Earth is about 4.5 billion years old. The Sun is just 4.57 billion years old. Humans have only been around between 3.5 and 4.5 million years—a very short time.

- By many estimates, in 200 million years, the Earth will become too hot for humans, and in 500 million years, the oceans will evaporate. In another 5 billion years, the Sun will expand to encompass Mercury, Venus, and maybe what is now the Earth's orbit. The Earth may have moved to a wider orbit by then, in which case everything will freeze. But if not, everything will be vaporized.

- This seems to indicate that not only us, but also our children if we have them—and their children if they have them—and all of history, and all traces of life on Earth will eventually be obliterated. Everyone is going to die, but we live as though we won't. This unspoken fantasy of immortality keeps us from being connected to one another. We imagine that it's going to protect us, but it leaves us more vulnerable.

- We don't notice that we're part of a larger order, or a larger ecosystem. We don't notice that we're subject to the same rhythm of birth and death as all other beings. The alternative—realizing that we're in this together—can really unite us. And mindfulness practice helps with this, in part by simply seeing it all changing before our eyes.

- A lot of meditators do hospice work, and some health-care workers are trained in mindfulness meditation so that they can better be with people who are dying. One way that mindfulness meditation helps us do this is to bring home impermanence. The ability to discover and pay attention to the fact that death is real—that everything is falling apart—makes us not so shocked by it. And it allows us to approach these moments with so much more equanimity.

- The Buddha said that mindfulness of death was the most important meditation practice you could do, because it's what can fully liberate preoccupation with the self. And it brings us back most powerfully to appreciating the present moment.

- There are many such practices in the Buddhist tradition. A very simple contemplation that we can revisit during any day is to simply bring up the following thoughts: Death is inevitable, and we don't know when we'll die. Notice how thinking about this reorients your attention.

- Another very simple and poignant practice is to imagine yourself on your deathbed surrounded by the people you love most. Once you conjure up that image, just imagine saying good-bye. It's intense, but it's very real.

- As we explore these various practices, we realize that we're not actually afraid of dying, because we haven't experienced it and we have no idea what it's going to be like. Instead, we're afraid of the idea of dying—of all of our thoughts and fantasies about it. Who knows what it will actually be like? So, what can we do? We can certainly take refuge in the present moment. So many things that we fear lose their fearsomeness when we can be with them in the present.

- The other thing that we remember is that we're in this together. This is part of simply being alive as a being. It can be helpful to put energy into whatever helps you identify with something larger than yourself—including nature or animals; friends, family, or community; a spiritual teacher; or a religious figure.

- It's said in the Zen tradition that if we can die the big death, which is letting go of the sense of separate self, then there's no need to fear the literal death, because nothing's being lost. These practices can help us not just with our own death and illness, but they can also help us with the death and illness of others.

Suggested Reading

Halifax, *Being with Dying*.

Kumar, *Grieving Mindfully*.

Rosenberg, *Living in the Light of Death*.

Siegel, *The Mindfulness Solution*, chapter 10.

Questions to Consider

1. In what ways throughout your life, and even today, have you found yourself living for the future?

2. Spend a few moments considering the five subjects for frequent reflection found in Buddhist traditions. How might you live today differently if you were fully aware that change—including illness, death, and loss—were inevitable?

befriending the changes: A brief meditation on the impermanence of the body that is useful when we're finding ourselves struggling with the challenges of aging.

Growing Up Isn't Easy—Facing Impermanence
Lecture 20—Transcript

Some years ago, I had the privilege of visiting Wat Tham Suea, the Tiger Cave Temple, in Krabi, Thailand. And this monastery could best be described as a death theme park. Everywhere in the place, there were real human skeletons, skulls on the table, in the ways in which we used to have ashtrays on the tables and other sorts of places.

And the monks used to perform spiritual autopsies. What would happen is the townsfolk, if they'd lost a loved one, they would bring the body to the monks so that the monks could dissect him or her. And the monks weren't dissecting the bodies to gain medical knowledge, they were doing it to see what the body's made of, to see that it's just flesh and bones, to see that the body is made up of meat, essentially.

Now these monks and nuns were not a gloomy lot. They seemed buoyant, and happy, and very engaged in life. And what they explained was they were focusing on death continuously so that they could remember to appreciate this moment in this day, and that they could remember not to be living in the future, but to be living in the now.

Sometime after visiting the Tiger Cave Temple, I heard Drew Faust, the president of Harvard University, giving a lecture. And before she became an administrator, she was a Civil War historian. And she was describing how in the American Civil War, we had more deaths than in all of our other wars combined.

The really interesting thing, to my mind, was she said that all of that death brought about a shift in the culture, a shift in our attitude toward death, and that people started to adopt an attitude that it was important every day to think about our own death. And the purpose for thinking about our own death was so that we could appreciate today.

So what can we learn from the monks and nuns at the Tiger Cave Temple or from the Americans during the Civil War? We can learn that we would actually be happier if we could embrace the law of impermanence rather than struggling so hard to repeal it. And there's actually laboratory research to support the reports of the monastics and the historians.

Researchers at the University of Kentucky and Florida State University studied 432 undergraduate volunteers. And they randomly assigned half of them to write about their own death and half to write about dental pain, which they thought was an unpleasant but not threatening topic.

They then gave them all sorts of psychological tests to look into their mood. And they used tests to try to gauge what was going on unconsciously. They gave them word stems and asked them to do a kind of sentence-completion or phrase-completion exercise. And what they found was that the death and dying group was actually happier on the unconscious measures than was the group that had written about dental pain.

Now mindfulness practices can also help us to become more aware of impermanence. And in this lecture, we're going to look at how to use them to do this and how we can have greater well-being as a result. But since most of us don't usually like to focus on this, it can be a little bit of a difficult topic. But I invite you to come along, approach it with an open heart and mind, and see what you discover as you look a little bit more carefully perhaps into this idea of impermanence in everyday life.

Let's start with the challenges of aging. Where will you be in 100 years? Think about it for a second. It's likely that we'll all look pretty similar and we'll all be doing pretty much the same thing. And on the way, we're going to face all sorts of changes. Some of these changes are going to be rough. It would nice not to be fighting them all. Indeed, as the Zen master Suzuki Roshi put it, "One purpose of our [mindfulness] practice is to [actually be able to] enjoy our old age."

Remember our earlier discussion about *Necessary Losses*, the book by Judith Viorst about our difficulty facing changes? It starts with giving up the diapers, then the crib, going to school, and like that. The later stages can be harder still—our kids leaving home, our parents dying, retiring—even though many of us might look forward to that, a lot of people have trouble because we lose our identity. We lose our social role. And then the really hard stuff, things like our spouse dying, the body falling apart, entering into assisted living, maybe even finding ourselves in a hospital bed.

Clearly, we need some help. And luckily, mindfulness practice can be a resource. It can help us to see things as they actually are, rather than our fantasies about them, to loosen our preoccupation with a separate self, which has its difficult trajectory, and to experience the richness of the moments, because that's what we actually have despite all of our fantasies to the contrary.

A remarkable amount of the time, we're thinking about the future. And we're imagining that this future is going to bring us some form of happiness. Like to find happiness, I'm going to lose weight. Or I'm going to get rich. Or I'm going to get in shape. Or I'll find my true love. Maybe even I'll meditate more, get enlightened, or find God.

And we have much shorter goals. I'm really looking forward to the weekend when I'll have a day off. I'm really looking forward to next week when I'm going to get to spend time with my kids. Or just, even in the midst of the meal at the restaurant, I'm really looking forward to eating at that new place across town with the great new food.

We have all sorts of fantasies about what will make us happy someday, but of course, these become increasingly dubious as the number of possible somedays diminishes. And as we get older, we do the math. We realize that they're diminishing.

Now, we're not the first to discover that this orientation has limitations. The central legend of the Buddhist tradition speaks to this. The Buddha was born as a prince. So his dad was a king of a small kingdom that was in what was then northern India and is now the south of Nepal. And when the child was born, the custom of the day was to invite the Brahmans, the wise men, to come and evaluate the new infant.

Now, they didn't have Apgar scores back then, but what they did look for were 32 signs of greatness. And, indeed, when the Brahmans came, they found those 32 signs. And they said what it meant was this infant was either going to become a great worldly leader or a great spiritual leader.

The dad, hoping that he would take over the reins of the kingdom, thought, how do I make sure that he becomes a great worldly leader? He thought, I know. I'll make sure he doesn't become a spiritual teacher. What makes people become spiritual teachers? Well, the pain and suffering of the world.

So the dad set out to shield him from that. And he created an environment to shield him. They had a winter palace when it was cool, a summer palace when it was warm. And they pretty much kept the boy from going out on his own. Whenever they'd go into visits into the town, everything was kind of sanitized. It's like nowadays when the Olympics come to a city, and they take the homeless people and they give them somewhere else to stay for the time being. It was like that.

And the boy grew up with all of the luxury that was possible in those days. But as he became older, he became more curious and he kind of wanted to sneak out on his own. And he convinced his chariot driver to take him on an unauthorized trip outside of the palace gates.

On the first of these trips, he spied an old man. And he asked the chariot driver, "Gosh, what's that?" And the chariot driver said, "Well, that's old age." And the prince said, "Well, who does that happen to?" And the chariot driver says, "Well, that happens to, I guess, the lucky ones."

On a second trip, he saw a sick man. And he said, "Oh my, what's that?" "Well, that's illness." "Oh, who does that happen to?" "I'm afraid that happens to most everybody."

On the third trip, he saw a corpse. He said, "What is that?" "Well, that's death." "Who does that happen to?" "Well, that really does happen to everybody."

And then finally on the fourth trip out, he saw a wandering sadhu, one of the ascetic seekers of the time, a spiritual man. And he asked the chariot driver, "What's that?" And the chariot driver said something like, "Well, that somebody trying to figure out how to deal with the things that we've seen on our other trips."

So the prince was quite set back by this. He was no longer content in the palace, no longer content with luxury, because he had a sense that it was all impermanent, that it wasn't going to last. And he told his father, "I have to leave. I have to seek some way to deal with this." And his father said, "No, no, please don't go." And the prince said, "Well, I won't go if you can promise me three things." Father says, "Sure, just ask."

So the prince said, "I won't leave if you can promise me that I won't grow old, I won't get sick, and I won't die." And his dad said, "Gosh, I'm sorry. I can't promise that."

He said, "OK, I'll stay with just two things. Just promise me I won't get sick and I won't die." Dad said, "Sorry, I can't do that either."

"OK, I'll stay if you just promise me one thing, that I won't die." Dad said, "No, sweetheart, I'd love to, but I can't." When the dad couldn't promise, he left the palace and began his spiritual quest.

So what did the prince learn? Well, he went through an ascetic phase. We talked about that before, where he learned these concentration practices and tried to starve his body to get rid of desire, to find peace. But that didn't work. And then eventually he set off, and he started practicing mindfulness.

And what did he discover? He discovered that everything changes, all things are interdependent, our trying to grasp or hold onto changing phenomena causes endless suffering, all we actually experience is the present moment, and our thoughts, however much they occupy our attention, are not actually reality. And it's precisely these insights that are essential in dealing skillfully with illness and aging. Because we see that it's actually thoughts about illness and aging more than the moment-to-moment experience of these events that distresses us so much.

My dog sadly died of cancer last year. And when we received the diagnosis, we were told by the vet that she had somewhere between one and nine months to live. It was an interesting time. She actually lived 13 months, and we were very grateful for that. But the thing that struck me most was that my dog was completely OK having cancer. She got to eat some bread with her medication. And I guess because she wasn't in a great deal of pain, she was fine, because she wasn't thinking about it.

My wife, my kids, and I had a lot more trouble. We kept thinking about her diagnosis, anticipating her deterioration, and thinking, oh gosh, she's not going to be with us very long. So it's actually our thoughts about ourselves and our loved ones as these separate selves that make the life cycle feel so difficult.

Now, mindfulness practice can help us to loosen our identification with these thoughts. And there's some practices we can do to do this. We can be involved in sitting, and every time a thought comes, just label it, thinking, thinking, or planning, anticipating. We can watch the thoughts come and go like clouds across the sky or ripples in a pond. And then we can see how they're dependent on our feeling states, as much as they also help to determine our feeling state. And doing this helps us to see how unreliable they are and how they cause all this unnecessary suffering.

Mark Twain, who's a keen observer of both the mind and human behavior, he reflected near the end of his life on this. This is what he said. "I'm a very old man and have suffered a great many misfortunes, most of which never happened."

So one way to work with illness and aging is to practice stepping out of the thought stream and participating more fully in this moment. Of course, while stepping out of the thought stream can help us to appreciate the moments of our lives, thoughts are not likely to stop entirely. So this leaves us with two broad options to manage these thoughts, to manage our awareness of impermanence. We can either use denial and distraction, which is probably most people's preferred approach, or we can practice identifying with something larger than me and mine.

The problem with denial and distraction is it's a very unreliable solution. Reality keeps threatening to invade our consciousness. We become constantly stressed trying to keep out realization of illness and aging. How many times can we reassure ourselves? Well, I won't get cancer, I didn't smoke. Or, I won't have a car accident, I'm a careful driver.

So the alternative is to identify with something larger than me, and it's really the better option. And mindfulness practices help us to do that. They help us to notice that all of these thoughts are just thoughts. The sense of me is actually constructed by the thought. And we're actually part of this interconnected world in constant change and flux.

The Buddhist tradition emphasizes facing this reality as a path to happiness. And one of the exercises that's prescribed are five subjects for frequent reflection. Now, these are kind of hard because they're things we don't like to think about, but I invite you to join me in reflecting on them for a moment.

This is what we're to remember. I'm sure to become old. I cannot avoid aging. I'm sure to become sick. I cannot avoid sickness. I'm sure to die. I cannot avoid death. All things dear and beloved to me are subject to change and separation. And I'm the owner of my actions. I will become the heir to my actions.

People who are willing to work with these kinds of thoughts will often write them down and post them in prominent places, just to remind us every day. Think about what a day would be like at work, for example, if you had these posted on your desk. Or what a day around the house would be if these were on the fridge every time you went to them. It starts to shift our perspective a bit.

Now, of course, this can be a difficult practice. Our resistance, our tendency for distraction and denial, while it ultimately causes greater suffering, we do it for a purpose. We tend to grasp onto these kinds of defenses because we find it hard to be with these experiences. But as we do continued practice, we start to discover, as one meditation put it, that it's actually wiser to contemplate the law of impermanence rather than trying so hard to repeal it.

Of course, timing matters. If you're in a time in your life where you're already overwhelmed and it's unstable, it's probably not the best time to go headlong into these impermanence practices. But if you're not in a crisis, and you're feeling a little bit more secure in that sense, and you're game to push your meditation practice further, you can join me in a meditation, which can help to really increase our awareness of what it's like to go through the changes.

This is befriending the changes. Try imagining your body, looking at yourself naked in the mirror, as it was 10 years ago. Recall what your hair looked like, what your weight looked like, what the quality of your skin was like. Can you vision it?

And now picture your body, naked in the mirror, as it is today. Again, your hair, your physique, your weight, your skin.

And now see if you can play this forward, and imagine what your body will look like 10 years from now. How will your hair look? How will your face look? What will be the quality of your skin? What do you imagine your physique will be like?

And then, imagine going further. Imagine your body 10 years after that, 20 years from today. Do the math. Figure out about how old you'll be 20 years from today. What would your body look like? How would your hair be? How would your face be? What would the skin be like? And what would your physique be like?

And see if you can hold that image with a kind of loving kindness, as though it were really OK to go through all of these different changes.

I always find this exercise difficult. Even if I can accept my body at the moment, it's really hard to acknowledge its trajectory. But as the old adage goes, "Age isn't a problem. It's a question of mind over matter. If you don't mind, it doesn't matter." So if we can make friends with these changes, we're going to be a lot happier.

Now, for some of us, even harder than facing aging is facing death. After all, all things change. The house we grew up in doesn't last forever. Neither does a mountain, a course of a river, ultimately the whole planet. But it's amazing that this surprises us.

I find it helpful to step back and get a really big-picture perspective on this. I looked it up. The Earth is about four-and-a-half billion years old. The Sun is just 4.57 billion years old, little bit older. Humans have only been around between three-and-a-half and four-and-a-half million years—a very short time.

But here's the ringer. By many estimates, in 200 million years, the Earth will become too hot for humans. And in 500 million years, the oceans will actually evaporate. In another five billion years, the sun will expand so much as to encompass Mercury, Venus, and maybe what's now the Earth's orbit.

Scientists aren't quite sure what is going to happen. The earth may have moved to a wider orbit by then, in which case everything will freeze. But if not, everything will be vaporized.

So what does it all mean? If not only us, but our children if we have them, and their children if they have them, and all of history, and all traces of life on Earth will eventually be obliterated.

Well, a Zen master was once asked, "What's the most amazing thing that you've experienced in all of your life of introspection, of practice, of teaching?" And he said, "The most amazing thing I've seen is that everybody is going to die and yet we live as though we won't." And this unspoken fantasy of immortality actually keeps us from being connected to one another. We imagine it's going to protect us, but it leaves us more vulnerable. We don't notice that we're part of a larger order, a larger ecosystem. We don't notice that we're subject to the same rhythm of birth and death as all other beings. It's really pretty silly. You'd think we'd get it by now. There's a basic principle. If you don't want to die, don't be born.

The alternative, realizing that we're in this together, can really unite us. And mindfulness practice helps with this, in part by simply seeing it all changing before our eyes.

I mentioned before that I was in India not long ago. And I was at the banks of the Ganges watching a cremation. And I've been to a number of funerals in my country, in the United States, and seeing a body cremated with a relative watching the body burn up brings home the reality of this in a way that we don't quite get, or I don't quite get, as vividly in funerals here.

And one day I wandered into a park. And this park had a little science museum in the back, a kind of bizarre place. It had various animals that were in formaldehyde and a few diagrams of how the life cycle works. And then there was a human skeleton. And above the human skeleton, written in English and in Hindi, was this sign. It said, "Please see toward me. I was as you are. You have to be as I am. Hence, love all." And it was very moving. I've remembered it quite vividly.

Now, it's not an accident that a lot of meditators do hospice work. There's a wonderful program run by Roshi Joan Halifax—she's a Zen master in Santa Fe—that trains health-care workers in mindfulness meditation so that they can better be with people who are dying. And one way that mindfulness meditation helps us to do this is to really bring home impermanence.

There's a famous Zen teaching story of a novice monk who has gotten the privilege of being able to clean and sweep in the master's private quarters. And he's doing a careful job, and he's trying to do the best he can. And then he turns and he knocks over this vase, and the vase shatters into a million pieces. And the vase was extremely precious. It had been there for hundreds of years, irreplaceable.

And he's thinking, oh my god, how am I going to tell the master? He squirrels up the courage. He goes to talk to the master. And he says, "I have to tell you, something terrible has happened." He says, "Please, tell me." He says, "You know that precious vase? I knocked it over, and it broke into a million pieces." And the master says, "Oh, that's OK." And the monk says, "Aren't you upset? I thought you'd be so angry." And the master said, "Well, you see, to me, the vase was already broken."

It's this ability to really discover, to pay attention to the fact that death is real, that everything's falling apart, that then makes us not so shocked by it. And it allows us to approach these moments with so much more equanimity.

The Buddha said that mindfulness of death was the most important meditation practice you could do, because it's what can fully liberate preoccupation with the self. And it brings us back most powerfully to appreciating the present moment.

And there are many such practices in the Buddhist tradition. The five subjects for frequent reflection that we talked about a few moments ago, that's one useful daily practice. A very simple contemplation we can revisit during any day is to simply [meditate on] two lines: Death is inevitable, and we don't know when we'll die. [It is] very interesting just to bring that up in the course of the day and notice how it reorients our attention.

Or another very simple and poignant practice: Imagine yourself on your deathbed surrounded by the people you love most coming to your side. Can you conjure up that image? And just imagine saying goodbye. It's intense, but it's very real.

A particularly elaborate practice is found in a central Buddhist text, the Satipaṭṭhāna Sutta. And here's an abridged version just to give you an idea of how one can do this kind of work.

> A monk reflects on this very body, from the soles of the feet on up, from the crown of the head on down, surrounded by skin and full of various kinds of unclean things. In this body, there are head hairs, body hairs, nails, teeth, skin, flesh, tendons, bones, bone marrow, kidneys, heart, liver, spleen, lungs, intestines, feces, bile, phlegm, pus, blood, sweat, fat, tears, urine.

> Or again, as if you were to see a corpse cast away in a charnel ground, picked at by crows, vultures, and hawks, by dogs, hyenas, and various other creatures. A skeleton smeared with flesh and blood, connected with tendons. And then a skeleton without flesh or blood connected with tendons. And then just the bones detached from their tendons, scattered in all directions. Then the bones whitened, then later decomposed into a power.

> And he applies this to his very body, this body, too. Such is its nature. Such is its future. Such is its unavoidable fate.

It's pretty intense, but it's also potentially pretty liberating.

One of my favorite cartoons is from *The New Yorker*. And it's got a guy reading the obituary page. And if you look at the various titles to the obituaries, they say things like, "Two years older than me," "One year younger than me," "Three years older than me," "My age on the dot." I don't know if you've ever read the obituaries, but when I have, the same kinds of thoughts come to my mind.

A friend of mine actually uses this to good advantage. Whenever he's going to give a talk and he's dealing with the usual public speaking anxiety, he just writes in bold letters on the front page of the talk, soon dead. It tends to put these things in a bit of perspective.

As we explore these various practices, we realize that we're not actually afraid of dying, because we haven't experienced it and we actually have no idea what that's going to be like. Instead, we're afraid of the idea of dying, of all of our thoughts and fantasies about it. Who knows what it will actually be like? So what can we do? Well, we can certainly take refuge in the present moment. This is what we have. I often think when I'm having more senior moments, and I start to feel, oh my gosh, I'm losing my memory. I'm losing my cognitive abilities. And I think, well, even if it gets a lot worse, maybe I can practice being in the present more and it won't be so bad. Because so many things that we fear actually lose their fearsomeness when we can be with them in the present.

And the other thing that we remember is that we're so in this together. This is part of simply being alive as a being. So it can be helpful to put energy into whatever helps you to identify with something larger than yourself—nature, animals, friends, family, or community, a spiritual teacher, or a religious figure. It's said in the Zen tradition that if we can die the big death, which is letting go of the sense of separate self, then there's no need to fear the literal death, because nothing's being lost.

Now, these practices can help us not just with our own death and our own illness, but they can help us to work with that of others. A friend of mine came to visit me who lives on the west coast. And she had remarried later in her life and had really a nice second marriage. And they were married for maybe a year-and-a-half when her husband was diagnosed with cancer. And it was one of these fast-moving cancers, and it was only a matter of months before he passed away.

And we had corresponded a little bit, but this was the first time that we were meeting face-to-face. And she's a very psychologically awake person. She's a meditator. She had been crying. She had been feeling all the different feelings, really mourning his loss.

But then we were sitting in a restaurant, and she said,

> You know, I want to tell you some experience I have, which a lot of people won't understand. Sometimes, like right now, when I'm sitting here talking with you, there's simply the sights and sounds of you, of the restaurant, the feelings in my body.

> And I realize the only difference is that if my husband were still around, I would conjure up the thought, "My husband's waiting for me on the west coast." And now I conjure up the thought, "My husband's no longer there on the west coast." It's only the thought that's different. The moment-to-moment experience of life is very much the same. And you know, sometimes I feel it's really OK.

So it seems that facing aging and death, while difficult, can also be tremendously liberating. And one of the ways it frees us is by helping us to develop wisdom, a core purpose of mindfulness practice in its context in Buddhist psychology.

In the next lecture, we'll look at what scientists, psychologists, and philosophers say about what wisdom is, and how mindfulness practice can help us to develop it.

Toward a Science of Wisdom
Lecture 21

W isdom is important for virtually all of life's pursuits. Wisdom is valuable for everyone, but we particularly notice its presence or absence in leaders—including political leaders, spiritual leaders, and leaders within families. In fact, there seems to be an inverse relationship between thinking of oneself as wise and actually being wise. In this lecture, you will learn what scientists, psychologists, and philosophers say about what wisdom is and how mindfulness practice can help us develop it.

What Is Wisdom?
- Scientists are starting to grapple with the ancient question of what wisdom is and how it can be developed. They're even trying to identify which brain structures support it.

- Simply by reflecting about wisdom, you may find yourself becoming a little bit wiser. This is in part because wisdom involves maintaining a certain perspective toward life, and exploring what wisdom is and isn't seems to help us develop that perspective.

- Almost every language has a word for "wisdom." It is the highest human virtue across diverse cultures. Until recently, modern psychologists, and even philosophers, had hardly touched the subject. In fact, they've had a very difficult time even agreeing what it is. It is something that is understood by virtually everyone across cultures but is difficult to define.

- Given the historical paucity of psychological literature on wisdom, scientific psychologists have had to start pretty much from scratch to study it. They began by seeking an operational definition—a way of identifying what wisdom is and isn't.

- They have taken two broad approaches to operationalizing it. One way they have tried to define it is to discover implicit models, which involves asking people to call to mind a wise person and then describe his or her characteristics. They've done this with subjects from many different cultures. The other way psychological scientists have tried to define wisdom is by looking to ancient cultures. We find quite a variety of perspectives there.

- In addition to implicit theory research and searching the world's wisdom traditions, some scientists have attempted to develop laboratory models for studying wisdom. The most developed of these are from Paul Baltes and the Berlin Wisdom Project, which was conducted at the Max Planck Institute for Human Development in Germany. Researchers generated hypothetical vignettes, or thinking-aloud exercises, and asked subjects to reflect on them. Then, they analyzed the kind of considerations subjects used to respond.

- This is quite similar in methodology to a well-known work by Lawrence Kohlberg that was used to study stages of moral development. While Kohlberg's conclusions have been critiqued for their gender bias, his methods were very innovative. Kohlberg would pose an ambiguous moral problem to people, and then he would see how they respond to it. The participant's answer wasn't critical for measuring the subject's stage of moral development; what mattered was what principles the person used to come up with his or her answer.

- Baltes and his colleagues factored and analyzed the results of hundreds and hundreds of these sorts of exercises. They found that wisdom involved five factors.

1. Factual knowledge

2. Procedural knowledge

3. Life-span contextualism

4. Value relativism

5. Awareness and management of uncertainty

- The Berlin Wisdom Project's five factors are very individual oriented—they come from an individual psychology perspective. Other investigators have included more of an emphasis on concern for others or the greater social good, coming to the same conclusion in Buddhist psychology that wisdom and compassion are inseparable.

Developing Wisdom
- The intention to grow wiser seems to help. In addition, involvement in introspective pursuits helps. So, we might assume that mindfulness meditation, psychotherapy, and being involved in the arts should help.

- Mindfulness practice, by increasing awareness of our own reactions to each moment of our lives, would support using all of our activities as paths to greater wisdom. In fact, we have reasons to believe that it works precisely this way.

- Some of the evidence comes from neurobiological studies. Psychiatrists Thomas Meeks and Dilip Jeste factor analyzed the literature on wisdom and found six factors, or components. Note that this list overlaps with, but has more interpersonal elements than, the factors found by the Berlin group.

  1. Prosocial behavior/attitudes

  2. Social decision making/pragmatic life knowledge

  3. Emotional homeostasis

  4. Reflection/Self-understanding

5. Value relativism/tolerance

6. Acknowledgement of/dealing effectively with uncertainty/ ambiguity

- Meeks and Jeste then tried to identify parts of the brain that have been shown to be active when people exercise each of these faculties. Each one has a putative neurological substrate, and they have several regions in common.

- Also, all six components of wisdom are related conceptually to meditative practice, and there is particularly strong overlap with neurological changes we see in meditation and three of the wisdom factors or components: prosocial attitudes, emotional homeostasis, and self-reflection/self-understanding. In other words, parts of the brain that are active when we're demonstrating these three components are parts of the brain that are activated during meditation practice.

- These findings are pretty complicated and, at this point, very tentative. They're complicated in part because neurobiologically, wisdom is perhaps our most top-down process. It integrates, regulates, and draws on so many different inputs and cognitive faculies. But the findings nonetheless suggest that meditation practice may help us become wiser.

- Robert Sternberg is the leading research psychologist currently studying wisdom. He differentiates between general wisdom and personal wisdom. Personal wisdom involves how wisely we conduct our daily affairs and interpersonal interactions, as opposed to the more general wisdom we display in our thoughts and attitudes toward larger problems.

- Sternberg is fond of pointing out that many otherwise wise thinkers and leaders seem to be lacking in personal wisdom. In their personal lives, they often seem to act foolishly. For example, Martin Luther

King, Jr., was notoriously unfaithful to his spouse, and the Buddha left his wife and child to pursue enlightenment.

- Of course, these actions can be interpreted differently—perhaps they did these things in service of a greater good. We don't know the particulars or understand the larger causes. In fact, it would be a sign of wisdom on our part to consider these possibilities. But it would also seem that just because a person is wise in one area, it doesn't guarantee wisdom in all realms.

- Perhaps this is also true of enlightenment, which overlaps extensively with wisdom as a construct. Wisdom in Buddhist psychology is the awareness of three marks of existence: *anicca* (impermanence), *dukkha* (unsatisfactoriness), and *anatta* (no enduring, separate self). In Buddhist psychology, deeply understanding these realities is synonymous with having wisdom.

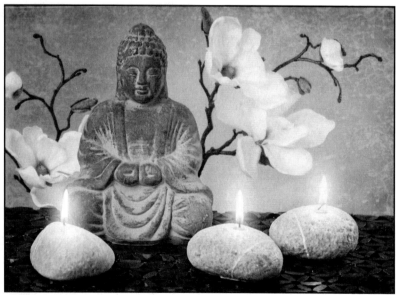

In Buddhist psychology, wisdom and compassion are inseparable.

- Mindfulness practices are designed to bring us insight into these three marks of existence. The following are eight skills that mindfulness practices foster and that can contribute to our developing wisdom. Of course, to develop these, we need to practice doing formal meditation, as well as informal mindfulness practices, regularly.

  ○ Stepping out of the Thought Stream: By returning our attention repeatedly to moment-to-moment sensory experience, we gain perspective on our thought processes. We see how thoughts are conditioned by family and culture and how they change with moods and circumstances. We also see our intellectual defenses at work—the resistance that arises in response to unsettling thoughts and our urges to maintain comforting ideas or interpretations. Stepping out of the thought stream supports the ability to entertain multiple perspectives, by not believing in particular thoughts. We can even gain firsthand insight into how the mind constructs a seemingly stable reality out of the ever-changing flux of experience.

  ○ "Being with" Discomfort: The capacity to step back and resist the urge for immediate personal comfort is necessary if we're going to act in the interest of the greater good. This is only possible if we can get beyond our instinctual habit of seeking pleasure and avoiding pain. In addition, this involves not identifying with our discomfort as being about "me."

  ○ Disengaging from Automatic Responses: Whether our automatic responses are instinctual or conditioned through reward and punishment, modeling, and/or classical or operant conditioning, mindfulness practices help us disengage from our automatic responses. We want to be able to observe stimulus-response processes in microscopic detail so that we can experience the arising of a sensation, thought, or feeling, followed by the urge to act in response to it, finally followed by overt behavior. We want to develop the ability to pause, take a breath, and evaluate whether or not the action would actually lead to desirable results.

o   Transpersonal Insight: This is direct insight into *anatta*. This is closely related to what later Buddhist traditions refer to as *shunyata*, or "emptiness." Mindfulness reveals that all experience is in constant flux. Our minds relentlessly generate words to organize this flux into what we take as conventional reality. This dissolves the barrier between "me" and "mine" and "you" and "yours," leading to compassion, another cornerstone of wisdom.

o   Moment-to-Moment Observation of the Mind's Antics: This illuminates our defenses. We see how we often project onto others, but we have difficulty seeing them clearly. With mindfulness practice, we see all of the stereotyping, judging, jealously competing, idealizing, denigrating, and other not-so-noble things that are part of human interpersonal interactions.

o   Seeing How the Mind Creates Suffering for Itself: The mind is forever making comparisons and judgments, struggling to get things right and then keep them from changing. Attempts to cling to pleasant moments and avoid or push away unpleasant ones inevitably fail, causing endless distress. We see the impossibility of winning consistently.

o   Embracing Opposites: Our dearly held views of reality—"I'm smart," "I'm stupid," "I'm kind," "I'm mean"—are merely mental constructions. Mindfulness practice helps us tolerate the views of others and find cooperative solutions to conflicts. It allows us to embrace different levels of reality simultaneously.

o   Developing Compassion: Several definitions of wisdom include compassion. Mindfulness practices reveal how interconnected we all are. We learn to abide peaceably in the midst of our own suffering, see that everyone else also suffers, and spontaneously feel like helping others.

Suggested Reading

Hall, *Wisdom*.

Siegel and Germer, "Wisdom and Compassion."

Sternberg, *Wisdom*.

Sternberg and Jordan, *A Handbook of Wisdom*.

Questions to Consider

1. What, in your opinion, are the most important qualities of a wise person?

2. What most gets in the way of your acting wisely in your life?

Toward a Science of Wisdom
Lecture 21—Transcript

I hope you've been able to find the time to develop some regularity in your formal and informal meditation practice. And I hope you've been experimenting with different combinations of various practices, including breath awareness, walking meditation, eating meditation, and loving-kindness practices and that you've been able to see their different effects firsthand.

The more we practice, the more mindfulness becomes our new normal. Rather than being a special state that we experience during or just after meditating, we naturally start to savor more, to smell the roses in our everyday lives, and to spend less time stuck in the narrative thought stream. There are a few things you could try that will help to support your efforts to establish a regular mindfulness practice and to have it be a central part of your life.

If you haven't already done so, try to pick a regular time and a regular place for formal meditation practice. After a while, just sitting down in your special spot at your special time will evoke a bit of cue-dependent learning. It'll make you feel a little bit more mindful. It's like reentering a church or a temple—just being there shifts our attitude. You may also find it helpful to find one or more meditation buddies, other folks who are involved with the practice, or members of a meditation group with whom you can touch base. Feeling part of a larger meditation community is a time-honored way to support the practice.

I've been fortunate to be part of such a community for some decades, and it's been enormously helpful. In fact, the theme of this lecture arose out of a conversation that I had with one of my meditation buddies.

I was talking with my friend and colleague Chris Germer because he and I were going to co-direct a psychotherapy conference in which we had invited the Dalai Lama to join a large group of psychotherapists. And we started thinking, what would be an appropriate topic? We stepped back and thought, what would we want to see ourselves if we were, at this late stage in our careers, to seek a psychotherapist for ourselves? And we realized we wouldn't be so interested in knowledge of the latest techniques, nor even a grasp of current research findings. We would, however, want someone who was wise, who had a sense of how to live life well, and who was compassionate, who was caring, interested in our welfare in an accepting, nonjudgmental way.

We were struck in talking about this that, despite all of our years of training and despite our strong wish for a psychotherapist who was wise and compassionate, neither of us had had any formal training about how to develop either wisdom or compassion. So we set about investigating what's known about how wisdom and compassion might actually be cultivated.

We've already discussed some ways to use mindfulness techniques to develop compassion, both for ourselves and others. Now, let's turn our attention to the other wing of the bird or the other wheel of the cart to wisdom, because it turns out that wisdom isn't just important in a good psychotherapist, but it's important in virtually all of life's pursuits.

Wisdom is valuable for everyone. We particularly notice its presence or absence in leaders. The leaders we most revere have wisdom in large measure. Take a political leader like Nelson Mandela, who, even after being incarcerated for so many years, worked for reconciliation with his former jailers. Or a spiritual leader like the Dalai Lama, who speaks quite regularly about the communist Chinese government that has, after all, exiled him and pretty much tried to wipe Buddhism out of Tibet. And he calls them "my friends, the enemy." And all of us know what it's like to be around a wise mom or dad or a wise grandparent. They're enormously helpful in everybody's lives.

Now, in some ways, I'm a little nervous giving this lecture because it feels kind of presumptuous. Teaching about wisdom suggests knowing something about it. And there seems to be an inverse relationship between thinking of oneself as wise and actually being wise. We see this throughout the world's wisdom literature. Confucius—and most others after him—said, "Anyone who thinks he or she is wise probably isn't." Still, it's worth exploring.

As you'll soon see, scientists are starting to grapple with the ancient question of what wisdom is and how it can be developed. They're even trying to identify which brain structures support wisdom. And I think you'll find, as I have, that simply by reflecting about wisdom, you may find yourself becoming a little bit wiser. This is in part because wisdom involves maintaining a certain perspective toward life. And exploring what wisdom is and isn't seems to help us to develop just that perspective.

So what is wisdom? Well, almost every language has a word for it. And it's seen typically as the highest human virtue across diverse cultures. But until recently, modern psychologists—and even modern philosophers—have hardly touched the subject. In fact, they've had a very difficult time even agreeing what it is. When we look at the giants of psychology, we see very little. Freud hardly mentions the term. Jung discusses wisdom archetypes—the wise old man, the wise old woman—but he doesn't describe wisdom itself or speculate on how to develop it.

The first glimmers we get are really from Abraham Maslow. And you may recall he identified a hierarchy of human needs, from basic survival to more noble and sublime pursuits. And he probably contributed the most. He talks about self-actualizing individuals, and these self-actualizing individuals embrace reality and facts rather than denying truth. They're spontaneous, and they focus on problems outside of themselves. They can accept their own human nature with all its shortcomings. They're accepting of others, and they lack prejudice. And these are glimmers of some of the components that we might begin to think, "Ah, those sound like features of wisdom."

Erik Erickson was the first to address wisdom in any detail. You know, Erikson was a fellow who was the first theorist really to outline in detail stages of development, from early childhood through old age. And he described wisdom as the outcome of successfully negotiating the eighth and final stage of human development, what occurs between around age 65 and onward. And he called that "integrity versus despair." And what he was looking at was the idea that people, when they get older, typically reflect back on their life. They see how they've lived it. And they come away with either a sense of fulfillment from a life well-lived or a sense of regret or despair over a life misspent. So that's another feature we can look for as we begin grapple with what wisdom may be. Does our life feel like it's being well-lived?

Now, George Vaillant, a Harvard psychiatrist who conducted the Harvard Study for Adult Development that followed a cohort of Harvard men for decades beginning with their undergraduate years, he thought that wisdom was about having mature defenses—basically, ways of coping with thoughts and feelings that were more mature and didn't get people in trouble as opposed to the immature ones that cause trouble. As I look at Vaillant's formulation, it's not a very high bar because wisdom basically means finding ways to cope with our impulses and feelings that aren't too destructive, but they include fooling ourselves as long as the fooling of ourselves doesn't hurt others.

So given this historical paucity of psychological literature on wisdom, scientific psychologists have had to start pretty much from scratch to study it. And they began by seeking an operational definition, some way of identifying what "wisdom" is and what it isn't. They've taken two broad approaches to operationalizing it. The first is to discover what are called *implicit models*. And the way they do that is to ask people to call in mind a wise person and describe his or her characteristics. And they've done this with subjects from many different cultures.

We can try this together right now. Take a moment to think of someone you know or have known that you consider to be particularly wise. They don't have to be completely wise in all areas, just wiser than most folks. Got someone? Now, list a few of the ways in which their wisdom is expressed. What wise things have you seen them do? Take a moment to think about this. Perhaps there's some incident or interaction that stands out as a particularly wise one. Now, if you were in a research study, I'd ask you to write down your responses. We'd collect them from many different people, and we'd looked for commonalities. We'd try to develop an implicit model for wisdom.

The other way that psychological scientists have tried to define "wisdom" is by looking to ancient cultures. And here we find quite a variety of perspectives. I'll give you a little bit of a historical overview so you could see how broad the different approaches have been over history.

One of the earliest Western writings about wisdom comes from Mesopotamia in 3000 B.C. "If we are doomed to die, let us spend." I think a lot of people use that same philosophy with their credit cards today. But as we step back, we may think, well, that may not be the highest possible expression of wisdom. And we start to see that one person's wisdom might be another person's folly.

A thousand years later, around 2000 B.C., we find this from the ancient Egyptians: "Be not puffed up with thy knowledge, and be not proud because thou are wise." Here we're echoing Confucius. This thing that we see over and over, that thinking we're wise is probably a sign of not being so wise.

And then, 1,600 years later in ancient Greece—around 400 B.C.—Socrates points out that "the narrow intelligence flashing from the keen eye of a clever rogue is not wisdom." And this becomes very interesting because this is one of the differentiations between intelligence and wisdom, because it is possible to be quite, quite smart but not wise in the least.

A little later in ancient Greece, Aristotle put forth the idea of the golden mean—this idea that wisdom involves finding balance in the various aspects of our lives. And then, the later Hebrew and Christian texts, they veer off in a different direction in which wisdom is revelation from God and adherence to faith is the path to wisdom—you just think about Job's struggle in the Old Testament. So in the Western biblical tradition, wisdom included knowing our place in the world, accepting that much is beyond our capacity to understand, and remaining faithful to God.

Now, surprisingly, modern Western philosophers haven't explored the topic much at all. A notable exception is John Kekes, who's frequently quoted by the contemporary scientists studying wisdom. And Kekes emphasizes wisdom's characterological aspect in a way that resonates with Socrates—this separation of intelligence from wisdom. He says, "A fool can learn to say all the things a wise man says and to say them on the same occasions, but this isn't real wisdom." And we know that. We've been with people who are saying the right words, but we just sense that they're not really wise.

Now, wisdom looks quite different East and West. And this is one of the reasons why these implicit studies are helpful for us—because we start to see cultural differences. Compared with Eastern traditions, Western traditions have a greater emphasis on cognitive capacities involving knowledge and developing the skill to use that knowledge effectively in the world. The ancient Asian wisdom traditions typically have a different flavor. They generally emphasize inner transformation—the often transcendent aspect of wisdom that affects our cognitive, intuitive, affective, and interpersonal experience. And all of these aspects of wisdom are valuable.

Let me tell you a story. There's a Western guy who had gone off to Tibet, and he was studying with a great meditation master many years ago. And he was diligently following the practice—doing mindfulness practice and other practices—and his tooth started to hurt. And it got worse. And he was trying to be with the pain, very much in the way that we've discussed in earlier lectures, but it was really a rough ride.

So he asked to have an interview with the teacher to try to figure out how to handle this better. He waited. He got the interview. He explained to the teacher that he's trying so much to be present, but his tooth really hurts. It's so hard not to resist it. He said, "So what should I do?" And the teacher said, "I don't know. See a dentist." There's a real value to factual knowledge and procedural knowledge in addition to transcendent acknowledge.

Now, there have been some Western psychological and neurobiological scientists who have really tried to unpack what wisdom is and what's happening in the brain with wisdom. It turns out it's quite hard to study, and this is in part because it's multi-dimensional. It's much easier to study more elemental things, like the hearing threshold—above what level do we hear a sound—or what are peoples' reactions to various pleasant or unpleasant stimuli, or even to study biases and prejudices. These are all more elemental than wisdom.

So in addition to implicit theory research—asking people to identify and describe wise persons—and searching the world's wisdom traditions to try to get a handle on what wisdom might be, some scientists have tried to identify laboratory models for studying wisdom. The most developed ones of these are from Paul Baltes and the Berlin Wisdom Project, and this was done at the Max Planck Institute for Human Development and Education in Germany. And what they did was they generated hypothetical vignettes, thinking-aloud exercises, and asked subjects to reflect on them.

This is quite similar in methodology to a well-known work by Lawrence Kohlberg—you may have come across that if you ever took intro psych—that was used to study stages of moral development. And while Kohlberg's conclusions have been critiqued for their gender bias, his methods were very innovative. Kohlberg would pose an ambiguous moral problem to people. And then, he would see how they respond to it.

One of them—probably the most famous—is known as the "Heinz dilemma."

This is what a subject is told:

> A woman was near death from a special kind of cancer. There was one drug that the doctors thought might save her. It was a form of radium that a druggist in the same town had recently discovered. The drug was expensive to make, [and] the druggist was charging 10 times what the drug cost him to produce. [The druggist] paid $200 for the radium and charged $2,000 for a small dose of the drug. The sick woman's husband, Heinz, went to everyone he knew to borrow the money, but he could only get together about $1,000, which [was only] half of what it cost. He told the druggist that his wife was dying and asked him to sell it cheaper [to him] or let him pay later. But the druggist said: "No. I discovered the drug and I'm going to make money from it." So Heinz got desperate and broke into the man's store to steal the drug. … [The question is], should Heinz have broken into the laboratory to steal the drug for his wife? Why or why not?

Now, you may vote one way other. The "yes" or "no" answer wasn't what's critical for measuring the subject's stage of moral development. What mattered in Kohlberg's research was what principles the person used to come up with their answer. And this is what inspired Paul Baltes in the Berlin project to try using a similar approach to measure the development of wisdom. They presented subjects with a number of different vignettes and analyze the kinds of considerations the subjects used to respond.

Here's one of the classic ones. Try this yourself for a moment. A 15-year-old girl wants to get married right away. What should she consider and do? How might you respond to that? Can you think of a few thoughts or answers?

A wise answer in the Berlin Project's rubric would go something like this— well, on the surface, it seems easy. On average, marrying at age 15 isn't a great idea—but there are situations where the average doesn't fit. Maybe she has a terminal illness, or maybe she's just lost her parents, or perhaps she lives in another culture or another historical period with a very different value system. Also, you need to consider how—whatever you think—you need to talk to the girl in a way that considers her emotional state and her reactions. So you see that here a wise response considers many different angles. The unwise answer is pretty straightforward. No way. Marrying at 15 is really stupid. It's a crazy idea.

So Baltes and his colleagues factor analyzed the results of hundreds and hundreds of these sorts of things, these sorts of exercises. And they found that wisdom involved five factors. They did statistical processes to determine— what are the themes that pop up over and over?

The first is factual knowledge—having some sense of how the world works in terms of the facts of the matter. The second was procedural knowledge—having a sense of how processes unfold. The third was lifespan contextualism—can you look at this from the point of view of a big picture, of realizing that everybody's not at the same stage in their development? The fourth was value relativism—realizing that my values aren't necessarily your values and I shouldn't necessarily impose mine on yours. And the fifth was awareness and management of uncertainty. And if you think about those five, you may realize—yeah, well, it's true. People who we would turn to for help, people who we would think could be helpful and that we would trust as wise would manifest all five of these qualities.

Now, the Berlin Project's five factors are very individual-oriented. They come from a kind of individual psychology perspective. As we'll see in a few minutes, other investigators have included more of an emphasis on concern for others or the greater social good. And they come to similar conclusions to what we see in Buddhist psychology—that wisdom and compassion are inseparable.

Now, perhaps the favorite research question of the Berlin Project and others who have tried to study wisdom is this—does wisdom increase with age? Many people wonder about that. The answer is a resounding "sometimes." There's actually no evidence across quite a few different studies that wisdom steadily increases with age. On average, young adults actually look as wise as elders. Seems strange, right?

Well, there's a reason for that. They found a plateau of wisdom-related performance through much of middle and old age. And in fact, wisdom begins to decline around age 75 probably along with cognitive decline. If there's such a thing as a peak, Baltes said it's somewhere in your 60s where you've had the maximum life experience without serious cognitive decline.

Now, it doesn't mean that there aren't some extraordinarily wise folks at different ages or that it can't increase over the lifespan, it just doesn't necessarily grow when we average it all out. The reason is because some people, as they grow older, grow wiser, and others grow more foolish. Take a moment to think of older people you know. Some are definitely wise. They're flexible. They see the big picture. They don't sweat the small stuff. They care about others. They're not self-preoccupied.

Others seem to cling more tightly to what's good for me and mine and narrow beliefs. They kind of circle the wagon. And these folks are very resistant to change. They're very intolerant toward competing views. They tend to be close-minded and prejudiced, have everybody divided up into groups of good and bad. They're kind of like—if you remember the old sitcom *All In the family*, they're like Archie Bunker, the bigoted star of that program who had something to say about all those other people.

So what might help us grow wiser? Well, the intention to do so seems to help. So just listening to this lecture is probably a good idea. Also, involvement in introspective pursuits help. We can assume from this that mindfulness meditation, psychotherapy, being involved in the arts, all these kinds of things can help.

In fact, in one study, clinical psychologists did particularly well on measures of wisdom. And I know that sounds suspect. You think, oh, yeah. A psychologist studying psychologists. They think psychologists are wise. But this study was actually conducted by research psychologists who are often very critical of their clinician colleagues because they think the clinicians are too unscientific.

Now, mindfulness practice, by increasing our awareness of our own reactions to each moment, would help to support all of our activities as paths to greater wisdom. In fact, we have reasons to believe that it works in precisely this way.

Some of the evidence comes from neurobiological studies. Two psychiatrists, Thomas Meeks and Dilip Jeste at the University California in San Diego, factor analyzed the world's literature on wisdom. And they came up with six factors or components. You'll see that these overlap with what we have from the Berlin group: prosocial behavior and attitude—so caring about others; social decision-making and pragmatic life knowledge—that's kind of knowing how things work among people; emotional homeostasis—that's having some equanimity and balance; reflection and self-understanding, being able to think about—what am I doing here? What are my motives? Value relativism and tolerance—we've seen that before; and acknowledgement and dealing effectively with uncertainty and ambiguity—we've seen that as well.

Now, Meeks and Jeste tried to then identify parts of the brain that have been shown to be active when people exercise each of these faculties. And each faculty has a putative neurological substrate. And they have several regions in common—the dorsal lateral, orbital frontal, and ventral medial prefrontal cortex, the anterior cingulate, amygdala, and the limbic striatum. Don't worry about the names. What's important is that all six components of wisdom are related conceptually to meditative practices. And there's a particularly strong overlap with the neurological changes we see in meditation and three of the wisdom factors or components. In other words, they change the same parts of the brain. And these are prosocial attitudes, emotional homeostasis—having balance or equanimity—and self-reflection and self-understanding.

In other words, the parts of the brain that are active when we're demonstrating these three qualities—caring about others, having emotional homeostasis, and reflecting and having self-understanding—are the same parts of the brain that are activated during meditation practice. Now, the findings are complicated, and they're still tentative. They're complicated in part because wisdom is so complex—it draws on so many different parts of the brain—but the findings, nonetheless, suggest that mindfulness practice may be a way to get wiser.

So stepping back, looking at all of these things together, can we come up with an overarching touchstone for wisdom drawing from all these different inputs? Many scientists say yes, that wisdom is, in essence, concern for the effects of our behavior both near and far in the short and long term. That's easy to remember. It's just concern for the effects of the behavior near and far in the short and long term.

The opposite—concern for the effects of behavior, just short term, and only for me or mine—we might call "foolishness." And of course, it's quite possible for a person to be wise in some areas and foolish in others. Robert Sternberg is the leading research psychologist currently studying wisdom, and he differentiates between general wisdom and personal wisdom. Personal wisdom involves how wisely we conduct our daily lives and interpersonal interactions, as opposed to the more general wisdom we display in our thoughts and attitudes toward big-picture problems. And he's fond of pointing out that many otherwise wise thinkers and leaders seem to be lacking in personal wisdom. In their personal lives, they often seem to act foolishly. For example, Martin Luther King was notoriously unfaithful to his spouse. Socrates didn't support his family—he abandoned them to hemlock. And even the Buddha left his wife and child to pursue enlightenment.

Now, of course, these actions can be interpreted differently—perhaps in the service of the greater good—and we don't know the particulars. In fact, it would be a sign of wisdom to consider these possibilities. But it would also seem that just because a person's wise in one area, it doesn't guarantee wisdom in all realms.

So wisdom in Buddhist psychology involves awareness of three marks of existence: of *anicca* (impermanence), of *dukkha* (of unsatisfactoriness) and of *anatta* (the sense of no enduring or separate self). We discussed these earlier in the context of absolute truth. In Buddhist psychology, it's deeply understanding these realities that's synonymous with having wisdom. And such awareness would lead us to the principles we've been discussing from a Western perspective, culminating in concern for the effects of actions near and far, short and long term. And mindfulness practices are actually designed to bring insight into these three marks of existence.

Let's examine some ways in which they do this. Here are eight different skills that mindfulness practices foster which can contribute to our developing wisdom. Of course, to develop these, we need to practice formal and informal meditation regularly, which is one of the reasons I've been encouraging you to do so.

First, they help us develop wisdom by stepping out of the thought stream. By simply returning our attention to moment-to-moment sensory experience, we gain perspective on our thought processes. And we see how they're conditioned by family and culture, and they change with our moods and circumstances. We also see our defenses at work, how we resist certain thoughts and cling to others. And this helps us to maintain multiple perspectives, which we've seen is such a central part to most definitions of wisdom. And we can even gain firsthand insight into how the mind constructs a seemingly stable reality out of the ever-changing flux of experience.

Second, mindfulness practices help us to be with discomfort. The capacity to resist the urge for immediate comfort is necessary if we're going to act in the interest of the greater good. Because otherwise, we just compulsively do what I need and I want right now. So much as our muscles become stronger by lifting weights in the gym, we become stronger at tolerating discomfort and not having to do what's good for me in the moment with mindfulness practice.

Third, they help us to disengage from our automatic responses, whether these are instinctual responses biologically hardwired or conditioned through reward and punishment. What happens is we want to be able to observe the stimulus response processes in a microscopic detail so that we don't have to act on them, so we can see a sensation arising, followed by a thought or feeling, followed by the urge to act, and finally, moving into overt behavior. But we have the ability to pause, to take a breath and not necessarily do the thing that immediately we have the urge to do.

A friend of mine suggests that we use the acronym WAIT. This is actually designed for psychotherapists, but any of us can use it. It's W-A-I-T. It stands for, "Why am I talking?" And at so many moments when we start in talking, WAIT—thinking, why am I talking?—can help us to take a more wise perspective on the matter.

Fourth is transpersonal insight. And this is direct insight into *anatta*. What we've discussed before is the fact that there's no independent separate self here, and it's closely related to what later Buddhist traditions refer to as *sunyata*, or emptiness. It's simply the direct intuitive experience of the interconnectedness of all things. And as we step out of the thought stream and we see this, then the barrier between me and mine and you and yours starts to dissolve. And that naturally leads to compassionate action.

Fifth is moment-to-moment observation of the mind's antics. That's really seeing all of the crazy things that we do to try to make ourselves feel better— stereotyping, judging, jealously competing, idealizing, denigrating, all the not-so-noble things we do with other people—we see these more clearly with mindfulness practice.

And then, we see all the ways the mind creates suffering for itself. We've been discussing these throughout the course—all of the ways in which we try to get things just right and cling to the pleasant and avoid the unpleasant.

Now, seventh is embracing opposites. Our dearly-held views of reality—I'm smart, I'm stupid, I'm kind, I'm mean—they're merely mental constructions. And the more we see these, the more we can embrace different peoples' views.

And then, finally, there's the other wing of the bird. And we've talked about how mindfulness practices help us to develop compassion, and compassion and wisdom are inseparable. Once we have wisdom, if it's combined with compassion, that makes us act ever more wisely in the world.

As the 11th-century Indian sage, Atisha put it, "The supreme goal of the teachings is the emptiness whose nature is compassion."

In our next lecture, we're going to look at other potential benefits of mindfulness practice from the perspective of Buddhist traditions. We're going to look at how it can help us to awaken to the psychological freedom which is sometimes called "enlightenment."

The Promise of Enlightenment
Lecture 22

The arrival of Buddhist teachings in the West is having an important impact: Buddhist teachings are changing Western psychology, and Western science and culture is changing Buddhist teachings. In this lecture, you will learn about the potential benefits of mindfulness practice from the perspective of Buddhist traditions. Specifically, you will learn how mindfulness practice can help us awaken to the psychological freedom known as enlightenment. Buddhist psychology is profound in its implications: Grasp a little, and you'll experience a little enlightenment; grasp a lot, and you'll experience a lot of enlightenment.

Buddhist Psychology

- Buddhist teachings are not a religion in the Western sense. Rather, they are this 2,500-year-old tradition of introspection evolved into a system for psychological understanding and treatment. Nonetheless, it's a profoundly spiritual practice—at least in one way of understanding the word.

- Attending to one's experience is probably as old as humankind. But doing it in a deliberate and structured way seems to have particularly strong roots in the religious traditions of ancient India, where it's been going on for thousands of years.

- There was an ancient view in the time of the Buddha that informed his understanding—a view that we see in many of the ancient Hindu texts. The view is that conscious awareness is embedded in a sensory system that yields pleasurable and painful experience. Pain is inevitable, and lasting pleasure is unattainable.

- Furthermore, they realized in the Buddha's day that humans have trouble seeing themselves and their world clearly, and this results in what's called *dukkha*, or dissatisfaction. In Buddhist psychology, no explanation is offered for how this came to pass. Unlike in some other religious traditions, there's no reason for humankind's predicament, and there's nobody around to provide salvation—only an understanding of how suffering is caused through desire and ignorance and how it could be resolved.

- In Buddhist tradition, desire is the deep, hardwired compulsion to pursue pleasure and avoid pain, while ignorance is the unconscious and unexamined nature of our attitudes and assumptions about who we are and the world we inhabit—especially the assumption of being a separate itself. Together, desire and ignorance shape how we construct our reality from one moment to the next, trying with only limited success to find satisfaction.

- Western cultures tend to embrace and honor reason to govern human nature. We see this in our systems of law, social philosophy, even psychology. The ancient Asian traditions were skeptical about reason. They were concerned that it may just be a rationalization for pursuing desires. And they also doubted revealed truth, because they wondered how we know that the first person got it right. The emphasis, instead, is on discovering for oneself, through direct experience. We can find this critique of reason in the West as well.

- The ancient Indian traditions used asceticism and meditation instead of reason. They developed a science of inner inquiry, not outer measurement. Asceticism deprives the mind of what it wants so that we can see the operation of desire more clearly, and meditation allows clear and keen observation, shedding light on processes that are either too subtle or too ubiquitous to notice much of the time.

- The illuminating power of restraint involves resisting, at least for a moment, whatever our urge is. Whether it's to have a drink, visit the refrigerator, or check our smartphone, that moment's resistance illuminates what's happening in the mind at the moment.

- Using asceticism and meditation, the ancient sages discovered that we don't actually see reality, but we construct it. Western cognitive scientists say the same thing. Buddhist psychology stresses how this happens moment to moment. They say that the mind is a world-building organ that makes order out of chaos, and we construct reality out of all of this data streaming in at breakneck speed.

- They also point out that we spend a lot of time defending illusions. We fear illness and death, and we try not to think about it. We also see other people as objects to fulfill our desires, rather than part of a superorganism that we participate in. And there are all sorts of suffering results.

- One of the reasons that we can't see clearly is because perception is a means to an end. It's a means to pursuing pleasure and avoiding pain. So, our perceptions are distorted by our desires.

- Many of our psychological defenses aren't against instincts; instead, they are to buttress our sense of self. They keep us from noticing that there's no one home, that there's just this moment-to-moment changing experience. But these very defenses help us feel like we're a self cut off from our direct experience and from one another.

The Mindfulness Cure

- The Buddha saw himself as a physician, and mindfulness was his principal healing technique. He set out very detailed practice instructions. He liked to make numbered lists to help his followers remember various instructions.

- The Buddha's formula began with mindfulness of body, feeling, and mind. First, the idea was to begin by paying attention to body sensations in four postures: sitting, standing, lying down, and walking. He also suggested being mindful of the breath and whatever other body sensations arise and noticing when they're absent and when they're present.

- Next, he suggested mindfulness as a feeling—to notice whether any experience was pleasant, unpleasant, or neutral and to distinguish the feeling response from sensation. The idea was to notice the feeling reactions to images and thoughts as well as the body sensations.

- The next step was to be mindful of the mind. This meant noticing the arising of what we call the three "poisons" or "fires": greed (trying to hold on to things), hatred (trying to push things out of awareness), and delusion (zoning out).

- The Buddha provided detailed instructions about how to be mindful of all of the different contents that arise in the mind. He suggested noticing the five hindrances: sense-desire, aversion, indolence, restlessness, and doubt. The task is to observe all of these different elements in the mind when they're present, when they're absent, or when they're just arising.

- He also suggested noticing the five aggregates: materiality (sense contact), perception, feeling, formations (intentions and dispositions), and consciousness. The task is to observe these aggregates as continually arising and passing away, noticing the lack of any unifying agent (self) who sees, feels, and thinks. Instead, there is just this flux of experience.

- In addition, we are supposed to notice the six sense spheres: how the eye sees, the ear hears, the nose smells, the skin touches, the tongue tastes, and the mind thinks. The task is to notice how desire arises out of each of these senses—that we're always craving more of one sense experience or trying to pull back from another.

- Finally, the Buddha suggested noticing the seven factors of awakening: concentration, mindfulness, investigation present, energy, joy, tranquility, and equanimity. The task is to notice when all of these qualities are present, absent, or arising. Here, unlike the hindrances, we're working to cultivate these factors.

Enlightenment
- Mindfulness of these events in consciousness is said to lead to enlightenment. The waking up that the Buddha said can happen if

we follow this course is that greed, hatred, and delusion fall away. Pleasure and pain remain, of course. But pleasure doesn't create the desire for more pleasure, and pain isn't met with aversion or resistance. So, we don't get caught in compulsive or addictive behaviors anymore.

- Rather, the awakened person moves through the world responding to events as they emerge with wisdom and compassion. Lives become an expression of generosity, which is the lack of greed; kindness, which is the lack of hatred; and understanding, which is the lack of delusion.

- There are a number of pitfalls along the path to awakening. Some involve what we might call spiritual materialism. We have this remarkably robust tendency to compare ourselves with others. In fact, it's said to be the last neurotic pattern to fall away before complete enlightenment.

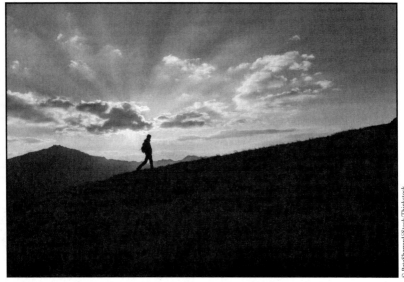

Enlightenment, or psychological freedom, can be achieved through Buddhist psychology.

- As we start working on this path, thoughts like "look how selfless I am!" arise, and we can start getting hooked on the enlightened role. It's also very easy to become attached to some of the positive effects of mindfulness. We start to crave clarity, and we start seeking higher states of consciousness. Worst of all, we start feeling superior to others that we imagine are less awake or aware than we are.

- The path is not really about getting somewhere. This is very paradoxical. Even though there's a pathway to awakening, the way we tread this path is by simply being in the moment and working on accepting what's going on right now.

- Different Buddhist traditions emphasize different aspects of the path, and they use different techniques to try to create the transformation of mind that occurs. Mindfulness practice is actually one of several, but it's usually considered the foundational practice.

- There are dangers along the path to waking up. Some people experience a sense of fragmentation, dissolution, or aggrandizement. Because of these possible difficulties in traditional practice, some mindfulness practices were kept pretty esoteric.

- People can get into trouble if they have sudden awakenings without the foundations of maturity. This can happen during intensive meditation practice. It can even happen when they're in proximity to a guru, or a spiritual teacher. People can even get into trouble with the mania of bipolar illness. There's also the danger of interpreting one's experience narcissistically.

- In addition, people become very attached to getting high. Some of these states can feel really energizing and illuminating, and we can start to see awakening as a state of consciousness, or a state of mind, rather than a stage of development. Nowadays, it's better to be a decent human "being with" limited spiritual awakening than someone with profound awakening but limited maturity who has difficulty getting along with others.

- It's possible to have spiritual awakenings in all sorts of traditions and not to advance very far developmentally. When people like this get into challenging situations, they can regress from their enlightened position to a much more immature position.

- What's missing from Buddhist psychology—from this path to enlightenment? Traditionally, these are solitary practices that were developed by monks, nuns, and hermits. So, there was very little examination of projection, interpersonal skills, or systemic phenomena. And advanced practice often didn't prepare practitioners very well for interpersonal life.

- Unless we practice in interpersonal contexts, our interpersonal issues are likely to remain unresolved. So, we need to cultivate interpersonal awareness, affect tolerance, and restraint by practicing interpersonally. And realizations that are developed in one realm may not translate to other realms.

Suggested Reading

Batchelor, *Buddhism without Beliefs*.

Goldstein and Kornfield, *Seeking the Heart of Wisdom*.

Kornfield, *After the Ecstasy, the Laundry*.

Olendzki, "The Roots of Buddhist Psychology."

Questions to Consider

1. What are some of the pitfalls of pursuing mindfulness practice as part of a spiritual path? How have you encountered these challenges?

2. How do you imagine an enlightened person would act in everyday life? Do you think that enlightenment is a thoroughgoing transformation, touching all aspects of a person's life, or do you suspect that people can be more or less enlightened in different realms at different times?

The Promise of Enlightenment
Lecture 22—Transcript

There's an ancient prophecy that says, "When the iron bird flies, and horses run on wheels, the Dharma will come to the land of the red faces." This prophecy has been widely and uncritically assumed to mean that, at the time of airplanes and motorized transport, the Dharma, or Buddhist teachings, will make its triumphal entry to the West.

The prophecy actually probably had other symbolic meanings. The land of the red faces were how the Chinese characterized Tibetans. And the iron bird may refer to the 700s, when Buddhism became established in Tibet. Still, the arrival of Buddhist teachings in the West is having an important impact. It's changing Western psychology, and Western science and culture is changing Buddhist teachings.

The central legend of the Buddhist tradition reveals a lot about its heart. You remember the story—after his father couldn't promise the young prince that he wouldn't grow old, get sick, or die, he left home. And he followed an ascetic route. He mastered all manner of concentration practices, studying with the greatest teachers of the time. He became a strict ascetic, went down to eating one grain of rice, or one sesame seed, a day. But still, it didn't work. He still felt he was suffering. He was struggling with desires, struggling with the realization of the challenges of the life cycle.

So he started eating again and taking care of his body. And then he committed himself to sit for 49 days and nights—actually committed himself to sit as long as it took, but it took him 49 days and nights. And as it's described the classic text, the demon Mara tried to distract him from his efforts. First, he sent beautiful, seductive maidens, then horrible, frightening, and disgusting images. This is how, in the language of the time, the arising of intense pleasant and unpleasant mental contents in the mind were described. Finally, the young prince felt that he understood. He had found a pathway to happiness.

Initially, he thought people weren't going to believe him. He thought, this is too odd, too different from the way most people live. But then he saw some children playing, and they inspired him to teach. And he taught the children his first lesson. And they seemed to get it, so he went on to teach more broadly.

And as he traveled around India at the time, people were struck that he was somehow different. He was unusually happy. And they would ask him, using the language of the time, "What are you? Are you a god, a spirit, or a ghost?" And he said, "No, I'm just a man. I just woke up." And the word Buddha, in the language of the time, simply means "to have woken up," like waking up from a sleep, or waking up from a dream. And this awakening that he had is what we've come to appreciate as enlightenment.

He went on to say, "I can show you how to do it." But when he was asked religious questions, he eschewed them. He said he teaches about the origins of suffering and its alleviation because that's all enlightenment is.

So Buddhist teachings were not a religion in a traditional or in a Western sense—rather, they were this 2,500-year-old tradition of introspection evolved into a system for psychological understanding and treatment that has, at its goal, waking up. Nonetheless, we'll also see that it's a profoundly spiritual practice, at least in one way of understanding the word.

Now, attending to one's experience is probably as old as humankind. But doing it in a deliberate and structured way seems to have particularly strong roots in the religious traditions of ancient India, in the forest and plains along the banks of the Indus and the Ganges rivers because there, it's been going on for thousands of years. They found clay statues of men sitting in Lotus posture that are at least 4,000 years old, predating the Buddha by many, many centuries. I just visited some of those places in India. Remarkably, a lot of people are still threshing rice and making bread just as they did back then.

Now, there was an ancient view in the time of the Buddha that informed his understanding. And it's a view that we see in many of the ancient Hindu texts. And this is that conscious awareness is embedded in a sensory system which yields pleasurable and painful experience. Pain is inevitable, and lasting pleasure is unattainable. Furthermore, they realized back in the

Buddha's day that humans have trouble seeing themselves and their world clearly, and this results in what's called *dukkha*, or dissatisfaction, as we've talked about before.

Now, in Buddhist psychology, no explanation is offered for how this came to pass. Unlike we have in some other religious traditions, there's no reason for humankind's predicament, and there's nobody around to provide salvation—only an understanding of how suffering is caused through desire and ignorance, and how it can be resolved.

So what exactly are desire and ignorance as they're used in this tradition? Well, desire is the deep, hard-wired compulsion to pursue pleasure and avoid pain. And ignorance is the unconscious and unexamined nature of our attitudes and assumptions about who we are and the world we inhabit. It's essentially the assumption and the belief in being a separate self. Together, desire and ignorance shape how we construct our reality from one moment to the next, trying with only limited success to find satisfaction.

Now, Western cultures tend to embrace and honor reason to govern human nature. And we see this in our systems of law, social philosophy, even psychology. The ancient Asian traditions were skeptical about reason. They were concerned that it may just be a rationalization for pursuing desires. And they also doubted revealed truth because they said, "Well, how do we know that the first person got it right?" The emphasis, instead, is on discovering for oneself, through direct experience, what is.

We can find this critique of reason in the West as well, and our wisest philosophers seem to talk about it. My favorite is a line from Ben Franklin. He said, "So convenient a thing it is to be reasonable creature, since it enables one to find or make a reason for everything one has a mind to do."

So if not reason, what? Well, the ancient Indian traditions used asceticism and meditation instead. They developed a science of inner inquiry, not outer measurement. Asceticism deprives the mind of what it wants, so we can see the operation of desire more clearly. And meditation allows clear and keen observation, shedding light on processes that are either to subtle or too ubiquitous to notice much of the time.

I mentioned earlier the illuminating power of restraint. This is, for example, if anger arises, and I just stay with the feeling of anger happening in the body, I will actually know that anger in a more subtle, in a more nuanced, in a more vivid way than if I simply enact it and start yelling or screaming. So resisting, at least for a moment, whatever our urge is, whether it's to have a drink, visit the refrigerator, check our smartphone, or yell at our partner, that moment's resistance actually illuminates what's happening in the mind at the moment.

And what the ancient sages discovered using asceticism and meditation, was that we don't actually see reality—we construct it. This is exactly what Western cognitive scientists say as well. And Buddhist psychologies stress how this happens moment to moment. They say the mind is a world-building organ. It makes order out of chaos, and we construct reality out of all of this data streaming in at breakneck speed.

They also point out that we spend a lot of time defending illusions. We fear illness and death, and we try not to think about it. We also see other people as objects to fulfill our desires, rather than part of a superorganism that we participate in—and all sorts of suffering results. One of the reasons we can't see clearly is because perception is a means to an end and it's a means to pursuing pleasure and avoiding pain. So our perceptions, as we've discussed earlier, are distorted by our desires.

They also say that many of our psychological defenses aren't against instincts—they're not because we can't tolerate a sexual urge, or an aggressive urge, as psychoanalysts have viewed it—but they are to buttress our sense of self. They are to keep us from noticing that there's no one home, that there's just this moment-to-moment changing experience. But these very defenses that help us to feel like we're a self cut us off from our direct experience and from one another.

So the Buddha saw himself as a physician. And mindfulness was his principal healing technique. And he set out very detailed practice instructions. He liked to make numbered lists to help his followers to remember the various instructions. Here are few of his lists.

The Buddha's formula began with mindfulness of the body, of feeling, and of the mind. And the idea was to begin by paying attention to body sensations and to do those in four postures—we've discussed these before—sitting, standing, lying down, and walking. He also suggested being mindful of the breath and mindful of whatever other body sensations arise, and to notice when they're absent and when they are present.

Next, he suggested mindfulness of feeling. And the idea was to notice whether any experience was pleasant, unpleasant, or neutral. And to distinguish the feeling response from sensation—he wanted us to dismantle the building blocks from which we derive a sense of self so that we could live in the world without that profound sense of self. And the idea was to notice the feeling reactions not only to body sensations but also to images and thoughts.

The next step was to be mindful of mind. And this meant noticing the arising of what we call the *three poisons*, or the *three fires*. We discussed these in working with addictions. This is greed (trying to hold onto things), hatred (trying to push things out of awareness), and delusion (basically, zoning out).

And the Buddha provided detailed instructions as to how to be mindful of all of the different contents that arise. You'll notice we've already looked at many of these in exploring the application of mindfulness to life's difficulties. Here are the other elements. He said, notice the five hindrances. Notice sense desire; notice aversion, pulling back; notice indolence, which is the word for, kind of, zoning out; notice restlessness, when we're having trouble being present; and notice doubt, when we're thinking, ah, forget that meditation practice, it doesn't work. And the idea is to observe all of these different elements in the mind when they're present, when they're absent, or when they're just arising.

He also suggested noticing what are called the *five aggregates*. And we've talked about these—noticing that, well, everything begins with sense contact; and then it's organized into perception; and then we add a feeling tone to that; and then we develop these intentions, or dispositions, these characteristics of our personality over time; and that all of this is going on in what we experience in consciousness. And the task is to observe that these are things continually arising and passing, but there's no unifying agent. There's no self. There's nobody who actually sees, feels, and thinks—just this flux of experience.

And then we are supposed to notice exactly how the eye sees, the ear hears, the nose smells, the skin touches, and notice how sense desire arises out of each of these senses, that we're always craving more of one sense experience or trying to pull back from another.

And then, finally, he said keep an eye on the seven factors of awakening—some of these we've looked at—whether, in any moment, is concentration present? Are we attentive to what's going on? Is mindfulness present? Are we open to what's going on? Is investigation present? Are we curious about what's going on? Is our energy level at an optimal level? Are we awake and engaged, but not overwrought? Can we experience the joy of moment-to-moment experience, at the same time that we experience a kind of background tranquility? And can we experience equanimity? And the task is to notice when all of these qualities are present, absent, or arising. And here, unlike the hindrances, we're trying to work to cultivate these things because these factors of mind help us to wake up. They help us to become enlightened.

So what exactly is this enlightenment? Well, this waking up that the Buddha said can happen if we follow this course is that greed, hatred, and delusion—hanging on to things, pushing things away, and zoning out—fall away. Pleasure and pain remain, of course. Some experiences are pleasant. Others are unpleasant. But pleasure and pain doesn't create the desire for more pleasure. We don't cling to it so much. And pain isn't met with a version of resistance. So we don't get caught in compulsive or addictive behaviors anymore. Rather, the awakened person moves through the world responding to events as they emerge with wisdom and compassion. Lives become an expression of generosity, which is the lack of greed, kindness, which is the lack of hatred, and understanding, which is the lack of delusion.

Now in the typical artistic depiction, we see the Buddha sitting in full Lotus meditation posture. And in the awakened posture, it looks like this. He's got the monk's bowl, which uses for eating. And he's touching the earth, invoking the earth to be a witness to his supreme realization. And in the traditional text, this is called *highest perfect alignment*. And it's said that it can come about suddenly, and even that it can be irreversible.

Different traditions talk about this a little bit differently. In the Zen tradition, they talk about stages. So they talk about *kenshō*, which is seeing one's true self, basically, seeing the interconnectedness of all things, seeing how desire, and clinging to desires, causes suffering. But *kenshō* can come in a flash, but it can go away quite easily. And we can get caught in our usual delusions again. But *kenshō* leads to satori, which is a profound understanding and awakening. And that is supposed to be irreversible. Our attachment to pursuing pleasure is gone, never to return.

Now, my colleagues and I, who are working in Western psychology and doing these practices for years, wonder whether this is how it really works, or if, more typically, there's a waxing and waning of delusion, and waking up, delusion, and waking up. Might people also become enlightened in some areas and not in others, like with any other skill and talent? We'll return to that question in a moment.

Now there are a number of pitfalls along this path to awakening. Some involve what we might call *spiritual materialism*. We have this remarkably robust tendency to compare ourselves with others. In fact, it's said to be the last neurotic pattern to fall away before complete enlightenment. So as we start working on this path, and we start doing our mindfulness practice, and we start becoming somewhat wiser, thoughts arise like—hey, look how selfless I am? I'm more selfless than you are! And we can start getting hooked on this idea of enlightenment, or the enlightenment role.

It's also very easy to become attached to some of the positive effects of mindfulness. We start to crave clarity because it really feels nice to have a sense of non-attached clarity. We start seeking higher states of consciousness because they feel so much better than being caught in our struggles. And, worst of all, we start feeling superior to others that we imagine are less awake or aware than we are.

So this path is not really about getting somewhere. There's a great story in which the monks are sitting down in a group and the Buddha is addressing them. And one monk raises his hand a little bit timidly, and he says, "Please, I understand the path, and it makes a lot of sense, and I want to follow it. But how long does it take to get enlightened?"

And with the Buddha says is he says, "Imagine a mountain made out of solid rock. And it's [I'm making this up] 10 cubits high by 10 cubits wide by 10 cubits deep." And he says, "Imagine that every 50 to 100 years, a small bird trailing a silk handkerchief brushes across the top of that mountain. Oh, monks, in as many years as it will take that bird to wear down that mountain, that's how long it takes to become awakened."

Now why is the Buddha telling such a distressing and discouraging story? Well, most people understand this as an admonition not to get hooked on getting anywhere else. This is very paradoxical. Even though there's this pathway to awakening, the way we tread this path is by simply being here and working on accepting what's going on right now.

A friend of mine, Bill Morgan, who has been one of my meditation buddies for all these years, he did his dissertation research on the lifelong experience of meditators. And he found, typically, they had three stages. The first was ambition. They were working hard, thinking they were getting somewhere, working to reach enlightenment. The second stage was a crisis. Uh-oh, it's not going to work. Basically, I'm still crazy after all these years. The third stage was acceptance—that it's about the process, not the goal. It's really being accepting of what's going on in the present.

My own experience is that having the concept of awakening is useful as a motivator, but, basically, we have to come back to being in the present. Joseph Goldstein, who is a wonderful meditation teacher, described an experience where he went off to India to practice. And he spent six months in a silent retreat and experienced all manner of awakening. He felt a sense of interconnectedness with all beings, the thought stream got quieter. He was much less concerned with the various kinds of desires that usually preoccupied him. It was really a lot of states of bliss. But he had to come back to the States to deal with some business. And he did that. But he was eager to get back his retreat in India.

Well, when he returned to India, he described the next six months as feeling like twisted steel. He kept trying to get back in the rhythm, kept trying to get back into accepting the present moment, but everything felt wrong. He felt like he wanted to be different. He was uncomfortable. Everything felt wrong. And he said it took in nearly six months to realize that, whoops, he had lost track of the instruction. The instruction was to be with whatever is here—to basically be with twisted steel. And when he could be with the feeling of twisted steel, then the practice started to transform again.

Now, this can be a big disappointment. A lot of us enter meditation practice, psychotherapy, or whatever self-improvement program hoping that we're going to get a whole new personality. I won't have to deal with my longings, my fears, my jealousy, my neurosis—that's all going to go away. But what we get instead is a new relationship to them. We wind up making friends with ourselves as we are. And, ironically, this actually leads to being much more comfortable, and we don't need a new personality anymore. We're no longer so judgmental about the one that we have.

So we basically arrive here. There's a wonderful cartoon that shows two monks meditating. And one is clearly older than the other. And the older one is scowling and upset about something the younger one has done. And he turns to the younger one. He says, "Nothing happens next. This is it." We're on a journey to nowhere. The spiritual aspirations start to fall away as we settle more and more into the unfolding of ordinary experience.

In the Buddhist tradition, they use the image of a raft. And they say, "If you were crossing a river, and you used a raft, would you keep carrying the raft after you went?" They say, "No." So you would let go of the raft. The thoughts of enlightenment and the like are simply tools along the way, nothing that we have to hold onto.

Now different Buddhist traditions emphasize different aspects of the path. And they use different techniques to try to transform or create the transformation of mind that we've been discussing. Mindfulness practice is actually one of several, but it's usually considered the foundational practice.

In Soto Zen, for example, which is a southern school in the southern part of Japan they pay a lot of attention to just doing bare attention, or just sitting, which is not so much concentration practice; it's more like open monitoring.

In Rinzai Zen, they do koan practices. You've probably heard of these. These are things like, what is the sound of one hand clapping? Or why is a mouse when it spins? The idea is to contemplate these, and what's going to happen is they will sort of short circuit our reasoning process, and we'll no longer be able to be so caught the thought stream because we won't trust it so much. In Tibetan traditions, they do all sorts of devotional practices—prostrations and devotion to revered teachers, all to help let go of self-concerns.

Now there are dangers along the path to waking up. These practices are designed to dismantle or deconstruct our conventional sense of self, so sometimes people get into trouble. And a friend of mine actually, Willoughby Britton at Brown University, is currently studying adverse events in meditation practices—particularly the problems that come up when people sit long intensive retreats of many months.

Some people experience a sense of fragmentation, like they're noticing the multiple selves, and they start to get scared about this. They start to feel— oh no, I can't find myself—and they get very anxious. And this is difficult. Other people will experience a sense of dissolution, like, I don't know where I end and where you begin. And while this is ultimately, in a sense, a goal, if it happens in the sense of I don't know if I'm angry or you're angry at the moment, it can be quite confusing. And some people become aggrandized. They start to think, wow, I'm having all of these insights. I must be quite special.

Because of these possible difficulties, in traditional practice, these things were kept pretty esoteric. In fact, mindfulness practice, as we're doing it in the West, was reserved for people who had already worked out a lot of life's problems and knew about how to live an ordinary life well.

Carl Jung, who studied the world's mythologies, he says that, across world traditions, across various mystical traditions, you sort of see a pattern that worldly accomplishments—finding out how to make a living, how to take care of yourself, perhaps having and raising a family—they're kind of reserved for the first half of life, under age 35. And introspection and spiritual practice is more for the second half. And this suggests that, indeed, you kind of have to become a somebody before you become a nobody. You have to establish a conventional sense of self before we go into dismantling it.

I remember reading this when I was in college, and 35 seemed really old. And I felt rather advanced having taken up meditation practices and other introspective disciplines as a teenager. Little did I understand, then, how much of what I thought of as spiritual accomplishment, or even enlightenment, might actually be understood as plain old maturity.

And we can get into trouble if we have sudden awakenings without the foundations of plain old maturity. People ran into this a lot with psychedelic drugs, where they suddenly had an experience of the interconnectedness of all things, and the fluid and transient nature of what we think of as self, but sometimes they get scared by that, and they can have what we think of as bad trips.

This can happen during intensive practice, as I mentioned, the adverse effects of meditation. It can even happen when we've got proximity to a guru, to some kind of spiritual teacher, because some people who have advanced a lot on these kinds of paths emanate a kind of loving presence that can be a little scary for people to be around because they don't sort of look like ordinary people. They're fully present.

People can even get into difficulty with the mania of bipolar illness. Sometimes people who are manic, who are not in the depressed stage, but in the over-excited stage, have spiritual insights. And these spiritual insights can be very destabilizing for them.

There's also always the danger of interpreting our experience narcissistically. I often joke with psychotherapists that if a patient who has taken up mindfulness practices comes into your office and says, "Wow, doc, it is so profound, I've discovered that I'm god—and they say, and so are you, and so is my sister, and my wife, and everyone else," that's great. That's simply a realization of the interconnectedness of all things. If, on the other hand, your patient comes into the office and says, "I'm god, and other people aren't," then you have a problem. So any situation in which we start to interpret what's going on as an indication of our specialness is probably having gotten off the path to enlightenment.

The other thing that happens is people become very attached, as I mentioned, to, basically, getting high. Some of these states can feel really energizing and really illuminating. And we can start to see awakening as a state of consciousness, or a state of mind, rather than as a stage of development. So we keep going for these feelings of being energized, and high, and seeing it all as interconnected, as opposed to the somewhat more mundane work of figuring out how to get along with people well as though we really appreciate our interdependence.

My friend and meditation teacher Jack Kornfield has a book with a wonderful title that addresses this. It's called *After the Ecstasy, the Laundry*. Nowadays, I think, you know, it's better to be a decent human being with limited spiritual awakening than someone with profound awakening but limited maturity who has difficulty getting along with others.

Now, it's possible to have spiritual awakenings in all sorts of traditions and not to advance very far developmentally. And when people like this get into challenging situations, they can regress from their enlightened position to much more immature positions.

What's missing from Buddhist psychology? What's missing from this path to enlightenment? Well, traditionally, these are solitary practices that were developed by monks, nuns, and hermits, and other renunciates. So they didn't spend a lot of time examining the interpersonal world. They didn't look at interpersonal skills. They didn't look at the ways in which, what we call in psychology, *systemic phenomena*—the way in which our embeddedness in a particular community, or our family system, or that kind of thing—shapes our experience. And they didn't look at the kind of psychological defenses we get caught in as human beings, which is projecting onto others. For example, thinking that somebody else is feeling something that really, I experienced either in myself, or with another person. So these advanced practices don't necessarily prepare practitioners very well for interpersonal life.

There's a story about this, about a great meditation master, who is in a hermitage. And the town's folks were having increasing difficulty. And they thought, we really need guidance from somebody with great wisdom. So they went up to ask him, "Would you please come down and teach?" And he said, "Nah, you know, that's not my thing. I do solitary practice."

And they visited him on several occasions and begged him to please come down. Eventually, he said, "OK." He came down. And he started coming down the mountain with the people who, in a very respectful way, were honoring him and so glad he was going to come down to share his teachings. And as they were wending their way through the marketplace, he got jostled by an old woman and suddenly, he was like this [raises fist]. The old reactions were right there, right back.

The point of the story is, unless we practice in interpersonal contexts, our interpersonal issues are likely to remain unresolved. So we need to cultivate this awareness in the rough and tumble of regular daily life, not just on the meditation cushion. And realizations that are developed in one realm may not translate to the other realm.

This may be a reason why we have this remarkably common problem that I mentioned previously. A lot of times, Asian meditation masters will come to the West, and they are unaccustomed to our more relaxed sexual mores. And they wind up having sex with their students, causing emotional trauma and disrupting communities. It seems that they haven't worked out their advanced understanding in the context of interpersonal life. Now as Western psychotherapeutic traditions are meeting the ancient Buddhist traditions, it's expanding the application of these ancient insights to interpersonal life.

Buddhist psychology is profound in its implications. Grasp a little, and you'll experience a little freedom, a little awakening. Grasp a lot, you'll experience a lot of freedom, a lot of enlightenment. And they're compatible with many aspects of other spiritual traditions as well. It doesn't have to be a Buddhist-only path. Indeed, there are many paths to awakening.

If you find Buddhist psychology intriguing, learning more about it is another way to further establish and deepen your mindfulness practice. You might consider attending a class at a local meditation center where you can get support for your practice and have opportunities to discuss the more radical implications of the practice with other meditators.

While it needn't be a Buddhist center, a lot of these Buddhist meditation centers, these days, at least in the West, operate with a strong spirit of *ehipassiko*—come and see for yourself. We'll offer these teachings, we'll let you know what others have found over the last 2,500 years, but then you look in the laboratory of your own mind to see what you discover to be true.

In our next lecture, we're going to address an aspect of practice it's essential for supporting mindfulness but has often been left out of our Western work, and particularly, Western psychotherapies—and this is ethical behavior. We're going to look at why it's been neglected, and how it can help us to become more aware, and more fulfilled, and to have a deeper practice. Thanks for listening.

Mindful Ethics as a Path to Freedom
Lecture 23

This lecture will address an aspect of practice that is essential for supporting mindfulness but that has often been left out of Western psychotherapies: ethical behavior. In this lecture, you will learn why it has been neglected and how it can help us be more aware and fulfilled. When we commit unethical acts, in fantasy or in reality, paying mindful attention to the whole process can transform our behavior. Being mindful of the moment-to-moment experience of unethical behavior can help us act more ethically.

The Role of Ethics in Buddhist and Western Psychologies

- In Buddhist psychology, ethical training is a critical component of the Eightfold Path. It's the foundation of a treatment plan designed to create well-being. In Western psychology, ethics have been seen as more the province of religious traditions. "Scientific" psychology likes to distinguish itself from religion with its strong ethical focus. Furthermore, therapists often see ethical strictures as a source of psychological distress.

- Psychotherapists put a lot of effort into trying to help their patients feel comfortable with sexual and aggressive feelings, wants, and impulses of all sorts that may not be socially sanctioned. They work hard to help their patients or clients not view their inner experience as sinful. So, many therapists avoid ethical discussions that they worry will make people less comfortable with these aspects of their mammalian nature.

- At it's extreme, mental health researchers and professionals may associate morality with sexual inhibition, dishonesty, and inability to freely express needs and wants, threatening a hallmark value of many modern societies: individual freedom.

- Recent research developments are challenging this position. We're discovering that there's a bilateral relationship between morality and well-being: Happier people act more ethically and more ethical behavior leads to greater happiness.

- While in all Buddhist traditions people are encouraged to behave ethically, contemporary Buddhist psychology emphasizes a kind of "personal research" approach. It's actually close to the kind of approach taken in Western psychology and psychotherapeutic traditions. It is about developing an empirically derived ethics—not one passed down in doctrine or from a divine source but, instead, one that comes from an attitude of *ehipasiko*, or an attitude of "come and see for yourself."

- The idea is to examine in your own experience what happens when you act ethically and what happens when you don't. The goal is to be a lifelong learner, developing ever-increasing moral sensitivity and greater capacity to live in alignment with this awareness.

- This is actually one understanding of the law of karma that we find in both Buddhist and Hindu traditions. Karma has often been viewed as though there is some system keeping track of our good and bad behavior, rewarding us with good fortune for ethical behavior and punishing us for unethical behavior.

- Another view, held by many Buddhist traditions, sees it as simply the law of cause and effect. It is the observation that certain actions tend to lead to suffering for ourselves and others, while others tend to alleviate this suffering. We're charged with discerning which is which.

- In Buddhist framework, morality is actually the behavioral manifestation of good reality testing. As our vision becomes clearer, we naturally act more ethically.

Deriving Morality Empirically
- One way in which we might embark on deriving morality empirically is by considering some traditional ethical guidelines,

but using them as tools of inquiry rather than hard-and-fast rules. These are sometimes described as "training wheels" that we can use until wisdom and compassion develop sufficiently to guide our action.

- In the Buddhist tradition, there are five ethical precepts, or training guidelines for lay practitioners. (Monks, on the other hand, have hundreds of detailed rules designed to both support their meditation practice and keep the community harmonious.) While sometimes treated as prohibitions, many Buddhist traditions see the five precepts more as guidelines for living skillfully. They frame a discipline, which when undertaken, helps to calm and focus the mind, allowing for the development of what has been called moral sensitivity.

- Thich Nhat Hanh's formulation of these is to pair restraint, the traditional prohibition, with ethical action. It starts with the first of the five precepts, which is restraint from killing. He expands this to include compassionate action, reverence for life, and working to prevent others from killing.

- The second traditional precept is restraint from stealing. This is expanded to mean concern for equity and generosity; not possessing anything that should belong to others; sharing our time, energy, and material things with those in need; and working to stop social injustice.

- The third precept involves sexual misconduct. Of course, this is defined differently in different cultures, but it basically means skillfulness with sexual energy and protecting the safety and integrity of individuals, couples, families, and society. It also involves respecting my commitments and the commitments of others.

- The fourth precept is restraint from lying. This simply involves using honest and skillful speech. (Right speech is one component of the Eightfold Path.) This includes cultivating loving speech, deep listening, and refraining from uttering words that can cause division or discord.

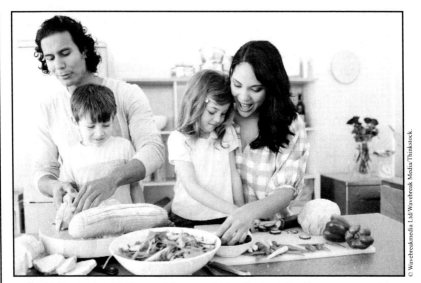

Ethical behavior can be learned from one's family, but it has been neglected in modern times.

- The fifth is restraint in using intoxicants. The positive formulation of this is to simply be aware of consumption and consume in a way that cultivates good health, both physical and mental, for myself, my family, and my society. It involves practicing mindful eating, drinking, and consuming of all sorts, including avoiding the consumption of toxic food and drink and also toxic TV programs, magazines, books, films, and conversations.

- In the Buddhist tradition, these ethical precepts are part of a threefold training. Buddhist training requires attention and effort in three dimensions: concentration (*samadhi*), insight (*prajna*), and moral action (*sila*). These are interdependent; each one potentiates the other two.

- Undertaking the precepts creates a calming, settling effect in one's life that aids concentration. Greater concentration leads to more insight, which in turn deepens and refines our understanding of and ability to embody the moral precepts. *Sila* (morality practice) pushes and develops our understanding, while also being an expression of our understanding.

- Each precept represents a continuum, offering the opportunity to attend, practice, and learn with increasing refinement in wisdom and skillful means. Practicing with the precepts involves reflection, intentionality with behavior, and awareness of cause and effect.

- Practice involves taking care with a light touch. Most of us discover that precepts are actually impossible to keep—which helps cultivate humility. So, we undertake five precepts knowing that we'll regularly fail, and we commit to paying attention to what happens when we keep, or don't keep, the precepts.

- Each time, we learn more about the causes, conditions, and outcomes of our behavior. We need willingness to begin again, time after time—much like trying to simply be with the breath in meditation practice.

How Do Ethical Violations Cause Suffering?

- Most people discover that violating the precepts leads to a lot of personal suffering. There are many levels of suffering, and they can be arranged from coarse to subtle. At a very coarse level, there is fear of external consequences. "I'll get caught and punished"; "people will judge or reject me."

- A little subtler is the feeling of not living up to what psychologists call the ego ideal, which is the ideal self-image. This is somewhat variable across cultures. Many of us think of ourselves as "bad" for having, or acting out of, lust, greed, anger, or jealously.

- More subtle yet is noticing the suffering of others and feeling empathy or compassion. Also quite subtle is noticing the stress or tension associated with pursuing desire. All unethical behavior involves pursuing desire—for example, killing to enjoy the taste of meat or vanquishing an enemy or stealing to enjoy having something that doesn't belong to us, or lying to enjoy either being seen in a positive light by others or getting material gain.

- Notice that tension, or lack of peace, is associated with all of these. Meditation can be quite painful after unethical action. Ultimately, seeing that the fruits of unethical behavior (getting the ill-gotten goods) isn't sustaining. It doesn't feel deserved, is transient, and perturbs the mind.

- This empirical approach is, of course, different from what we see in many cultural traditions. As such, we can feel uneasy approaching ethics with so much value relativism. To deal with this, it can be useful to step back and look at the various ways that we humans organize ourselves to create greater harmony.

- Often, we employ a notion of sin, and we use this notion to try to get one another to act ethically. Implicitly, problematic behavior is understood to be the end point of a chain of events. We're often taught to try to cut off unethical behavior as early in the chain as possible.

- The chain begins with sensory experience—seeing, hearing, touching, tasting, or experiencing some mental content. This leads to the desire to increase pleasure or decrease pain, which in turn gives rise to an urge or impulse, which ultimately gives rise to the behavior. To gain control over our behavior, we're often taught to interrupt this chain of events as early as possible.

- To at least some extent, we've almost all been encouraged to limit tempting sensory inputs. Usually, this is most pronounced around sexuality. We learn not to stare at others we might find to be attractive, and we might learn to dress modestly to not tempt others. At a little later stage in the chain, we attempt to interrupt the sequence by trying to clamp down on the urge or impulse when it has already arisen—to declare the urges as sinful.

- Many of us learn a mix of these first two approaches. The first approach leads to living in fear of certain stimuli. We experience tension or constriction as we work to keep sensations and perceptions out of awareness. The second approach creates fears of losing control. What if we were to give in to a forbidden impulse? People can become afraid of all sorts of urges, including sexual attraction toward the wrong partner; desires for money, power, or status; and temptations to lie or steal.

- A third approach, for which mindfulness practice can lend support, is to notice and accept stimuli in our environment, notice and accept the urges that arise in response to those stimuli, but be able to freely choose whether or not to act on those urges.

- How can we work mindfully with sinful thoughts and feelings? We begin by reflecting on how different cultures approach a problem, and we recognize how they all naturally strive for moral behavior—including social harmony and justice.

- So, it becomes a practical challenge: How can we best ensure our own ethical behavior? Might it be okay to maintain ethical behavior but allow not-so-ethical-seeming sensations, feelings, thoughts, and urges into awareness?

- Mindfulness—awareness of present experience with acceptance—can help us notice and accept these sorts of mental contents. And, paradoxically, it seems that if we can accept such mental contents, we're actually less likely to act on them.

- This is because when we get to know our wishes and reflect on their likely consequences, they're less likely to take us by surprise. Many people are afraid to do this, fearing that if we give our minds too much leeway, our behavior will get out of control. But, in reality, just the opposite happens: We gain more freedom of choice.

Hanh, *Creating True Peace.*

———, *For a Future to Be Possible.*

Morgan, "Compassion and Wisdom."

———, "Practical Ethics."

Questions to Consider

1. What are the five ethical precepts for lay practitioners in Buddhist traditions? Do they make sense to you as guidelines for living life?

2. Which precepts do you find most challenging to adhere to? What happens in your mind, and in your relationships, when you don't adhere to one or more of them?

Mindfulness Practice

ethical reflection: A useful practice to support developing mindful ethics.

five in five: A program for integrating the five ethical precepts of Buddhist traditions into our lives, by focusing on one precept each week for five weeks.

Mindful Ethics as a Path to Freedom
Lecture 23—Transcript

In Plato's *Republic*, Socrates argues that the just man is happy and the unjust man is miserable. And he goes on to say that the best and most just character is the happiest. Contemporary research seems to back this up.

Using data from the 2005 to 2006 world values study, Henry S. James, an economist at the University of Missouri, found that people living in the four largest economies of the Western hemisphere—that's the US, Canada, Mexico, and Brazil—who don't justify unethical actions have higher reported well-being than those who justify them.

Controlling for other factors that have been shown to predict happiness and well-being, these folks came out ahead in terms of happiness. And pretty much all of the world's religious and philosophic traditions agree that behaving ethically is an essential ingredient in living life well.

Yet people in modern societies often view conventional ethical codes with some suspicion, as though they are vestiges of pre-scientific, even oppressive orthodoxies. Well, it turns out that mindfulness practice can offer a useful middle way between these views. Without blindly accepting moral doctrines passed down from bygone eras, mindfulness practices can help us to develop and live by an empirically derived ethical code, and this code has the potential to form a foundation for personal as well as societal well-being.

Mindfulness practices can help us to discover that ethical action isn't a zero-sum game. Acting in a way that respects the rights and desires of others can actually make each of us feel freer and happier ourselves. It's another example of a theme we've discussed before: that by practicing restraint, we can actually find a new freedom.

Here's how the Dalai Lama put it:

> It is in everybody's interest to do what leads to happiness and avoid that which leads to suffering. And because, as we've seen, our

interests are inextricably linked, we are compelled to accept ethics as the indispensable interface between my desire to be happy and yours.

Let's look a little bit at the role of ethics in Buddhist as well as Western psychologies. In Buddhist psychology, ethical training is seen as the critical component of the Eightfold Path. It's the foundation of a treatment plan that's designed to create well-being. After all, it's been said that it's hard to have a good meditation session after a day of raping, pillaging, and stealing.

In Western psychology, ethics have been seen as more the province of religious traditions. In fact, scientific psychology likes to distinguish itself from religion with a strong ethical focus. And furthermore, therapists, in particular, see ethical strictures as a source of a lot of psychological distress.

Psychotherapists generally put a lot of effort into trying to help their clients or patients feel comfortable with sexual and aggressive feelings, with wants, longings, impulses of all sorts that may not be socially sanctioned, and that may violate ethical codes. They work hard to help their patients or clients not view their inner experience as sinful. So many therapists avoid ethical discussions and they worry that these discussions would actually make people less comfortable with these inner aspects of their mammalian nature. At its extreme, mental health researchers and professionals may associate morality with sexual inhibition, with dishonesty, with the inability to freely express needs and wants. They see them as threatening a hallmark value of many modern societies, which is individual freedom.

Recent research developments, though, are really challenging this position. We're discovering that there's a bilateral relationship between morality and well-being. Happier people actually act more ethically, and more ethical behavior actually leads to greater happiness.

While in all Buddhist traditions, people are encouraged to behave ethically, contemporary Buddhist psychology emphasizes a kind of personal research approach. And it's actually close to the kind of methodology or approach we would take in Western psychological or psychotherapeutic circles.

So this is about developing an empirically derived ethics, not one passed down in doctrine from a divine source, but rather one that comes from an attitude of *ehipassiko*, of come and see for yourself. The idea is to examine in your own experience what happens when you act ethically and what happens when you don't. The goal is to become a lifelong learner, to develop an increasing moral sensitivity and a greater capacity to live in alignment with what you discover.

This is actually one understanding of the law of karma that we find in both Buddhist and Hindu traditions. Karma has often been viewed as though there's some system keeping track of our good and bad behavior, rewarding us with good fortune for ethical behavior, and punishing us with bad fortune for unethical behavior. Another view, which is held by many Buddhist traditions, sees it as simply the law of cause and effect.

It's the observation that certain actions lead to suffering for ourselves and others while other actions tend to alleviate this suffering. And we're then charged with discerning which is which. In the Buddhist framework, morality is actually the behavioral manifestation of good reality testing. It's said that if our vision becomes clearer, we will naturally act more ethically. The Dalai Lama says that with increased insight, we will see that due to the fundamental interconnectedness, which lies at the heart of reality, your interest is also my interest.

So how might we embark on deriving morality empirically? One way is by considering some traditional ethical guidelines, but to use them as tools of inquiry rather than as hard and fast rules. These are sometimes described as "training wheels." They're rules that we might consider until we develop, through our mindfulness practice, sufficient wisdom and compassion that ethical action flows naturally.

In the Buddhist tradition, there are five of these training wheels, if you will— five ethical precepts. And these are training guidelines for lay practitioners. The monks actually have hundreds of detailed rules that are designed both to support their meditation practice and to keep the community harmonious and intact. While these rules have sometimes been treated as prohibitions, many Buddhist traditions see them more as guidelines. They frame a discipline, which when undertaken, helps to calm and focus the mind, allowing for the development of what's been called *moral sensitivity*.

Thích Nhất Hạnh, the Vietnamese Zen teacher, has a particularly nice formulation of these because what he does is he pairs the restraint, the traditional prohibition, with the ethical action that might be encouraged. Let me give you an example. It starts with the first of the five precepts, which is restraint from killing. And he expands this out to include compassionate action generally, reverence for life, and working to prevent others from killing.

The second traditional precept is restraint from stealing. And this is expanded out to mean concern for equity and generosity generally—not possessing anything that should belong to others as well as sharing our time, our energy, and material things with those in need—to work to stop social injustice.

The third precept involves sexual misconduct. And of course, this is defined differently in different cultures, but it basically means skillfulness with sexual energy. And thinking about—is my activity here protecting the safety and integrity of individuals, of couples, of families, and of society? It also involves respecting my commitments and the commitments of others.

The fourth precept is restraint from lying. And we can see this as simply using honest and skillful speech. You may recall that right speech is one component of the Eightfold Path. And this includes cultivating loving speech, and deep listening, and refraining from uttering words that can cause division or discord.

The fifth—and we talked about this earlier—is restraint in using intoxicants. The positive formulation of this is to simply be aware of consumption, and consume in a way that cultivates good health, both physical and mental, for myself, my family, and my society. And to practice mindful eating, drinking and consuming of all sorts, including to avoid the consumption of toxic food and drink, and also toxic other things like toxic TV programs, magazines, books, films, even toxic conversations.

So it's interesting to begin trying to live a life using these training wheels, considering these issues every time we engage in an action. In the Buddhist tradition, these ethical precepts are part of a threefold training. And the three dimensions are concentration or *samadhi*, which is learning to focus so we notice what's going on; insight or *prana*, which is seeing the way things work; and these moral actions, which is called *sila*. Now each one of these potentiates the other two. So undertaking the precepts, following these training wheels, if you will, creates a calming, settling effect in one's life that actually aids concentration and opens the door to wisdom.

Greater concentration leads to more insight, which in turn deepens and refines our understanding of and ability to embody the moral precepts because if we really see our interconnectedness, we are more likely to see when our behavior is causing suffering. The *sila*, or morality practice, pushes and develops our understanding while also being an expression of that understanding. It's both. It's kind of, we work the practice, and the practice works us simultaneously.

Now, these precepts aren't absolute rules. Each one represents a kind of continuum, offering the opportunity to attend, practice, and learn with increasing refinement in wisdom and skillful means. Practicing the precepts involves constantly reflecting, being intentional with our behavior, and being aware of cause and effect.

We want to do this with a light touch. This isn't about beating ourselves up for violating the rules. Most of us discover that the precepts are impossible to keep. It cultivates a lot of humility. No, we may not go out robbing banks or stealing cars, but there are little ways in which we might take what's not freely given. We might be a teacher and use somebody else's idea without crediting him or her, for example. So we understand that undertaking these five precepts is something that we do knowing that we're going to regularly fail, and we commit to simply paying attention to what happens when we keep them and what happens when we fail.

And each time, we learn more about the causes, conditions, and outcomes of our behavior. We need a willingness to constantly begin again, time after time. Very much like we do when we're doing the breath awareness training, and each time the mind wanders off like a frisky puppy to some other thought, we gently bring it back to the present moment. Each time we start getting ourselves caught in some slightly unethical behavior, we notice its consequences and we try to come back to our goal. In fact, you know in Jewish tradition, sin, or *chet*, means "missing the mark." We just notice when we miss the mark and we come back.

Most people notice that every time they violate one of the precepts, there's a little bit of suffering that happens. There's a lot of popular wisdom supporting this. There's the line, "Oh, what a web we weave, when at first we do deceive." We know this. Once we start to lie, things get complicated quickly.

Or Mark Twain's wonderful observation, where he said, "You know, I just can't be a liar. I don't have a good enough memory." It's hard when we start to lie, because it's hard to remember who we told what to, and trying to get the story straight to not get into trouble.

So how do our ethical violations, both the little ones and the big ones, cause suffering? Well, there's a lot of levels to this, and we can think of these as being arranged kind of from the coarser to the more subtle. At a very coarse level, there is fear of external consequences. Uh-oh. I'll get caught and I'll be punished. Either I'll literally be punished—I'll be fined or sent to jail—or people will judge or reject me because they'll think I'm not an ethical person.

At the next, more subtle level, we feel badly because we're not living up to what psychologists call the *ego ideal*, which is our ideal sense of self-image, the image of who we think we're supposed to be, which is often formed in childhood by our parents either praising or admonishing us for various behaviors. And this, of course, can be very different across cultures, the ideals about how we're supposed to be. But many of us wind up feeling that we are bad if we either experience or act out of lust, or greed, or anger, or jealousy, or so many of the not so noble aspects of human behavior.

More subtle yet, and at a greater level of wisdom, we just notice the suffering of others and we feel empathy and compassion when we cause suffering to others. And at a very subtle level, we may notice that what we call stress

472

occurs every time that we start pursuing a desire in a way that might be harmful to others. And all unethical behavior involves pursuing desire.

If I'm violating the precept about killing—not murdering somebody, but maybe I'm just doing it to enjoy the taste of meat, or maybe to vanquish an enemy—it's pursuing a desire. Or stealing—taking some little thing— it's to enjoy having something that doesn't belong to me. Or lying, which sometimes is just bending the truth a little bit to enjoy being seen in a more positive light by others, or maybe getting some small material gain. And certainly sexual misconduct—that's about pursuing the pleasure of sex, or probably more often, the ego boost that it can bring. And with intoxicants, we talked extensively about this, it's about having relief from discomfort, or getting a high. We notice if we approach all these things mindfully, that there's a kind of tension, a kind of lack of peace associated with all of these. Meditation can be quite painful after unethical action.

Ultimately, we also see that the fruits of unethical behavior aren't very sustaining. It doesn't feel deserved. If you cheat on a test, or you get more money but you didn't deserve it, it doesn't feel so good. We see that these things are transient. The sexual pleasure that comes from sexual misconduct doesn't last very long. And most important, we see that all of these activities perturb the mind. And this empirical approach is, of course, very different from what we see in a lot of cultural traditions that have ethical rules that we need to follow. And because of this, we can feel uneasy approaching ethics with so much value relativism.

One way to deal with this, that I think of it myself, and I also try to help my patients think about it this way, is to step back and look at the various ways that we humans have organized ourselves to create greater harmony. Very often, we employ some kind of notion of sin. And we use this notion to get one another to act ethically. Now, implicitly we're understanding that problematic behavior is the endpoint of a chain of events. And often, we try to cut off this unethical behavior as early in the chain as possible. Let me explain.

The chain often begins with sensory experience—with seeing something, hearing something, touching, tasting, or experiencing some mental content.

And then it's followed by desire, right? We see it as pleasurable, and we want to increase the pleasure, decrease the pain. And that gives rise to an urge or impulse, which ultimately leads us to our behavior. So to gain control over the behavior, we can interrupt this chain at any point. But most cultures try to interrupt it very early on—they try to keep us from even having the sensory experience.

To at least some extent, we've all been taught or encouraged to limit tempting sensory inputs. It's kind of like putting blinders on a horse. We see this most around sexuality. We learn not to stare at others that we might find to be attractive if it might make them uncomfortable. And we learned to dress modestly so as not to tempt other people.

Now a little later stage in the chain, we try to interrupt the sequence by clamping down on the urge or impulse after it's already risen. And this is to declare our urge as sinful. In other words, if I notice myself wanting to take what's not freely given, or coveting my neighbor's wife, I interpret this is a sin and I try to shut it down when it arises. And many of us learn a mix of these two approaches—don't be tempted, don't go near the tempting thing; and then if you feel these feelings, try to shut them down.

Now, the first approach leads to living in a world where we're kind of afraid of stimuli. We experience a kind of tension or constriction whenever we get near something that might tempt us. The second approach creates all sorts of fears of losing control. What if I gave in to the forbidden impulse? I'd be a terrible person. And people can become afraid of all sorts of stimuli and urges. Certainly sexual attraction toward the wrong partner is a biggie. But so is desires for money, power, or status, or even temptations to lie or steal—again, not always in big ways; sometimes in very little ways.

Now, there's a third approach for which mindfulness practice can lend us support. And that's to simply notice and accept all of the stimuli in our environment (awareness of present experience with acceptance) and notice and accept the urges that arise in response to those stimuli (here too, awareness of present experience with acceptance) but then to be able to freely choose whether or not to act on the urges.

474

I was once teaching a workshop for a psychotherapist down in South Carolina, and an older woman came up to me, and she told me that she was a graduate of a very conservative evangelical seminary and she writes for *Christian Counseling Today*. And she was enjoying this class on mindfulness practice. And she was concerned that in her tradition, so many people rejected parts of their experience as sinful, and she realized that this is causing them a lot of unnecessary suffering, because people felt tormented by their inner experiences and were very often worried about being punished by God for having a thought or feeling.

And she thought mindfulness practices could help them to become more accepting of the contents of their minds as well as of themselves as people when they didn't behave ethically as they might want to, or when the contents of their mind weren't the most noble. The problem was, she didn't want it to seem like humanism, because in her tradition, that meant putting human reason above God's message, and that would be a problem. So we worked together to find ways to present mindfulness practice and acceptance of experience that would be consonant with scripture. And in this process, we looked for an approach that wasn't about violating or bending ethical principles, but it was about distinguishing between unethical feelings and impulses and unethical action. It was about determining where in the chain toward unethical behavior it's most skillful to interrupt the sequence to behave in a way that promotes wellness, rather than suffering.

So how do we do this? Well, one way I work with this clinically, very often, is by talking to my clients or patients about how different cultures approach this problem. And recognize that everybody wants, at some level, to be moral, and societies need us to be moral to have social harmony and justice. So it becomes a practical challenge. How can we best ensure ethical behavior? Might it be OK to maintain ethical behavior, but allow not so ethical sensations, feelings, and thoughts to emerge in consciousness?

I had a recent experience in my psychotherapy office that dealt with this. I've changed details to protect the gentleman's confidentiality. A patient of mine who is a mechanic in his mid-40s had fallen into a very painful depression, and he was having suicidal thoughts along with feelings of worthlessness. And we did the usual discussion of his safety and figuring out how he could check on his medications to make sure that they were optimal for his current status and his current situation. And then we began exploring his depression. With great difficulty, and with great sincerity, he asked me if he thought he'd need to kill himself if he ever had sexual feelings toward his goddaughter. And this is a perfect example of how, when we try to interrupt the chain of action early, we can create enormous suffering for ourselves.

Now that his goddaughter is getting older, he's noticing how pretty she is, and she's heading toward becoming a young woman. And he's terrified that this will lead to sexual thoughts or impulses. When he was a teenager, he had a few inappropriate contacts with younger girls, which until this session, he had never revealed to anyone, and about which he still felt very ashamed and very guilty. So he worried that if he ever felt a sexual impulse toward his goddaughter, that would make him so despicable, he couldn't go on living.

As we explored his thoughts and feelings, it became clear that he didn't have a distinction in his mind between the thought and feeling and the harmful action. It took some discussion, but he eventually felt enormously relieved to realize that he might actually accept these thoughts and feelings, even while being quite clear with himself that he would never act on them or harm his goddaughter in this way.

So mindfulness, awareness of present experience with acceptance can help us to do this. To simply notice and be with these thoughts and feelings when they come up. And paradoxically, it seems that if we can accept these contents, we're actually less likely to act on them. This is because when we really know our wishes, when we really know our impulses, and we really know our desires, and we can reflect on their consequences, they're less likely to come and take us by surprise. They're less likely to overwhelm us and move automatically into action. A lot of people are afraid of doing this because they're afraid that if they give their minds too much leeway, their behavior will get out of control. But in reality, just the opposite happens: We gain more freedom of choice.

We can try a little mindfulness exercise together to reflect on where in the chain we each focus in our efforts to behave ethically, and how to give ourselves more leeway to accept our not so noble impulses. And we can do this by bringing our attention to what happens if we entertain an unethical fantasy.

This is an opportunity for ethical reflection. Bring to mind an unethical impulse that you've had sometime in the past. It can really be anything. Maybe exaggerating a business expense on a tax return, or telling a white lie to get out of trouble or not hurt someone's feelings. Or maybe it involved bigger things, like infidelity or stealing, or maybe deliberately hurting somebody in a moment of anger.

Now develop the fantasy a little bit. What's the time? What's the place? Who else might be present? How would the environment be in the moment in which you're doing this not so ethical act? And then, what do you notice in the mind and the body when contemplating doing it?

Now imagine going through with it. Or, if this triggers a memory of an actual unethical act, something you actually did, recall what the experience was of going through with it. Now what do you notice in the mind and the body? What comes up?

Finally, imagine it's the next day, or the next week, and you're recalling your behavior. What then do you feel? What's the reaction?

This can be a very fruitful practice. The Dalai Lama says, "It is far more useful to be aware of a single shortcoming in ourselves than it is to be aware of 1,000 shortcomings in someone else. For when the fault is our own, we're actually in a position to correct it."

Paying mindful attention to the whole process in fantasy, or in reality, when we actually commit unethical acts, can transform our behavior. Just as eating meditation, where being mindful of eating leads us to snarf down less food, being mindful of moment-to-moment experience of unethical behavior can help us to act more ethically.

A good friend recently told me about what happened when he wasn't so mindful about his behavior. He had been a very shy, socially anxious boy and young man. Nonetheless, he was bright and an innovative thinker, and he felt inspired to teach in his field. So he managed systematically to overcome his inhibition through consistent, diligent effort, facing his fears repeatedly, getting in front of audiences and speaking, and he eventually got to the point where he was widely sought after as an excellent presenter.

He said that eventually he didn't feel self-conscious at all. It felt like the material he taught was simply flowing through him effortlessly—until the day he was on a business trip, met an attractive colleague, and went to bed with her. The problem was he happened to be married. And as the affair continued, his self-consciousness returned. He found that he was again preoccupied with what others would think of him, and he lost his whole sense of ease and freedom as a teacher that he had worked so hard to cultivate. It was a hard way to learn that it's indeed difficult to have a good meditation after a day of raping, pillaging, and stealing. (I'm being metaphorical, you know.)

So as we are mindful of ethics in daily life, we can all experiment with bringing mindfulness to every little ethical decision. The next time you feel torn as to whether or not to do something that you have some moral questions about, take a moment to breathe and check-in to what's happening right now. Ask—what's my intention in doing this? Try to take a deep sounding and rest with the reflection. Notice what feelings and associations arise. And as you emerge with awareness of your intention, appreciate it, and let it help guide your decision.

Now, most Buddhist traditions don't actually teach mindfulness of ethics in the way that I've been suggesting. Because they say that *sila*, or morality practice, is a necessary basis for beginning to practice mindfulness. But then again, the traditional approaches wouldn't prescribe mindfulness to work with psychological disorders in the way we've been talking about throughout the course either. They would first have the person live in the community and learn how to have a stable, productive life as a citizen, before teaching meditation.

So the Buddhist traditions typically suggest that you study and learn to follow ethical precepts before taking up mindfulness meditation. But in this more modern approach to it, the one that's done in modern Buddhist psychology, we use the mindfulness practice to illuminate ethical decisions. And here's a way that we can do this latter approach in a way that may suit our sensibilities quite well in the West.

This meditation my friend Stephanie Morgan came up with, and it's called the "five-in-five." Here's what you do. You choose one precept to focus on each week for five weeks. And you decide to focus on it in your personal life and your outside activities. For the first week, you choose one that you feel most aligned with, that's relatively easy to follow. In the last one, you work with the one that you find most challenging, that's the biggest stumbling block for you. And you try to arrange them in order of how easy they are to work with over the course of the five weeks.

Remember, the five classical precepts are restraint from and cultivating the opposite of killing. So, we're not going to kill and we're going to try to have compassionate action and reverence for life. This could mean not eating meat—something to consider. We're not going to steal. We're not going to in any way take things that aren't freely given to us, and this means concern for equity and generosity. We're going to try to avoid sexual misconduct. We're going to be skillful with our sexual energy, generally. That even might mean not flirting in a way that might cause damage to somebody else. We're going to try to not lie. We're going to be as honest and skillful in our speech as we can. And we're going to be mindful of our use of intoxicants, the awareness of consumption, and not consume things in a way that's going to perpetuate suffering.

Now, if you think of those five precepts, or the training wheels, if you will, how might you arrange them? Which is easiest for you to practice? Which comes naturally and doesn't require any effort at all? Which is harder? Which requires some thought and effort?

So you might start each day refreshing your intention to work with the practice of the week. Write it down somewhere where you can see it regularly throughout the day. And then reflect at the day's end. What causes and conditions made it more or less difficult to practice with the precept? Keep a light touch. Remember, we're working to refine our behavior, not to eliminate less-than-noble thoughts and feelings. And we're not going to get this perfect—we're going to fail regularly. Like all mindfulness practices, it's designed to increase your awareness of present experience with acceptance, not to turn you into some kind of saint.

So by exercising restraint, the impulse or desire for unethical behavior may be illuminated. Simply allow yourself to see what is.

In our next lecture, we're going to come back to examining how mindfulness leads to happiness and well-being. And we'll see how mindfulness practices can support pathways to well-being revealed by current research into the nature of happiness. We'll also see how this research is supporting the notion that ethical action is a cornerstone of living richer, more fulfilling lives. Thanks.

The New Science of Happiness
Lecture 24

The relatively new field of positive psychology seems to be confirming what ancient wisdom traditions have long suggested: There is a reliable path to well-being. And it involves living in the moment and being connected to and caring for others. Modern research is also confirming the ancient teaching that walking this path requires continued intention and effort. Otherwise, we just drift back to our set point. This is one of the many reasons why it is so vital to engage regularly in mindfulness practices.

The Pursuit of Happiness

- In recent years, a new field of psychology has developed that is focused on researching pathways to well-being, and what it is discovering about human happiness dovetails remarkably well with what we've learned through studying and practicing mindfulness.

- Clinical psychology developed after World War II essentially to treat all of the soldiers who were returning home from the battlefield with mental health difficulties. Its focus paralleled psychiatry—treating disorders.

- In 1998, after studying depression for many years, a leading psychologist named Martin Seligman coined a new term: positive psychology. And that initiated the formal study of the science of happiness. One of the first questions this new discipline investigated is, what are the ramifications of happiness, or well-being? How might it affect our health or capacity to be effective in our lives?

- They quickly discovered that happiness is indeed good for our health. Studies show that positive mental attitudes reduce the risk or limit the severity of cardiovascular disease, pulmonary disease, diabetes, hypertension, colds, and upper respiratory infections.

- Just as anger or sadness tends to bring about predictable cognitive and behavior patterns, such as loss of intellectual ability and limited life activities, happiness brings about the opposite. This is known as the broaden and build model, which was proposed by Barbara Fredrickson. She found that happiness boosts several aspects of cognition, including clarity, accuracy, creativity and concentration, and it supports our ability to play and our connection with others.

- The U.S. Declaration of Independence guarantees the right to life, liberty, and the pursuit of happiness. But there's a problem with pursuing it like it's some sort of fugitive. It turns out that people who are happy don't actually think about it a lot—they aren't pursuing it. This is the inverse of the paradox that occurs with so many symptoms of psychological distress: What you resist persists. Instead, this paradox is as follows: What you pursue flees. An alternative attitude is learning to let be and let go.

- Just as our bodies have set points in regard to our weight, we have set points for happiness. We have certain levels of well-being that we tend to return to after either positive or negative experiences— after good or bad fortune. There are a lot of things that everybody thinks work but don't. For example, almost everyone thinks that wealth, education or high IQ, and sunny days will make them happier, but this is not the case. Research shows that even being young doesn't work.

- What also doesn't work is indulgence and pleasure and status seeking. Almost everybody knows that some of these can cause trouble, including drugs or alcohol, sex, work, power, and food. Even achievement, which most people assume is a good thing, can fail us.

- On the other hand, asceticism and passivity—the opposite of an achievement orientation—generally don't work either. Ultimately, the Buddha had to find a middle way between pleasure seeking and asceticism. This middle way begins with finding balance between the two poles. It's not always easy to identify; it's easy to err in either direction.

Positive Psychology

- Positive psychology research suggests that the attitudes and activities that mindfulness practice engenders work to make us happy. And it starts with training the mind to "be here now."

- Practicing bringing our attention repeatedly to the present moment trains the mind to be in the present. And when the mind is in the present, it can appreciate moment-to-moment experience.

- When scientists have tried to identify sources of well-being that are not subject to the hedonic treadmill, one that comes up repeatedly is savoring. This is simply noticing and appreciating what's happening here and now.

- With mindfulness practice, we discover that to fully savor, we need to be willing continuously to let go. Otherwise, we can get caught in one of the more comic forms of *dukkha*, which is the mind's tendency to complain and to feel dissatisfied. It's called the *dukkha* of change or impermanence: As soon as we're no longer complaining that something is not to our liking—when our experience is just right—we realize that it won't last and start complaining about that.

- Mindfulness practice can help us savor experience in the moment, enjoying it in the moment while understanding its fleeting nature, allowing it to arise and pass like all phenomena, and knowing that it's impermanent. It's only by letting go, over and over, that we can find more lasting well-being.

- In recent years, there has been a shift in the field of positive psychology. In the early days, the emphasis was on how to experience pleasure, including savoring pleasure. Now, engagement is showing itself to be much more important for well-being.

- Psychologist Mihaly Csikzentmihalyi initiated and popularized the term "flow." In athletic terms, people often use the word "zone," as in being "in the zone," to represent a flow experience. In flow experiences, there's no hedonic treadmill, and we're experiencing gratification rather than pleasure. There's reduced self-consciousness, so we're not involved in a lot of self-referential thought. Flow occurs when our strengths engage challenges in an even balance. We don't necessarily feel pleasure, but we feel gratification.

- Mindfulness supports engagement by bringing full attention to what's happening in the present moment, by helping us step out of the thought stream, and by loosening our attachment to pursuing pleasure and avoiding pain.

Gratitude and Forgiveness

- Of all the specific interventions designed by positive psychologists, the most powerful involve gratitude. Fortunately, mindfulness practice also supports gratitude by helping us appreciate our interconnection. This helps us appreciate others' roles in our good fortune by reducing "selfing"—reducing our preoccupation with pride, with "me" being the star of the show—and by allowing us to open up and feel tender and vulnerable.

- Gratitude involves having a tender heart and being touched by the caring or help of another. One example of a gratitude intervention is a gratitude visit, which involves writing to someone to whom you feel gratitude, but whom you've never adequately thanked, and then visiting him or her. Research shows that doing this only once makes people measurably happier and less depressed one month later. Other studies found that just sending a letter, without a visit, also works.

- A close relative of gratitude is forgiveness. This, too, can be enormously freeing. When we can't forgive, we hold onto resentment. Forgiveness needs to be done thoughtfully, though.

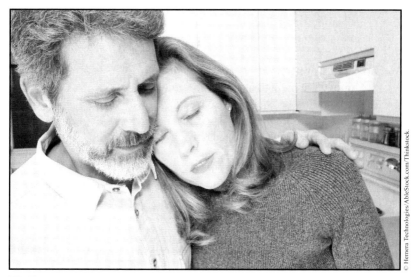

Mindfulness practice supports both gratitude and forgiveness.

- There are several potential pitfalls. Letting go of grudges before we're really ready can be counterproductive. Anger then festers. The premature closing down of affect eventually causes us to suffer symptoms as the feelings seek expression. Also, communicating forgiveness to someone who thinks he or she has done no wrong can lead to difficulties as the person rejects the forgiveness, interpreting it as containing an unfair accusation.

- But done at the right time, forgiveness can deepen well-being, and mindfulness practice can support forgiveness because it helps us see events through the lens of dependent origination. This is about asking what factors and forces led the other person to do what he or she did and asking, would I really have acted differently if I had the same genetics and the same environmental history as this person?

- As we learn to see our own thoughts, feelings, and behaviors as impersonal events, we see that others' actions are also impersonal events. We therefore blame less and understand the dynamics of the situation better. This leads to freedom from the past and the ability to open to relationships in the present.

Meaning and Connection
- Another area that has been shown not to be subject to the hedonic treadmill is meaning and connection. This means engagement for the benefit of something larger than ourselves. It's a positive-sum game—everyone gains, and nobody loses.

- Chris Peterson, a founder of the positive psychology movement, said that virtually all of the happiness exercises that have been tested and shown to be successful by positive psychologists make people feel more connected to others.

- There's a lot of research into meaning and connection that shows that performing acts of altruism or kindness increases happiness. For example, five acts per week showed very measurable gains. In fact, these acts are especially powerful if they are all done in a single day.

Suggested Reading

Gilbert, *Stumbling on Happiness*.

Seligman, *Authentic Happiness*.

Siegel, *The Mindfulness Solution*, chapter 11.

———, *Positive Psychology*.

Styron, "Positive Psychology and the Bodhisattva Path."

Questions to Consider

1. What are the avenues you usually pursue to find happiness? Are any of these subject to the hedonic treadmill (needing more and more to sustain a given level of well-being)?

2. How might you use the lessons of positive psychology research to focus your energies on more reliable pathways to fulfillment?

gratitude letter: A proven technique for generating well-being through cultivating gratitude.

The New Science of Happiness
Lecture 24—Transcript

Luckily, we humans have evolved the capacity to explore, experiment, and learn from our experience. And while our aversion to pain has both saved us from countless injuries and led us into all manner of distress, it's also led some pioneering individuals to find effective ways to work with it. In recent years, a new field of psychology has developed that's focused on researching pathways to well-being. And what it's discovering about human happiness dovetails remarkably well with what we've learned through studying and practicing mindfulness.

Clinical psychology developed after World War II, essentially to treat all of the soldiers who were returning home from the battlefield with mental health difficulties. And its focus paralleled psychiatry—treating disorders. The idea was to move people from negative five on the scale of well-being to neutral, to zero or normal.

In 1998, after studying depression for many years, a leading psychologist named Martin Seligman coined a new term, "positive psychology." And that initiated the formal study of the science of happiness. One of the first questions this new discipline investigated was—what are the ramifications of happiness or well-being? How might it affect our health or our capacity to be effective in our lives? They quickly discovered that happiness is indeed quite good for our health. There are many studies, my favorite one of which involves 678 elderly nuns. And these are women who many, many years ago, when they were 17 or 18 years of age and they entered the convent, had to write essays about their lives, about their aspirations, their feelings, their experience to date. And the psychologists went in and they acquired those essays and they rated them. They had ways to evaluate and code them for well-being when these nuns were young.

What they discovered was that those nuns who were optimistic or had a positive outlook in youth tended to have a positive outlook in old age. The striking finding was the top quartile in well-being lived 9.3 years longer than the bottom quartile. It turned out that a negative outlook or pessimism was a more powerful risk-factor for death than smoking or alcoholism. There have been many other studies that also show that positive mental attitudes reduce the risk or limit the severity of all sorts of difficulties, including cardiovascular disease, pulmonary disease, diabetes, hypertension, even colds and upper respiratory infections.

Why else be happy? you may ask. Well, just as anger or sadness leads to pretty predictable kinds of cognitive and behavioral patterns that are problematic, such as loss of intellectual ability and limited life activities, so happiness brings about the opposite. This has been called the "broaden-and-build model of well-being."

Barbara Frederickson, who studied this extensively, found that happiness boosts many aspects of cognition. It makes us clearer in our thinking. It makes us more accurate in various cognitive tasks. It makes us more creative. It improves our concentration. And it supports our ability to play and our ability to connect with others.

So clearly, happiness or well-being is a good thing. I mentioned earlier that the US Declaration of Independence guarantees the right to life, liberty, and the pursuit of happiness. But there's a problem with pursuing it like it's some sort of fugitive. It turns out that people who are happy don't actually think about it a lot—they aren't pursuing it.

It's kind of the inverse of the paradox we saw with so many different symptoms of psychological distress and physical pain, the idea that what you resist persists. Well, when it comes to well-being it turns out that what you pursue flees. Or, as my favorite refrigerator magnet which I have prominently displayed at home puts it, "let go or be dragged."

Now, many of you may be familiar with the concept of "set points." There was a discovery some years ago that we have set points for weight and that these are active when we try to diet, when we try to lose weight. It turns out that our bodies have a natural weight that they gravitate toward. Now, we can change this with effort. For example, if we want to lose weight, and we exercise regularly and we also restrict our calorie intake, indeed we'll move from the set point. We'll lose weight. Or, not that too many people want to do this, but if you wanted to gain weight, you could do that by being particularly gluttonous and sedentary. And you'd move off your set point. But as soon as we stop trying, we come back to our pre-existing set point. And this is set largely genetically, but also somewhat through our life experience of eating.

It turns out we also have set points for happiness. We have certain levels of well-being that we tend to return to after either positive or negative experiences, after good or bad fortune. Many people who have raised more than one child have seen this. We see, you know, some kids are just naturally happier. They roll with the punches. They see the bright side. And other kids are naturally more distressed. The negativity bias seems to be more powerful for them and they see trouble in everything that occurs.

Now, these set points don't determine everything. We can affect them, but it takes some consistent effort on our part to shift our set points. Because of our set points, we generally don't do such a good job of recognizing that things aren't as good or as bad as they seem. We tend to think that life events are going to determine our well-being but as it turns out, life events aren't all that important.

Sonja Lyubomirsky at the University of California, Riverside, and her colleagues have asked the question, "What determines our level of happiness?" And they found in group studies that 50 percent of the variance is simply genetic, has to do with those set points we're talking about. And those we're pretty much born with. Forty percent of the variance has to do with our attitude toward experience, what we do with the good or bad fortune that comes our way.

The really striking finding to my mind is that only 10 percent of the variance, a tiny slice of the pie, has to do with good or bad fortune. And this is really wild to think about, because when I watch my mind, my mind is always angling or scheming for how to maximize good fortune. I'll choose this restaurant instead of that one. It'll make me happier. Well, I'll dress this way instead of that way. I'll be more comfortable. I'm always looking for good fortune. And that's in the small ways and much larger ways as well. But it turns out that when we have good or bad fortune, we simply come back to our same level of well-being.

So we wind up being terrible at predicting what will make us happy. Many of the things we turn to in the pursuit of happiness are subject to what scientists call the *hedonic treadmill*, from the root word for hedonism, right? Pleasure. We need more and more of these things just to stay at the same level of well-being.

And there are a lot of things that everybody thinks work but don't. I'll share with you a few of them. Most everybody thinks—wealth will make me happier. If only I had more money. Well, the research about this is a little bit mixed, but in aggregate it says that once we meet basic needs, which in the developed world means a middle- to upper-middle-class standard of living, additional money simply doesn't help. And people who are very, very wealthy are certainly not any happier than people who are just comfortable. Of course, if you're at the low end of the scale and you're struggling to make ends meet, and you're worried about being able to feed your family, it definitely feels better to get to a level where you're not so panicked.

Education or high IQ don't work. This is very disappointing given all the effort that so many of us put into our educations. But we all know people who are really smart, really knowledgeable, and really, really unhappy.

Sunny days don't work, even though almost everybody thinks they help. And sunny days are a great illustration of how the hedonic treadmill works, because when we've had a stretch of either rain or snow or some kind of difficult weather and the sun comes out, yeah, we almost all feel better. And you walk around. You say, "Oh, everybody's smiling because the sun's out."

The issue is that if it's sunny continuously, every day, it doesn't work anymore. In fact, people in the upper Midwest, when they're surveyed, they believe that people in Southern California naturally would be happier because they have more sunshine there and more warmth. But it turns out they're not. In fact some of the happiest towns in America happen to be in the upper Midwest, where the weather is not very good and financially they haven't been doing that well. And it's because they have something else: They have a strong sense of community. We'll get back to that shortly.

So what you see with sunny days is what we see across the board with things that are subject to the hedonic treadmill. To move from our current level to a level of more feels pretty good. The problem is we habituate rapidly, and we habituate much more rapidly than most of us think.

Even being young doesn't work. Now most of us as we get older and we talked about changes in the body and we're not thrilled about those, right? Young bodies are kind of nice. But it turns out that people aged 20 to 24 are sad 3.4 days out of the month and people aged 65 to 74 are sad only 2.3 days out of the month, a very statistically significant and meaningful difference. And this is data gathered by our Centers for Disease Control here in the United States. There have been many other studies that point in the same direction.

The people studying positive psychology have been asking, well, why is this? And the best guess is that people over the age of 65 no longer believe that the things that are subject to the hedonic treadmill are going to work for them, so they don't get hooked on them in the same way and they wind up being happier.

Now there are other things that almost everybody goes for at some point or another but don't work very well in the long run. They're basically indulgence, pleasure-seeking, and status-seeking. Almost everybody knows that some of these can cause trouble. Too much drugs or alcohol, sex— particularly if it's not in a good relationship—too much work, even power and food, that if we go after these things for well-being, they feel good in the short run but in the long run, they don't go well.

Even achievement, which most of us assume is a good thing, can fail us. Joseph Campbell, student of the world's mythology, said, "Many people climb the ladder of success only to find that it is leaning up against the wrong wall." And you'll recall the story of my patient who sold his oil trading business for $30 million cash and still felt inadequate. He needed more.

On the other hand, asceticism, or passivity, the opposite of an achievement orientation, those doesn't work so well either. We can use as a case example the Buddha legend. You'll remember when his dad couldn't promise him that he wouldn't grow old, get sick, or die, he went out and he became a disciplined ascetic, went down to one grain of rice or one sesame seed a day. Didn't work. Ultimately, he had to find a middle way between pleasure-seeking and asceticism.

And this middle way begins with finding a balance between the two poles. It's not so easy to identify sometimes. There's a fun story about a Zen master who has one of his senior monks sitting by his side watching him all day long as the master gives counsel and advice and instruction to the other students. And the senior monk is watching carefully. He wants to learn from the master.

And by the end of the day, the senior monk has some grave misgivings. And he turns to the master. And he says, "You know, no disrespect, but gosh, your teachings are so contradictory. There's no consistency or coherence to them. Help me out here. It makes me wonder if you really know what you're talking about."

And the teacher says this. He says, "Ah, I get exactly what you mean. But this is how it looks from my perspective. I'm looking down this road. And I see one of my students and they seem to be falling into a ditch on the left. So I start yelling, 'Go right! Go right!' I see another student seems to be falling into a ditch on the right so I say, 'Go left! Go left!' I know it looks contradictory, but it's not contradictory if you see the road. This is about finding the middle path."

It's quite easy to err in either direction. The Buddha had an analogy for this. He said it's like tuning a lute, that when you're tuning a lute, if you tighten the strings too much, you can overdo it and—boing—they'll break. But if you don't do it enough, you don't get the note you want. And we're always finding our way really between indulgence and asceticism here.

So besides finding this balance, what else brings happiness? Well, not to shock you, but positive psychology research suggests that the attitudes and activities that mindfulness practice engenders, which we've been discussing throughout the course, actually work to make us happy.

And it starts with training the mind to be here now. Let me share with you a wonderful recent study that illustrates this. There's a graduate student named Matthew Killingsworth in Daniel Gilbert's lab at Harvard. Now, Dan Gilbert is a psychologist who studies fallacies about happiness. And Matthew Killingsworth devised a smartphone application. And this app would page people throughout the day. And you could volunteer to participate in the study; he got thousands of people to do this. And when the app paged you, you were to report on three things: what you were doing, how you were feeling, and where your attention was at the moment that you were paged. It turned out that it didn't matter what you were doing in terms of how you wound up feeling. What predicted people's sense of well-being or not was their attention. And if their attention was on what they were doing, they experienced more well-being.

Let me give you an example. It means that if somebody was washing the dishes when the app went off, or eating a gourmet meal, or even making love, but their mind was somewhere else, they tended to report a low level of well-being. But even something like washing dishes—if they were paying attention to it at that moment, they reported a high level of well-being. He also determined that minds wandered 46.9 percent of the time. And I suspect that's a very low estimate, because most of those people probably hadn't been practicing mindfulness and they didn't quite notice how mindless they are.

What Killingsworth didn't address was, how can we train the mind to be with experience in this way? How can we boost happiness? Well, you should have a pretty good idea of the answer at this point. By practicing bringing our attention repeatedly to the present moment, that trains the mind to be in the present. And when the mind is in the present, it can appreciate moment-to-moment experience.

When scientists have tried to identify sources of well-being that are not subject to the hedonic treadmill, one that comes up repeatedly is savoring. And this is simply noticing and appreciating what's happening here and now. Here's how the Buddha suggested we can learn to savor experience. You may recall that after his awakening he came across some schoolchildren. And they inspired him to teach. Well, he actually sat down and gave them a lesson. And here's what he said. "When you children peel a tangerine, you can eat it with awareness or without awareness. What does it mean to eat a tangerine in awareness? When you peel the tangerine, you know that you're peeling the tangerine. When you remove a slice and put in your mouth, you know that you're removing a slice and putting it in your mouth. When you experience the lovely fragrance and sweet taste of the tangerine, you're aware that you're experiencing the lovely fragrance and sweet taste of the tangerine."

With mindfulness practice, we discover that to fully savor, we need to be willing to continuously let go. Otherwise, we can get caught in one of the more comic forms of *dukkha*. You'll remember *dukkha* is the mind's tendency to always complain, to always feel dissatisfied. We've discussed it earlier. And this form of *dukkha* is called the "*dukkha* of change" or the "*dukkha* of impermanence." The way it works is as soon as we're no longer complaining that something is too warm, too cold, too sweet, too salty, or otherwise not to our liking, when we have a Goldilocks moment in which our experience feels just right, well, because we're thinking people, we realize that it won't last. And we start complaining about that. We start being upset that it's not going to last.

As William Blake advised in his famous poem called "Eternity," "He who binds to himself a joy does the winged life destroy. But he who kisses the joy as it flies, lives in eternity's sunrise." So how might we live in this eternity? Well, mindfulness can help, by helping us to savor experience in this moment, to kiss the joy as it flies, enjoying it in the moment, all the while understanding its fleeting nature and allowing it to arise and pass like all phenomena do, really knowing it's impermanent. When instead we cling to pleasure, we destroy its winged life. So it's only by letting go over and over, letting go or being dragged, that we can find more lasting well-being.

Now in recent years, there's been a shift in the field of positive psychology. In the early days, the emphasis was on how to experience pleasure, including savoring pleasure. Now, engagement is showing itself to be much more important for well-being. Let me explain what I mean by engagement.

Probably the best description of engagement comes from the work of Mihaly Csikzentmihalyi—a very difficult-to-pronounce name. He's a Hungarian psychologist—he's American, but of Hungarian descent—who works in Southern California. And he initiated and popularized the term *flow*. You may have heard of this before, about having flow experiences. And he studied what predicts flow experiences. In athletic terms, people often use the word "zone," being in the zone, to represent a flow experience. And this is what predisposes us to a flow experience.

In flow experiences, there's no hedonic treadmill. And we're experiencing gratification rather than pleasure, so there're certain characteristics to it. There's reduced self-consciousness, so we're not thinking all the time, "How am I doing?" We're not involved in a lot of self-referential thought. And it occurs when our strengths engage challenges in an even balance. And we don't necessarily feel pleasure, but we feel gratification.

Let me give you an example. If I'm skiing down the mountain and I'm in the zone or I'm having a flow experience, it may be really cold, I may be even being pelted with bits of snow or sleet, my quads might hurt. So it may not be pleasant in the sense of pleasurable versus not pleasurable sensations. But if I'm fully in the moment and the mountain is kind of at the right level for me so that I'm in the groove, I'm challenged, and I'm paying attention and I'm not worried about what everybody's going to think about me, I may find the experience to be very, very gratifying. And even if I go down that mountain the next day, it will be equally gratifying as long as I have this sense of engagement.

Now mindfulness supports engagement by bringing our full attention to what's happening in the present moment. By helping us to step out of the thought stream, we can get out of our own way. We can avoid Lolo Jones's problem that was brought about by her self-consciousness. And by loosening our attachment to pursuing pleasure and avoiding pain, so we can be with whatever's going on in the moment and not have to have it feel good, but we can be fully engaged.

Now, of all the specific interventions that have been designed by positive psychologists, the most powerful involve gratitude. Fortunately, mindfulness practice also cultivates gratitude. And it does this by helping us to appreciate our interconnection. This helps us to see others' roles in our good fortune. We no longer feel that we're necessarily the star of the show. There's less selfing and less preoccupation with pride, with me. By allowing us to open and feel tender and vulnerable feeling, we also feel more gratitude, because if you take a moment to think of a moment of gratitude you've had, it involves a kind of tender heart, a being touched by the caring help of another. And if we're tense, if we're rigid, if we're defended, we're not going to feel that so well.

Now there have been a number of gratitude interventions that have been shown repeatedly to have very big impacts on our sense of well-being. One is called the "gratitude visit." It involves writing a letter someone to whom you feel gratitude, but who you've never adequately thanked, and then visiting them and delivering the letter. Turns out that doing this only once makes people measurably happier and less depressed a month later. Later studies in fact found that it's not even necessary to deliver the letter, although that helps. Simply writing and mailing the letter also works.

Let's take a moment right now to imagine doing this. Who can you think of that has been helpful to you in some way but you've never adequately thanked? It could be a parent, a teacher, a relative, a friend. We all have folks like this. Just bring one to mind.

Who have you never adequately thanked? What would you wish to tell him or her? What would you want to thank them for?

And then imagine doing this: Imagine writing a letter and giving it to them. What feeling comes up? Can you sense the kind of tenderness in that? To fully reap the benefits of this, I encourage you sometime to actually write the letter, send it, and pay attention to how you feel.

A variation on the gratitude letter that you can try at any time is called the "gratitude journal." This is also part of Sonja Lyubormirsky's work. And she found out that asking people to simply write down what they're grateful for just once a week significantly increased the subjects' overall satisfaction with life over six weeks. And there was no change at all for a control group that was asked to write about something else. That doesn't take a lot. Just once a week sit down and write about something you're grateful for. Robert Emmons at UC Davis found that gratitude exercises improved physical health, raised people's energy levels, even relieved pain and fatigue. These are powerful.

Now a close relative of gratitude is forgiveness. And this too can be enormously freeing, because when we can't forgive, when we hold onto resentment, it's—I like this line—it's "like drinking a cup of poison and expecting the other person to die." Forgiveness, however, needs to be done thoughtfully. It takes a lot of strength actually to forgive. Mahatma Gandhi said this. "The weak can never forgive. Forgiveness is the attribute of the strong." And yet there are certain potential pitfalls. If we try to let go of grudges before we're really ready, it can be counterproductive. This is sometimes called in meditation circles a *spiritual bypass*. It's when we're actually still angry about something, still upset with somebody, but we're trying so hard to be a good person and loving and all interconnected that we fake it as though we're not. But it slips out in other ways. It slips out in passive aggressive actions, or it shows up in some symptom. We're trying so hard to keep the anger out of our awareness that we start getting stomachaches, headaches, and that kind of thing. In fact, generally, prematurely closing down on affects causes all sorts of stress and tension in the body as the tigers within threaten to roar and express themselves.

Another problem we can run into is if we communicate forgiveness to someone who thinks they haven't done anything wrong—that can create interesting problems. Of course, you go and forgive the person, they say, "What do you mean? I didn't do anything to hurt you. It was your fault." And you get into another whole problem. So it's useful if you're going to forgive somebody to be sure that they actually think that they need to be forgiven for something.

But done at the right time, forgiveness can really deepen our sense of well-being. And mindfulness practice can support forgiveness because it helps us to see events through the lens of dependent origination. We talked about this when discussing trauma before.

This is about asking what factors and forces led the other person to do what he or she did, and asking, "Would I really have acted differently if I had the same genetics and the same exact environmental history as this person?" And as we learn to see our own thoughts, feelings, and behaviors as impersonal events, we see that others' actions are also impersonal events. And this helps us to blame less and understand the dynamics—the forces and factors—that brought things about more. And it leads to freedom from the past and the ability to open into the relationship in the present. Nelson Mandela said this. He knew forgiveness was powerful. After all, he was able to forgive his jailers. And he said, "Forgiveness liberates the soul. … [And this is] why it's such a powerful weapon."

Now another area that's been shown not to be subject to the hedonic treadmill is meaning and connection. And this means engagement for the benefit of something larger than ourselves. It's a positive-sum game. Everybody gains and none lose. Chris Peterson, who was a founder of the positive psychology movement, he said virtually all of the happiness exercises that have been tested and shown to be successful by positive psychologists make people feel more connected to others. And we discussed the well-known suggestion of the Dalai Lama: "If you want others to be happy, practice compassion. If you want to be happy, practice compassion."

There's a lot of research into meaning and connection. Performing acts of altruism or kindness increases happiness. Five acts per week showed very measurable gains. So you've just got to do five nice things over the course of the week. And these are especially powerful if done in a single day. And there was a great study up in Toronto. It was published in the *Journal of Science*. And what they did was at the beginning of the day they gave people money. And they randomly assigned the folks into two groups. And one group had to take the money and spend it only on themselves. And the other group had to take the money and spend it only for the benefit of others. Guess which group was happier at the end of the day? Those who were thinking of others were feeling much better.

The relatively new field of positive psychology seems to be confirming what ancient wisdom traditions have long suggested. There is a reliable path to well-being, and it involves living in the moment and being connected to and caring for others. And modern research is also confirming the ancient teaching that walking this path requires continued intention and effort. Otherwise, we just drift back to our set point, which is why throughout this course, I've been encouraging you to take the time to practice mindfulness yourself.

People often ask me, "What resources are available to support and help deepen my practice?" And I'm happy to report that these days there are quite a few. We've been discussing throughout the course how different practices can help us when we're in different frames of mind. And you've already learned some basic practices of each type. But since we're all different from one another, it can be helpful to experiment with all sorts of variations on mindfulness practices.

I'll never forget when I first introduced the mountain meditation, which is one of your audio recordings, to a group of psychotherapists in Portland, Oregon. And a fellow raised his hand. He said, "You know, around here, our mountains explode." And about half the room said, "Yeah!" Or the woman who told me, "You know, I've always struggled with my weight, so I really don't like thinking of myself as a mountain." Now, luckily there are alternatives to almost every practice. For example, instead of imagining being a mountain, we can gain equanimity by becoming a scuba diver or an anchor resting beneath stormy seas. One resource for variations on mindfulness practice is a website I developed: It's mindfulness-solution. com. And there you can find, free of charge, audio downloads you can use to learn a number of other techniques, including the body scan, listening meditation, thought labeling, and different meditations to work with pain.

You can also find at the Mindfulness Solution website links to listings of meditation centers all over the world, where you can locate opportunities to learn from and practice with other people. Some of these follow Buddhist paths, while others are associated with different spiritual or cultural traditions. I hope you'll be able to check out these or other resources and use them to support your continued practice.

The Dalai Lama often tells a story that illustrates the power of lifelong efforts to develop mindfulness and compassion. It shows how these practices can lead to well-being even during very trying times. Here are his words.

A senior monk I know spent 17 or 18 years in a Chinese prison after 1959. In the 1980s he was released and able to join me in India. Once, when we were chatting about his experiences he told me that there had been dangerous moments during his imprisonment. I thought he meant threats to his life, but he said, "No, there were times when there was a danger of my losing compassion for my Chinese captors." This is an example of practice in action. He has since been examined by medical scientists who found he has no post-traumatic symptoms. He has physical pains, but no mental unease.

Now if mindfulness practice and the cultivation of compassion could see this monk through years of painful imprisonment, it can certainly help us to find well-being in lives that are sometimes a whole lot easier. It's exciting to be living in a time when the tools of science can be applied to our deepest and oldest quest for well-being, and to help us find paths for fulfillment. So I wish you and those you know and love continued fruitful journeys along this path, filled with many mindful moments. Thanks so much for joining me in the course.

Mindfulness Practices

Supplemental Audio Tracks
(~90 minutes total)

breath awareness practice (introduced in Lecture 2): A foundational formal meditation practice. This can be done initially as a concentration, or focused-attention, practice. Once some concentration develops, it can be expanded to be an open-monitoring, or choiceless-awareness, practice.

loving-kindness practice (introduced in Lecture 6): A foundational practice for cultivating acceptance, both toward the contents of our own minds and toward other people. This can also be expanded to include people who upset us at a given moment, which can help us connect with them.

mountain meditation (introduced in Lecture 8): A foundational equanimity practice designed to help us find stability and perspective when faced with instability in our emotional or external lives.

breathing together (introduced in Lecture 10): A powerful interpersonal practice that can help develop feelings of connection and mutual compassion with another person. It can be done either with a partner or by picturing a partner.

stepping into fear (introduced in Lecture 13): An exercise that we can use to develop experiential approach, rather than avoidance, when struggling with anxiety. This can help increase our capacity to bear anxious feeling, freeing us from the need to avoid activities that stir anxiety.

Practices Demonstrated within Lectures

apple meditation (Lecture 11): A version of eating meditation suitable for children that uses a vivid object of awareness and encourages reflection on the interrelated nature of all things.

befriending the changes (Lecture 20): A brief meditation on the impermanence of the body that is useful when we're finding ourselves struggling with the challenges of aging.

bell in space (Lecture 11): An easily accessed mindfulness practice for children. They can be given the instruction to count the bells (which may help younger children to remain attentive) or simply to listen to them.

breath awareness (Lecture 2): A brief version of a foundational formal meditation practice.

eating meditation (Lecture 3): A foundational practice that can be done either as a formal meditation (using a raisin or larger quantity of food) or as an informal practice (just paying attention to the process of eating during daily life).

equanimity phrases (Lecture 7): Simple reminders that can help us to "be with" another person who is in pain, even if we can't make that pain go away.

ethical reflection (Lecture 23): A useful practice to support developing mindful ethics.

five in five (Lecture 23): A program for integrating the five ethical precepts of Buddhist traditions into our lives, by focusing on one precept each week for five weeks.

giving and taking (*tonglen*) (Lecture 7): A compassion practice that can help us connect with a person or an animal that is suffering.

gratitude letter (Lecture 24): A proven technique for generating well-being through cultivating gratitude.

loving-kindness practice (Lecture 4): A brief version of this foundational practice for cultivating acceptance, both toward the contents of our own minds and toward other people.

loving-kindness practice for children (Lecture 11): An adaptation of this foundational practice for cultivating acceptance using language and imagery suitable for children.

mindful intoxication (Lecture 16): An exercise designed to increase our awareness of our use of intoxicants. This is not recommended if you've already learned that you have difficulty with an intoxicating substance and are trying to be abstinent.

R-A-I-N (Lecture 17): A brief practice designed to help us "be with" and investigate challenging emotional or physical states.

self-compassion letter (Lecture 7): An effective exercise for generating self-compassion, particularly when we're feeling shame about something we've done or a perceived shortcoming.

soften, soothe, allow (Lecture 7): A self-compassion exercise designed to help us find a loving relationship toward mental or physical pain that we find ourselves tending to resist.

stepping into fear (Lecture 13): A brief exercise to practice experiential approach, rather than avoidance, when struggling with anxiety.

three breaths (Lecture 11): A very brief exercise suitable for children to help them notice their experience in the present moment.

three-minute breathing space (Lecture 18): Developed as part of mindfulness-based cognitive therapy, this exercise can help us step out of the thought stream and bring our attention back to the sensations of the present moment at any time during the day. It's particularly useful when we're feeling stressed or overwhelmed.

urge surfing (Lecture 16): An exercise developed as part of the mindfulness-based relapse program designed to help us ride out urges toward unwanted behaviors, such as excessive drinking, overeating, gambling, or speaking unskillfully.

walking meditation (Lecture 3): A foundational formal meditation practice that can be done initially as a concentration, or focused-attention, practice. Once some concentration develops, it can be expanded to be an open-monitoring, or choiceless-awareness, practice. After spending some time doing formal walking meditation, we naturally find it easy to use walking as an informal practice whenever walking in daily life.

what defines me? (Lecture 4): A brief exercise that can help us see the domains or dimensions of our personalities we use to develop a sense of adequacy or self-esteem. Useful for loosening the grip of these preoccupations.

yes and no (Lecture 6): A simple, brief exercise that can help us see more clearly our tendency to resist contents of the mind and shift to a more accepting attitude.

Obstacles to Mediation Practice

To gain the benefits of mindfulness, it's important to practice regularly. Sometimes, we get discouraged when we encounter obstacles. The following are some suggested remedies to common difficulties you may encounter during sitting mindfulness meditation, such as the breath practice.

- **Sleepiness:** In Zen traditions, students are encouraged to try sitting at the edge of a very deep well or a high cliff! Less radical solutions include opening the eyes to let in light, which suppresses melatonin production and makes us less sleepy, or practicing standing up, or switching to walking meditation instead.

- **Physical pain:** Try initially bringing your attention to the discomfort, allowing the breath to be in the background. See if you can develop an attitude of curiosity or interest in the sensations rather than resisting them. The pain may transform by itself. Also, if you're sitting on a meditation cushion, raising the cushion will often keep the legs from "falling asleep," or becoming painful. But there's no need to be stoic; if you're very uncomfortable, feel free to change positions.

- **Restlessness:** Try bringing your attention to the sensations of restlessness—usually muscle tension in the body. See if you can develop an attitude of curiosity or interest in the sensations rather than resisting them. If they persist in making it difficult to continue meditating, try shifting to walking meditation.

- **Unwanted feelings:** Very often, feelings that we've pushed out of awareness at other times will return when we begin meditation practice. Try to open to those feelings as the combination of bodily sensations, thoughts, and images that they are. Simply attending to them with open curiosity will usually make them easier to bear and allow them to transform naturally.

Breath Awareness Practice

Now we'll do some breath awareness practice. And let's begin by finding a posture that feels relaxed and yet alert and dignified. While this practice can be done with either the eyes open or closed, most beginners find it easier to start with the eyes closed. So allow your eyes to shut gently. Should you find yourself dozing off or becoming dreamy, you may find it helpful to simply open your eyes to allow a bit of light in if your eyes have been closed. If you're quite sleepy, you can continue the practice standing up to encourage a little bit more wakefulness.

If you're sitting in a chair, you might imagine a string tied to the top of your head, gently elongating the spine, just pulling up toward the sky or toward the ceiling. That might mean not leaning up against the back of the chair. Just whatever posture works for you to feel like your spine is more or less erect and you're alert. If you're using meditation cushions, the same instructions apply, except you may want to make sure that the cushions are high enough so that your legs don't fall asleep too readily. And you'll notice that if all is going well, you're already breathing. The breath is happening by itself.

And just begin by turning your attention to the sensations of the breath. There are different places where the breath is traditionally observed. You might notice the rising and falling sensations in the belly with each breath, or perhaps more subtly, the sensations at the tip of the nose, where the air enters a little bit cool and leaves a little bit warm. And just see wherever the breath is most vivid for you. And bring your attention to that area of the body. And see if you can begin to follow the breath through its full cycles, from the beginning of an inhalation out to the end of an exhalation, and onto the next cycle.

Now, it would not be unusual for thoughts to enter the mind. That's OK; they're our friends. Simply allow the thoughts to rise and pass. But should your attention get hijacked by a chain of narrative thought such that you've lost contact with the breath entirely, in the moment that you notice that, congratulate yourself. That's a moment of mindfulness. And just gently and lovingly bring your attention back to the sensations of the breath.

We're not trying to control the breath in any way, so should you notice that the breath is short and shallow, that's fine. If it's long and deep, that's fine. We're simply using it as an object of awareness, working to cultivate awareness of present experience with acceptance and just accepting the breath however it presents itself.

This can feel a little bit like puppy training. The mind tends to scamper off. We gently bring it back to the sensations of the breath in this moment. It scampers off again. We gently bring it back again.

See if you can develop an attitude of interest or curiosity in the moment-to-moment sensations of each breath. Notice the texture and the feel of each in-breath and each out-breath.

As though there were nothing else to do, nowhere else to go—just this moment.

With each breath, practicing awareness of present experience with acceptance, opening to just whatever it is in this moment.

Should you notice that the mind is frisky or agitated or filled with all sorts of thoughts, that's fine—just practice being with a frisky and agitated, filled-with-all-sorts-of-thoughts mind. Should you notice that the mind is calm and focused and concentrated, that's OK—just be with a calm and focused and concentrated mind, as though it's all perfect just the way it is.

You may find that judgments enter the mind. Thoughts like, this is going well or this is going poorly, or I like this or I don't like this. Just notice that those are other thoughts and allow them to come and pass, like clouds passing through a vast sky. And then gently and lovingly bring your attention back to the moment-to-moment sensations of breathing.

Again and again, bringing the attention back to the present moment, to just what's happening here and now.

Trusting that each time we return our attention to the breath, we train the mind a little bit more to be able to be accepting of experience and to be in the present moment.

Seeing as some concentration develops, if it's now perhaps more possible to follow the breath through its full cycles from the beginning of an inhalation through the end of an exhalation, and then on to the next.

Should physical discomfort arise, perhaps an itch or an ache, that's a special practice opportunity. And you might experiment if the itch or the ache has some intensity to it, to allowing the breath to be in the background for a few moments and simply bring your attention to the itch or the ache as an object of awareness. And try not doing what we normally would, so try not scratching the itch or adjusting posture to resolve the ache. Instead, try just allowing the sensation to be the object of your awareness for a little while, and then return the attention back to the breath. You don't have to be stoic. If you're very uncomfortable, go ahead and make an adjustment. But try the experiment first.

It's impossible to fail at this project. Whatever you experience is OK. If you discover a mind that's busy and frisky and agitated, just be with a busy and frisky and agitated mind. If you find another kind of mind, be with that kind of mind. You really can't go wrong. Just continue to develop the intention to pay attention to what's happening moment by moment.

Now for the last few minutes of this practice, let's experiment with some other objects of awareness. So allow your breath to be in the background for a few moments and notice the sensation of contact between your body and the chair or the cushion and the floor. So just bring your attention to the sensations in the back of your legs, your buttocks, the soles of your feet, anywhere else where you're making contact. And notice that there's a symphony of sensations happening there, perhaps tingling or pressing. And just allow those to be the focus of your attention for a few moments.

And next, allow those sensations to be in the background and bring your attention to contact with the ocean of air we inhabit. Feel the air on your hands, your face, any other exposed areas. And notice the continuous subtle sensations of contact with air, perhaps noticing it at the tip of the nose where it enters cool and leaves warm. Just feel the air.

And next, join me in just listening. Listen to the sound of my voice, to any other sounds in your environment. Try listening as you might listen to a symphony—not labeling so much, as simply allowing all of the different notes to wash over you. Notice that there's always a symphony playing.

And then finally, if you've been practicing with your eyes closed, allow your eyes to open a little bit. And allow your gaze to cast down at about a 45-degree angle, and take in the visual field. Take it in as an artist might, noticing the colors, the textures, the forms—again, not labeling, just feeling and experiencing.

And then finally, let's shift from focused awareness or focused attention, where we're paying attention to one object at a time, to open the field of awareness now to everything. So allow the mind to notice the breath, the sensation of contact with the chair, the floor, the air, with sound, with sight. And see what it's like to be in the midst of this symphony of sensation. This is called *open monitoring* or *choice-less awareness*. Allow the attention to light on whatever predominates among all of these different sensory inputs.

Just feel it all moment by moment.

And now to bring us to a close, I'm going to ring a bell. And I want you to listen to the sound of the bell from the beginning of the ring until it trails off into space and you can no longer hear it. [Rings bell.]

And now just before you get up and move around, let yourself notice your environment and see if there are any features of the room or whatever space you're in that you can notice now that perhaps you hadn't noticed before. Just notice the colors, the textures, and as you get up and begin moving your body, see if you can maintain some continuity of mindfulness throughout the rest of your activities.

Loving-Kindness Practice

So this is a loving-kindness or, in Pali, *mettā* meditation. And it's helpful whenever the mind is more agitated, or particularly when it's in a critical frame. I want you to begin by bringing to mind some figure, some being, that you think of as being naturally loving and kind. It may be a living person who you know, a teacher, an elder. It may be a religious figure like Jesus, or Mohammed, or Moses, or the Buddha. It may be a spiritual leader like Mother Teresa or the Dalai Lama, or perhaps a world leader like Nelson Mandela or Martin Luther King. It can even be a pet, if there's a pet that you know who is naturally loving and kind, or perhaps a place in nature that just feels like it exudes love, peace, and kindness.

So bring to mind this loving being. And let's begin by sending good wishes toward this loving being. And you can use many different phrases. Here are some traditional ones: May you be happy. May you be peaceful. May you be free from suffering. So just try silently in your mind and in your heart repeating that. May you be happy. May you be peaceful. May you be free from suffering.

And it often helps a lot if you could take your hand and place one hand over your heart and the other hand over that hand, applying a little bit of warmth and pressure to the heart area as you wish well for this naturally loving being. So try it with the hands. May you be happy. May you be peaceful. May you be free from suffering. And see if you can feel a sensation of loving kindness toward this naturally loving being as you do this. Do it silently in your mind.

May you be happy. May you be peaceful. May you be free from suffering. And now imagine this loving being directing the same intention toward you. And you help them out with this by wishing the same for yourself, as though they're there wishing it for you. So it's May I be happy. May I be peaceful. May I be free from suffering. And again, you can leave the hand over the heart and another hand over that hand to add some warmth to the process. May I be happy. May I be peaceful. May I be free from suffering. And just breathe as you experience this intention for a few moments, repeating the phrases silently in your mind.

Should resistance to this come up, just allow that to be there. That's OK. We're not trying to force this. But just gently encourage this attitude of loving kindness, first toward the naturally loving other and then toward ourselves. May I be happy. May I be peaceful. May I be free from suffering.

Now as you do this, you can experiment with other phrases as well. Another traditional set is May I be safe. May I be healthy. May I live with ease. May I be safe. May I be healthy. May I live with ease. Just continue to allow yourself to breathe. And silently repeat whichever set of phrases seem best to touch your heart. May I be happy. May I be peaceful. May I be free from suffering. May I be safe. May I be healthy. May I live with ease.

And just continue working with the phrases, generating a little bit of loving kindness toward yourself, imagining the naturally loving being there wishing the same for you.

Some people find it feels more comfortable once you've done this for a bit not to use the whole phrases, but jut key words. So it could simply be happy, peaceful, free, or safe, healthy, ease. Feel free to experiment, the idea being just to have the practice involve generating some of this feeling, first toward the loving other and now toward yourself.

As though the loving other were holding you tenderly and sending you these wishes.

May I be happy. May I be peaceful. May I be free from suffering. May I be safe. May I be healthy. May I live with ease.

As you do this practice, you may sense a little softening or tendering— tenderizing of the heart. It can sometimes even open the door to feelings in the background. That's OK if those feelings arise, if there's a little bit of sadness, or a little bit tenderness. Just allow that to be in the background. And continue to bathe yourself with the loving kindness. Nothing to fear.

May I be happy. May I be peaceful. May I be free from suffering. May I be safe. May I be healthy. May I live with ease.

And now assuming you've been able to feel a little bit of this loving kindness intention toward yourself, bring to mind somebody you care about who you'd like to share this loving kindness with. It could be a friend, a family member, even an acquaintance, somebody who you feel you'd like to share this with or who could benefit from it. And hold this other person in your mind's eye. It could be an animal as well.

And begin wishing this for him or her. May you happy. May you be peaceful. May you be free from suffering. May you happy. May you be peaceful. May you be free from suffering. Or if you prefer, may you be safe. May you be healthy. May you live with ease. May you be safe. May you be healthy. May you live with ease. And you can experiment if you put your hands down with putting your hands back, one hand on the heart and the other over that hand as you wish well to this other person or being. May you be happy. May you be peaceful. May you be free from suffering. May you be safe. May you be healthy. May you live with ease.

And then take this same intention and direct it to a larger group, perhaps close friends, or family members, or your coworkers, some group that you'd like to develop some of this loving kindness feeling toward, or a group that you simply would like to wish well. And picture the group and send the feelings toward them. May you be happy. May you be peaceful. May you be free from suffering. May you be happy. May you be peaceful. May you be free from suffering. May you be safe. May you be healthy. May you live with ease. May you be safe. May you be healthy. May you live with ease.

And next again having the option of putting your hand over your heart and your other hand over that, let's practice sending the same impulse or wish out to a wider community. If you live in a city, perhaps everybody in the city, or if you live in a suburban community, everybody in the suburban community, or everybody in your rural area—just send this to the larger community of which you're a part. May you be happy. May you be peaceful. May you be free from suffering. May you be safe. May you be healthy. May you live with ease. And just continue repeating whichever phrases resonate for you silently as you imagine the whole community receiving it.

And now let's expand out to everybody in the country in which you live, so a vast array of different people, so many different types, so many different attitudes, all living in this complex ecosystem of a country together, wishing them all well. May you all be happy. May you be peaceful. May you be free from suffering. Or perhaps may you be safe. May you be healthy. May you live with ease—just wishing everybody in their diversity well-being, continuing to repeat the phrases silently.

And now expanding out even further, in your mind's eye and your heart, envisioning everybody in the whole world, in all the different countries, on all the different continents—the amazing, vast, diverse human family, and knowing that everybody is going through a combination of good and bad times, but nonetheless wishing them all well. May you all be happy. May you all be peaceful. May you all be free from suffering. May you all be safe. May you all be healthy. May you live with ease.

And now not limiting it to human beings, but to all sentient beings, to all beings that can feel pain, or pleasure, or safety, or distress, everywhere on the planet. May all beings be happy. May all beings be peaceful. May all beings be free from suffering.

And remembering—it's OK if other feelings come up, if the loving kindness doesn't always flow, just experimenting with the intention to see what happens. May all beings be happy. May all beings be peaceful. May all beings be free from suffering.

And to bring this to a close, I'm going to ring the bell. And listen to the sound of the bell from the beginning of the ring until it trails off into space and you can no longer hear it. [Rings bell.]

Mountain Meditation

This is the mountain meditation, and it's a nice equanimity practice. Find a posture in which you can sit with your spine more or less erect, and where you can feel solid and stable and well-planted. You can imagine a string tied to the top of your head, gently elongating the spine to help you to be alert and dignified. And I want you to imagine that you're a mountain. Perhaps you're in a mountain range with other mountains. Like all things, you change— but you change gradually in geologic time while things on and around you change a good deal more quickly.

And let's imagine that it's early spring. And flowers are coming up, baby animals are being born, the days are warm and comfortable. The nights are still somewhat cool. There's a great deal of activity, life bursting out everywhere. And some days are peaceful, sunny. Other days are pretty stormy, where winds whip around, perhaps thunder clouds come in where there's lightning and thunder and all sorts of activity. But then the clouds leave, it dries up and it becomes peaceful again. And as night goes to day and day goes to night, you notice that the days are continuing to get longer and the nights a little bit shorter. And it's getting warmer. Sometimes, now, it's quite hot in the afternoon. It still cools down at night. The animals are beginning to go through their changes: The babies are growing up a bit, maturing; the plants are becoming more firmly established, maybe moving from flowers to leaves.

And as night goes to day and day goes to night, the nights continue to get shorter and the days, warmer. And again, it changes. Sometimes, there are violent storms coming through; sometimes just gentle rains. Sometimes it's a little cloudy; other times there's brilliant sunshine. And as night goes to day and day goes to night, you notice that it's changing. And now the days, having been quite long, are getting a little bit shorter, and the nights a tad longer. Sometimes, it's kind of humid and languid in the afternoon, with buzzing of insects all over—not so much activity when it gets really hot, but then more activity around dusk and dawn. Birds are around everywhere, flying and chirping.

And as night goes to day and day goes to night, the days are getting shorter still and the nights longer still, until you start to notice it's not quite as warm in the afternoon, and at night, it cools down a bit. And the leaves are beginning to change just a little, first a tinge of orange here and a tinge of yellow. But as time progresses, the changes become more pronounced. And animals are starting to change their behavior. We start to see squirrels gathering up nuts and things for the coming winter. And night goes to day and day goes to night. And now the leaves are just gorgeous. They're just brilliant oranges and reds and yellows.

Sometimes, a storm comes through and it starts to blow the leaves off of the trees. But there are still many left. And then the sun comes out and the sky is brilliant and blue. And as night goes to day and day goes to night, now the nights are getting quite a bit longer and the days quite a bit shorter. And there's a real crisp in the air at night. And more of the leaves are falling, so that now on the ground there's just crunchy leaves to be found. And birds are beginning to thin out. Many of them seem to be going south for the winter.

And as the nights get longer still and the days shorter, one night it gets really quite cool. And a storm comes through and this time instead of rain, there's snow. And everything in the morning looks white. It melts—it's not that cold yet, but it's a harbinger of things to come. And as night goes to day and day goes to night, the changes continue. Until this time, a storm comes through and it's white and it sticks, because it just doesn't warm up that much during the day. And then another storm comes and there's another layer of white, until soon everything is quite frozen and it's not melting in the days at all. Even the streams have begun to freeze. And the animals now aren't seen so much—you just see footprints around. And not so many birds to be found.

And night goes to day and day goes to night, and some days are crisp and clear, with bright blue sky, and little icicles forming as the snow on the trees melts. Then they freeze solid at night. And now, the nights are quite long and the days are quite short. Very still in the night.

But as time continues to move on, the changes continue. And now the days are getting a little bit longer, and the nights a little bit shorter. And sometimes in the afternoon, there's a little bit more melting. First the icicles, then puddling appearing. It still freezes pretty solid at night. And sometimes the snow comes through as a blizzard, and everything is just white, white, white. But then it passes.

And after a little while, the nights are getting shorter and the days sufficiently long, so that there is real melting in the day. And one day, a storm comes through. And this time, it's not just white, but there's rain mixed in and it causes a lot of melting. And it seems virtually overnight that brown spots start to appear where the snow once was.

And now, night goes to day and day goes to night, and as the days get longer, more and more brown spots appear. And it doesn't take long before the brown starts to turn green. Little shoots appear, and the white retreats.

And now there's animal activity starting. At first, just a little, a few birds arriving. But as the days go on, there's more and more animals arriving. And more and more, the snow is retreating, until it's only left in the glaciated areas, in the shaded spots. And it's now pretty warm during the day and not so cold at night. And flowers are starting to come out. And you begin to realize that a full cycle has passed. A year has come and a year has gone. [Rings bell.]

Breathing Together

Let's do a breathing together exercise. It would be helpful for your partner to have had a little bit of exposure to meditation, perhaps having tried the breath awareness practice. Now, if you have a friend or a partner who you can do this with, who has some meditation experience his or herself, that works very well. And you can invite your friend or partner to join you in this.

If you don't have somebody you can do it with, then you can either conjure a mental image of another person, or even perhaps use a visual image, a photograph, or some other object that reminds you of the other person. And you might even do this with a pet, perhaps, if the pet's likely to be able to sit still with you for a while.

I'd like you to begin by facing you chair toward the image, or if you're doing it with another person, toward both of you, facing your chairs toward one another. And find chairs in which you can sit in an alert and dignified posture because we're going to begin by doing some breath practice together.

And we'll do this initially with the eyes closed. So find a comfortable posture in which you're able to sit in an alert and dignified way. And notice that you're both already breathing. And allow yourself to follow the cycles of the breath, from the beginning of an inhalation through to the end of an exhalation, and back onto the next in-breath.

And notice what it's like to be with your own breath, knowing that your partner, either present or as an image, is also there across from you, breathing, or being there as well.

To find an alert and dignified posture, you might imagine a string tied to the top of the head, gently elongating the spine. We're just sitting and breathing together.

Thoughts may enter the mind. That's fine. Allow them to come and go—including any thoughts of self-consciousness or awkwardness that may come up because you're doing this with another person or being. Allow them to freely enter and leave the mind as you return your attention again and again to the sensations of breathing.

We're just developing a little bit of concentration before moving on to other aspects of the practice.

Should judgments enter the mind—I like this, I don't like this, this is weird, this is good—just notice that all judgments are simply thoughts arising and passing like any other thought. And bring your attention back to the moment-to-moment sensations of sitting here together.

Now I invite you, if you're sitting with a live other person, to both open your eyes a little bit. And allow your gaze to cast downward in such a way that you can see your partner's breathing. If you're just being with an image of your partner, you can leave the eyes closed with the image. Or if you have a photo or something like that, you can open them. Or if you're with a pet or another being, you can open the eyes a bit. You want to simply observe the presence, and observe the breathing of the other.

So we're being aware of our own breath at the same time as being aware of the presence of the other, and perhaps his or her breath.

If you're doing this with a partner, it doesn't matter whether your breath synchronizes or doesn't—either way is fine. We're just breathing together.

We're practicing awareness of present experience with acceptance, including the awareness of being with another, and accepting the experience of being with the other.

And the next phase of this practice can be a little intense at first—especially if you're doing it with a live partner—because in a moment, I'm going to invite you to lift your gaze and look into your partner's eyes, and that can feel a little bit awkward or off-putting at first. And if it's too intense, feel free to come back down and just watch your partner's breathing, or even to close your eyes entirely.

But first, just try the experiment. Allow your eyes to open and gaze into your partner's eyes, and notice the sensations of breathing as you do this together. In some cultures, we only make eye contact when we're going to either fight or mate. And that's not what we're doing here—neither of those is—so it can feel a little awkward. But you may also find that you get used to it after a few moments.

So whether you're looking at your partner, or you've dropped your gaze a bit, I want you to consider that your partner, like you, was once a baby. And that your partner, like you, was once wholly dependent on caregivers for his or her well-being. And as a result, your partner, like you, probably had good days as a baby—days in which needs were cared for, days in which caregivers were responsive and present. And also some bad days— days perhaps where the caregivers weren't so attentive, or perhaps where you were sick or injured. And you, like your partner, went through infancy, alternating between states of pleasure and states of well-being, and states of discomfort or distress.

And like you, your partner then grew older, and eventually became a toddler. And started venturing out on his or her own, as you did. And here too, there were probably moments of joy, moments of excitement, moments of curiosity, moments of learning, as well as moments of frustration, moments of fear, moments of pain. And as a toddler, you and your partner both were very dependent on caregivers still. And there were probably times when they were responsive, and other times when they were not so responsive.

And then you, like your partner, grew older still, and perhaps reached an age of going off to school, with all that's entailed with that—the strangeness of other kids being around who you don't know, being away from mom or some other primary caregiver, having to deal with new grown-ups, having to deal with the challenges of learning things, and having some expectations about learning things. And you, like your partner, probably had moments of joy, moments of engagement, moments where this felt pretty good, and other moments where it was rough—feelings of loneliness, perhaps, or fear, or maybe anger if other children treated you poorly.

And perhaps your caregivers were able to provide comfort and nurturing, or perhaps not. Or perhaps some days yes and some days no. And you, like your partner, grew older still and became, say, a later–elementary school student, where suddenly there were all sorts of expectations—competition in the school yard, playing sports maybe. Where it was clear that some kids were faster learners than others, and where it was clear that some kids were more popular than others—and experiencing all the joys and sorrows that go with that. The moments of feeling good, of feeling capable, of feeling loved, and the moments of feeling alone, not so capable, not so loved. And depending, maybe you or your partner had caregivers who were attentive and responsive, or maybe they weren't so much. Or maybe they were on some days and not on others.

And then you and your partner grew older still and entered puberty. And the wild ride that that always is—the body changing, sprouting new parts, trying to figure out what my new identity's going to be. Usually peers taking on more importance—sometimes pulling away from parents or other caregivers. Sometimes feeling a lot of excitement, sometimes a lot of fear—all different feelings happening with the radical changes that happen as the body matures, and probably moments of joy and moments of distress associated with that.

And then you, like your partner, grew older still, and became an older adolescent, where issues of boyfriends and girlfriends, and independence, and what one's going to do with one's life often enter into the picture. And here too, there're so many opportunities for joy and excitement, and so many opportunities for sorrow, frustration, anger, and fear. It's a rough ride being a teenager.

And then at some point, both you and your partner probably began the process of leaving home. Maybe going off to college, or maybe going into the military, or going off to a job. Or maybe living at home while making some of those transitions, but still being more independent in the world, with all of the joys and sorrow that go with that. It's so great to be able to perhaps drive a car, or go places independently, perhaps form new and exciting relationships. But then all of the worries and the concerns about how is this going to be? Am I going to make it well on my own? Do I have what it takes?

And then you and your partner likely went through other developmental stages too—perhaps starting a family of your own, and all that's entailed with that. Now not only having to worry about your own well-being, but worrying about the well-beings of your partner, and your children if you've had children.

Perhaps you and your partner both went off to develop professions, careers, going to college, to graduate school even, maybe becoming licensed at something or another, with all of the joys and sorrows attendant on that—the good feeling about achievement, the bad feeling about making comparisons with others and not always coming out on top, concerns for how this is going to work out, and will I enjoy it or not. Maybe even greater concerns of will I be able to survive? Can I make enough money?

And somehow, through these stages, you and your partner came to this moment in time—to this particular moment of crossing paths in the life cycle. And if your eyes are open, take in what your partner looks like right now, at this moment, where you happen to be here together. And if you're working with a partner in your mind's eye, or a picture, or some other form, just take him or her in as he or she is now.

And of course, we have no idea what the future's going to bring, but it's possible that you and your partner will grow older still. And will go through other developmental stages. And at some point, both you and your partner will reach the end of this life cycle. You may know it. You may know that the end is near because you have a terminal illness, or just because you're very old. Or maybe it'll come suddenly without any preparation. But we can be certain that both we and our partner will reach the end of this life. And we'll have gone through this entire journey, the 10,000 joys and 10,000 sorrows—beginning as an infant, going through all the different stages, and then reaching an end.

So with awareness of being on this journey together, take one last look at your partner, if your eyes are raised. And then allow your gaze to come down again. If you're with an image of the partner, you can allow your eyes to close. If you're with a live partner, come back to experiencing your breath and your partner's breath.

And notice what it's like to breathe together, having gone on this little journey together and being on this life course together. Allow yourself to feel the breath again from the beginning of an inhalation to the end of an exhalation—breathing together.

And then allow your eyes to close completely. And come back into the sensations in what you call your body. And see if you can follow the breath through some full cycles, know that your partner is there, also going through the life cycle, following his or her breath. And allow yourself to feel some appreciation for the opportunity to be on this life cycle, and to have others on the life cycle with us as well.

And to bring this practice to a close, I'm going to ring a bell. And I invite you to listen to the sound of the bell from the beginning of the ring until it trails off into space and you can no longer hear. [Rings bell.]

Stepping into Fear

Now let's do a stepping into fear practice. And this practice is a little bit counter-intuitive because it's about increasing our capacity to be with fear. And most of the time, our natural temptation is to try to diminish fear, but this is instead going to be about moving toward fear, so that we're no longer afraid of fear.

So simply begin with the breath, and establish a posture in which your spine is more or less erect and you feel dignified and alert. And follow the breath through a few cycles.

It's going to be important to keep breathing throughout this exercise. And I want you to see if you can feel, or identify, a little bit of anxiety or fear somewhere in the body—it doesn't have to be a lot—but if you can feel a little tension or a little fear, I want you to see what you can do to increase that. Or you may be able to increase it by simply bringing your attention to the sensations of fear—to the bodily sensations. Or you may need to conjure an image that you know will help you to be anxious.

And what I want you to do is ramp the fear up, so it's at a level where you can really feel it. Doesn't have to be overwhelming, but you want it to be strong enough so you feel like you're challenged a little bit by working with it. This is like going to the gym, where you're lifting weights. You wouldn't want to pick weights that were so light that there was no challenge, nor that were so heavy that you're going to strain yourself. So try to ramp the fear up to a level where you can really feel it, and then we're simply going use the sensations of fear as the object of our awareness for some mindfulness practice.

Allow yourself to keep breathing. And let the breath be in the background as you feel the sensations of fear. Notice how they manifest in your heart, in your neck, and other muscles. Just feel all the sensations. Ah, my old friend fear, or anxiety—I know you. You've been with me from the beginning.

And we're not trying to do anything special. We're not trying to make it go away. We're just breathing with it. We're practicing befriending fear, so that it becomes just another sensation—just something else that we can turn our minds to, and practice awareness of present experience with acceptance toward.

So just keep breathing and feeling the fear.

Now it's important not to let it fade or slip away. That would be like putting down the weights too early. So if the fear starts to diminish, do whatever you need to do to keep it up, to keep it going at a good healthy level so you can continue practicing being with it. Just breathe the breath through full cycles as you feel the fear.

And keep breathing. Just notice all the body sensations that are associated with fear or anxiety. And notice that they can be our friends. They're just other sensations. They're not actually dangerous or threatening. It's just psycho-physiological arousal. I can be with that.

Just breathe and feel the fear. Again, if it starts to get elusive, if it starts to slip away, do whatever you need to do to bring it back. That could be just focusing on the anxiety sensations in the body, or maybe conjuring up new images and thoughts. We want to get a good workout here, to really make friends with the fear.

Don't forget to keep breathing. The breath becomes a kind of surfboard. It helps us to surf the waves of fear. Just feel each wave after each wave, as though being with fear were as natural as carefully tasting a gourmet meal, or smelling a flower, or petting a kitten—just another sensory experience.

Ah, fear. Again, try not to let it slip away. Try to keep it going so that you can really work with it. If the mind wanders away and you lose touch with whatever's fearsome, just gently and lovingly bring your attention back to the scary thought or image, so you can stay with it for just a little while longer.

Feel the fear in your heart, in your back—anywhere in the body where it's manifesting. Just keep breathing, and keep feeling it.

And now, having given yourself a good workout, allow the fear to reach its own level. So simply come back to the sensations of the breath. And if the fear wants to stay around, let it stay around. But if it wants to go, let it go also. Just don't push it away. Give it complete freedom to visit whenever it wants. And come back to the breath.

And follow the breath through a few cycles.

And then to bring this to a close, and to bring our attention back into the wider world, I'm going to ring a bell. And listen to the sound of the bell, from the beginning of the ring until it trails off into space and you can no longer hear it. [Rings bell.]

Bibliography

Batchelor, S. *Buddhism without Beliefs: A Contemporary Guide to Awakening.* New York: Riverhead Books, 1998. An examination of basic Buddhist teachings that can be observed through direct experience, contrasted with culturally determined beliefs widely held in Buddhist traditions.

Bays, J. C. *Mindful Eating: A Guide to Rediscovering a Healthy and Joyful Relationship with Food.* Boston: Shambhala, 2009. A guide to using mindfulness practices to improve eating habits and enjoy eating more fully.

Bien, T., and Bien, B. *Mindful Recovery: A Spiritual Path to Healing from Addiction.* New York: Wiley, 2002. A guide to using mindfulness practice as part of recovery from addictions.

Brach, T. *Radical Acceptance: Embracing Your Life with the Heart of a Buddha.* New York: Bantam Dell, 2003. A pioneering exploration of the "trance of unworthiness" by which we become trapped by self-critical thinking.

Brewer, J. A. "Breaking the Addiction Loop." In Germer, C. K., Siegel, R. D, and Fulton, P. R., eds. *Mindfulness and Psychotherapy.* 2nd ed. New York: Guilford Press, 2013. An academic exploration of the dynamics of addictive behaviors.

Brewer, J. A., Worhunsky, P. D., Gray, J. R., Tang, Y. Y., Weber, J., and Kober, H. "Meditation Experience Is Associated with Differences in Default Mode Network Activity and Connectivity." *Proceedings of the National Academy of Sciences of the United States of America* 108, no. 50 (2011): 20254–20259. A groundbreaking study showing the effects of meditation on default mode network activity and connectivity.

Briere, J. "Mindfulness, Insight, and Trauma Therapy." In Germer, C. K., Siegel, R. D, and Fulton, P. R., eds. *Mindfulness and Psychotherapy.* 2nd ed. New York: Guilford Press. A professional article outlining a mindfulness-oriented approach to trauma treatment.

Briere, J., and Scott, C. *Principles of Trauma Therapy: A Guide to Symptoms, Evaluation, and Treatment.* Thousand Oaks, CA: Sage, 2012. A professional text outlining a mindfulness-oriented approach to trauma treatment.

Brown, C. A., and Jones, A. K. "Meditation Experience Predicts Less Negative Appraisal of Pain: Electrophysiological Evidence for the Involvement of Anticipatory Neural Responses." *Pain* 150, no. 3 (2010): 428–438. A pioneering study showing how meditation tempers the anticipatory anxiety associated with pain responses.

Dahl, J., Wilson, K., Luciano, C., and Hayes, S. *Acceptance and Commitment Therapy for Chronic Pain.* Oakland, CA: New Harbinger Press, 2005. A professional text outlining how to use ACT to work with pain.

Davidson, R. J. "The Neurobiology of Compassion." In C.K. Germer and R.D. Siegel, eds. *Wisdom and Compassion in Psychotherapy: Deepening Mindfulness in Clinical Practice.* New York: Guilford Press, 2012. A review of recent findings on the neurobiology of compassion.

Davidson, R. J., Kabat-Zinn, J., Schumacher, J., Rosenkranz, M., Muller, D., Santorelli, S. F., … Sheridan, J. F. "Alterations in Brain and Immune Function Produced by Mindfulness Meditation." *Psychosomatic Medicine* 65, no. 4 (2003): 564–570. Classic study showing the shift from right prefrontal activation to left prefrontal activation in biotech workers who were trained in mindfulness practice.

Epstein, M. *Psychotherapy without the Self: A Buddhist Perspective.* New Haven, CT: Yale University Press, 2007. A very readable text by a psychiatrist about psychotherapy from a Buddhist perspective.

Forsyth, J., and Eifert, G. *The Mindfulness and Acceptance Workbook for Anxiety.* Oakland, CA: New Harbinger Press, 2007. A self-help guide to using ACT to work with anxiety.

Fulton, P. R., and Engler, J. "Self and No-Self in Psychotherapy." In. C. K. Germer and R. D. Siegel, eds. *Wisdom and Compassion in Psychotherapy: Deepening Mindfulness in Clinical Practice.* New York: Guilford Press,

2012. An insightful examination of the concept of no-self and its implications for psychotherapy.

Fulton, P. R., and Siegel, R. D. "Buddhist and Western Psychology: Seeking Common Ground." In C. K. Germer, R. D. Siegel, and P. R. Fulton, eds. *Mindfulness and Psychotherapy.* 2nd ed. New York: Guilford Press, 2013. A comparison of traditional Western psychotherapy and Buddhist teachings.

Gard, T., Hölzel, B. K., Sack, A. T., Hempel, H., Lazar, S. W., Vaitl, D., and Ott, U. "Pain Attenuation through Mindfulness Is Associated with Decreased Cognitive Control and Increased Sensory Processing in the Brain." *Cerebral Cortex* 22, no. 11 (2012): 2692–2702. Study demonstrating that meditators, when exposed to pain, have more activity in the insula—suggesting that they feel pain more—but less prefrontal activity, suggesting that they judge the pain less.

Garrison, K. A., Scheinost, D., Worhunsky, P. D., Elwafi, H. M., Thornhill, T. A., ... Brewer, J. A. "Real-Time fMRI Links Subjective Experience with Brain Activity during Focused Attention." *Neuroimage* 81 (Nov. 1, 2013): 110–118. Study showing real-time biofeedback of activation of the PCC.

Germer, C. K. "Mindfulness: What Is It? What Does It Matter?" In C. K. Germer, R. D. Siegel, and P. R. Fulton, eds. *Mindfulness and Psychotherapy.* 2nd ed. New York: Guilford Press, 2013. A conceptual overview of mindfulness and its role in health care.

———. *The Mindful Path to Self-Compassion: Freeing Yourself from Destructive Thoughts and Emotions.* New York: Guilford Press, 2009. Self-help guide to developing self-compassion.

Germer, C. K., and Siegel, R. D., eds. *Wisdom and Compassion in Psychotherapy: Deepening Mindfulness in Clinical Practice.* New York: Guilford, 2012. A professional text, inspired by a meeting with the Dalai Lama, exploring the implications of wisdom and compassion for psychotherapy.

Germer, C. K., Siegel, R. D., and Fulton, P. R., eds. *Mindfulness and Psychotherapy, 2nd Edition.* New York: Guilford, 2013. A detailed professional text examining the state of the art of mindfulness-oriented psychotherapy.

Gilbert, D. *Stumbling on Happiness.* New York: Vintage, 2007. A readable examination of how we so often pursue happiness where it cannot be reliably found.

Gilbert, P. *The Compassionate Mind: A New Approach to Life's Challenges.* Oakland, CA: New Harbinger Press, 2009. An examination of the role of compassion in psychological health.

———. *Overcoming Depression, 3rd Edition.* London: Constable Robinson and New York: Basic Books, 2009. A compassion-focused approach to treating depression.

Goldstein, J., and Kornfield, J. *Seeking the Heart of Wisdom: The Path of Insight Meditation.* Boston: Shambhala, 1987. A step-by-step guide to developing a mindfulness practice, including its implications for psychological awakening.

Goodman, T. "Working with Children." In C. K. Germer, R. D. Siegel, and P. R. Fulton, eds. *Mindfulness and Psychotherapy.* 2nd ed. New York: Guilford Press, 2013. A professional exploration of the use of mindfulness practices in child treatment.

Goodman, T., Greenland, S.K., and Siegel, D. "Mindful Parenting as a Path to Wisdom and Compassion." In Germer, C. K., and Siegel, R. D., eds. *Wisdom and Compassion in Psychotherapy.* New York: Guilford, 2012. A professional exploration of the use of mindfulness practices in child treatment, with an emphasis on developing wisdom and compassion.

Gunaratana, B. *Mindfulness in Plain English.* Somerville, MA: Wisdom Publications, 2002. A classic guide to developing a mindfulness practice.

Bibliography

Halifax, J. *Being with Dying: Cultivating Compassion and Fearlessness in the Presence of Death.* Boston: Shambhala, 2008. Guide to being with people who are dying written by a Zen master who trains hospice workers.

Hall, S. S. *Wisdom: From Philosophy to Neuroscience.* New York: Knopf, 2010. A very readable history of modern scientific attempts to study wisdom.

Hanh, T. N. *Creating True Peace: Ending Violence in Yourself, Your Family, Your Community and the World.* New York: Free Press, 2000. Another classic text by a Vietnamese Zen master about developing mindfulness and using it to promote peace.

————. *For a Future to Be Possible: Buddhist Ethics for Everyday Life.* Berkeley: Parallax Press, 2007. An examination of the five ethical precepts and their application to daily life.

————. *Peace Is Every Step: The Path of Mindfulness in Everyday Life.* New York: Bantam Books, 1992. A classic text by a Vietnamese Zen master about developing mindfulness and using it to promote peace.

Hanson, R. *Hardwiring Happiness: The New Brain Science of Contentment, Calm, and Confidence.* New York: Harmony, 2013. An examination of the negativity bias and ways to counteract it.

Hanson, R., and Mendius, R. *Buddha's Brain: The Practical Neuroscience of Happiness, Love, and Wisdom.* Oakland, CA: New Harbinger Publications, 2009. An overview of the negativity bias and our stress response and how meditation can help counteract it.

Harrington, A. *The Placebo Effect: An Interdisciplinary Exploration.* Cambridge, MA: Harvard University Press, 1999. Based on a conference at Harvard, this book examines placebo effects from multiple perspectives.

Harris, R., and Hayes, S. *ACT Made Simple: An Easy-to-Read Primer on Acceptance and Commitment Therapy.* Oakland, CA: New Harbinger Publications, 2009. An introduction to ACT.

Herman, J. L. *Trauma and Recovery*. New York: Basic Books, 1992. A classic text on approaching trauma recovery in stages—establishing safety first.

Kabat-Zinn, J. *Full Catastrophe Living: Using the Wisdom of Your Body and Mind to Face Stress, Pain and Illness*. New York: Dell, 1990. An introduction to mindfulness practice, the MBSR program, and stress-related health issues.

———. *Wherever You Go, There You Are*. New York: Hyperion, 1994. A collection of short meditations, each a page or two long, that can support mindfulness practice.

Kabat-Zinn, M., and Kabat-Zinn, J. *Everyday Blessings: The Inner Work of Mindful Parenting*. New York: Hyperion, 1998. A pioneering book on mindful parenting.

Kornfield, J. *After the Ecstasy, the Laundry: How the Heart Grows Wise on the Spiritual Path*. New York: Bantam, 2000. An exploration of the pitfalls of transcendent mystical experiences not grounded in ethics and compassion.

———. *A Path with Heart: A Guide through the Perils and Promises of Spiritual Life*. New York: Bantam, 1993. A comprehensive exploration of using mindfulness practices to resolve emotional difficulties, complete with many innovative exercises.

Kramer, G. *Insight Dialogue: The Interpersonal Path to Freedom*. Boston: Shambhala, 2007. An innovative look at interpersonal mindfulness practices.

Kumar, S. *Grieving Mindfully: A Compassionate and Spiritual Guide to Coping with Loss*. Oakland, CA: New Harbinger Press, 2005. An examination of how to use mindfulness practices to work through losses.

Lazar, S. "The Neurobiology of Mindfulness." In C. K. Germer, R. D. Siegel, and P. R. Fulton, eds. *Mindfulness and Psychotherapy*. 2nd ed. New York: Guilford Press, 2013. A professional overview of what we now know about changes in brain function and structure induced by mindfulness practices.

Lazar, S., Kerr, C., Wasserman, R., Gray, J., Greve, D., Treadway, ... Fischl, B. "Meditation Experience Is Associated with Increased Cortical Thickness." *NeuroReport* 16 (2005): 1893–1897. Classic study showing that certain brain regions of experienced meditators don't thin with age.

Levine, P. A., and Frederick, A. *Waking the Tiger: Healing Trauma, the Innate Capacity to Transform Overwhelming Experiences.* Berkeley, CA: North Atlantic Books, 1997. Mindful approach to working with trauma by focusing on bodily sensations.

Linehan, M. M. *Cognitive-Behavioral Treatment of Borderline Personality Disorder.* New York: Guilford, 1993. Classic step outlining dialectical behavior therapy.

Lucas, M. *Rewire Your Brain for Love.* New York: Hay House, 2012. An integration of insights into mindfulness practice, attachment theory, and the negativity bias designed to help readers establish successful, loving relationships.

Martin, J. *The Zen Path through Depression.* New York: HarperCollins, 1999. A guide to "being with" depressive feelings as a way to work through them.

Morgan, S. P. "Compassion and Wisdom: Growing through Ethics." In C. K. Germer and R. D. Siegel, eds. *Wisdom and Compassion in Psychotherapy: Deepening Mindfulness in Clinical Practice.* New York: Guilford Press, 2012. A professional exploration of the role of ethics in psychotherapeutic practice, emphasizing the roles of wisdom and compassion.

———. "Practical Ethics." In Germer, C. K., Siegel, R. D, and Fulton, P. R., eds. *Mindfulness and Psychotherapy.* 2nd ed. New York: Guilford Press, 2013. A professional exploration of the role of ethics in psychotherapeutic practice.

Neff, K. "The Science of Self-Compassion." In C. K. Germer and R. D. Siegel, eds. *Wisdom and Compassion in Psychotherapy: Deepening Mindfulness in Clinical Practice.* New York: Guilford Press, 2012. A professional exploration of the role of self-compassion in psychotherapy.

————. *Self-Compassion: Stop Beating Yourself Up and Leave Insecurity Behind*. New York: William Morrow, 2011. A book for general audiences by the research psychologist who developed the idea of self-compassion as well as scales to measure it.

Olendzki, A. "The Roots of Buddhist Psychology." In C. K. Germer, R. D. Siegel, and P. R. Fulton, eds. *Mindfulness and Psychotherapy*. 2nd ed. New York: Guilford Press, 2013. A particularly clear and concise description of the basic principles of Buddhist psychology.

Orsillo, S. M., and Roemer, L. *The Mindful Way through Anxiety: Break Free from Worry and Reclaim Your Life*. New York: Guilford Press, 2011. A self-help guide to using mindfulness practices to work with anxiety.

Peltz, L. *The Mindful Path to Addiction Recovery: A Practical Guide to Regaining Control over Your Life*. Boston, MA: Trumpeter, 2013. A guide to using mindfulness practice to work with more serious addictions.

Pollak, S. M., Pedulla, T., and Siegel, R. D. *Sitting Together: Essential Skills for Mindfulness-Based Psychotherapy*. New York: Guilford, 2014. A professional guide to using different mindfulness practices under different circumstances that contains a wide variety of practices with suggestions for their application.

Roemer, L., and Orsillo, S. M. "Mindfulness and Acceptance-Based Treatment of Anxiety." In C. K. Germer, R. D. Siegel, and P. R. Fulton, eds. *Mindfulness and Psychotherapy*. 2nd ed. New York: Guilford Press, 2013. A professional exploration of the use of mindfulness practices in anxiety treatment.

Rosenberg, L. *Living in the Light of Death: On the Art of Being Truly Alive*. Boston, MA: Shambhala, 2000. An insightful guide to working with the realities of aging and death.

Segal, Z. V., Williams, J. M. G., and Teasdale, J. D. *Mindfulness-Based Cognitive Therapy for Depression, 2nd Edition*. New York: Guilford Press, 2012. The classic text outlining MBCT.

Bibliography

Seligman, M. E. P. *Authentic Happiness: Using the New Positive Psychology to Realize Your Potential for Lasting Fulfillment.* New York: Free Press, 2002. The classic text outlining the field of positive psychology.

Shapiro, S. L., and Carlson, L. E. *The Art and Science of Mindfulness: Integrating Mindfulness into Psychology and the Helping Professions.* Washington, DC: American Psychological Association, 2009. A professional text exploring the integration of mindfulness practices into psychotherapy.

Shubiner, H., and Betzold, M. *Unlearn Your Pain, Second Edition.* Pleasant Ridge, MI: Mind Body Publishing, 2012. A self-help guide to using mindfulness practice to work with chronic pain disorders.

Siegel, R. D. "East Meets West." *Psychotherapy Networker* 36, no. 5 (Sept./ Oct. 2011): 26. A discussion of the current relationship between Western psychotherapy and mindfulness practices.

―――. *Mindfulness for Anxiety.* American Psychological Association Master Therapist Video Series. Washington, DC: APA, 2012. A professional video demonstrating the use of mindfulness practices to work with anxiety.

―――. *The Mindfulness Solution: Everyday Practices for Everyday Problems.* New York, Guilford, 2010. A book for general audiences explaining how to develop a regular mindfulness practice, tailor it to your individual needs, and use it to work with a wide variety of psychological and interpersonal challenges. This book expands upon many of the topics discussed in the course.

―――. "Psychophysiological Disorders: Embracing Pain." In Germer, C. K., Siegel, R. D, and Fulton, P. R., eds. *Mindfulness and Psychotherapy.* 2nd ed. New York: Guilford Press, 2013. A professional exploration of the use of mindfulness practices to treat chronic pain.

Siegel, R. D., ed. *Positive Psychology: Harnessing the Power of Happiness, Personal Strength, and Mindfulness.* Boston: Harvard Health Publications, 2011. A report prepared for general audiences reviewing current findings in positive psychology, including the relationship among happiness, mindfulness, and self-compassion.

Siegel, R. D., and Germer, C. K. "Wisdom and Compassion: Two Wings of a Bird." In C. K. Germer and R. D. Siegel, eds. *Wisdom and Compassion in Psychotherapy: Deepening Mindfulness in Clinical Practice.* New York: Guilford Press, 2012. A detailed conceptual exploration of what exactly are wisdom and compassion.

Siegel, R.D., Urdang, M.H., and Johnson, D.R. *Back Sense: A Revolutionary Approach to Halting the Cycle of Chronic Back Pain.* New York: Broadway Books, 2001. A self-help guide blending functional restoration rehabilitation with mindfulness practice to recover from chronic back pain, neck pain, and other stress-related problems.

Sternberg, R. J. *Wisdom: Its Nature, Origins, and Development.* New York: Cambridge University Press, 1990. The pioneering text exploring the scientific study of wisdom.

Sternberg, R. J., and Jordan, J., eds. *A Handbook of Wisdom: Psychological Perspectives.* New York: Cambridge University Press, 2005. An anthology providing an overview of the scientific study of wisdom.

Styron, C. W. "Positive Psychology and the Bodhisattva Path." In Germer, C. K., Siegel, R. D, and Fulton, P. R., eds. *Mindfulness and Psychotherapy.* 2nd ed. New York: Guilford Press, 2013. A professional exploration of the relationship between the findings of positive psychology and the idea of a bodhisattva path—commitment to the well-being of others.

Surrey, J. L., and Jordan, J. V. "The Wisdom of Connection." In C.K. Germer and R.D. Siegel, eds. *Wisdom and Compassion in Psychotherapy: Deepening Mindfulness in Clinical Practice.* New York: Guilford Press, 2012. A professional exploration of the implications of mindfulness for relationships, with an emphasis on developing interpersonal wisdom and compassion.

Surrey, J. L., and Kramer, G. "Relational Mindfulness." In C. K. Germer, R. D. Siegel, and P. R. Fulton, eds. *Mindfulness and Psychotherapy.* 2nd ed. New York: Guilford Press, 2013.

Tillich, P. *The Eternal Now.* New York: Charles Scribner's Sons, 1963. A classic text on the difference between loneliness and solitude.

Williams, M., Teasdale, J., Segal, Z., and Kabat-Zinn, J. *The Mindful Way through Depression.* New York: Guilford Press, 2007. A self-help guide to using mindfulness practices, along with cognitive behavioral techniques, to work with depression.

Internet Resources

www.mindfulness-solution.com. This website offers free audio recordings of variations of the practices presented in this course, as well as additional mindfulness practices. It also contains links to listings of meditation centers all over the world, where you can locate opportunities to learn from and practice with other people. Some of these follow Buddhist paths, while others are associated with different spiritual and cultural traditions.

www.backsense.org. This website offers charts that are useful for following a mindfulness-based program to work with chronic pain disorders.

Notes

Notes

Notes

Notes

Notes

Notes

Notes